ICD-9-CM Diagnostic Coding and Reimbursement for Physician Services

2006 Edition

Anita C. Hazelwood, MLS, RHIA, FAHIMA
Carol A. Venable, MPH, RHIA, FAHIMA

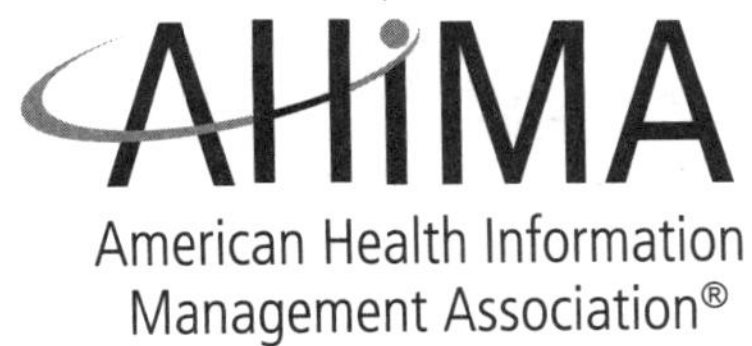

This book includes ICD-9-CM changes announced in the CMS Hospital Inpatient Prospective Payment Systems Proposed Rules, as published in the May 4, 2005 *Federal Register* available at http://www.access.gpo.gov/su_docs/fedreg/a050504c.html. Any additional changes to these codes may be obtained at the CMS Web site or in the Final Rule for IPPS in the *Federal Register* when it is available (usually in August). The official ICD-9-CM addenda are available at: http://www.cdc.gov/nchs/datawh/ftpserv/ftpicd9/ftpicd9.htm#guidelines.

Material quoted in this book from ICD-9-CM Official Guidelines for Coding and Reporting is taken from the April 2005 updated version.

ISBN 1-58426-151-X
AHIMA Product No. AC201205 (without answers)
AHIMA Product No. AC201205K (with answers)

Mary Stanfill, RHIA, CCS, CCS-P, Reviewer
Marcia Loellbach, MS, Project Editor
Melissa Ulbricht, Editorial/Production Coordinator

*AHIMA strives to recognize the value of people from every racial
and ethnic background as well as all genders, age groups, and sexual
orientations by building its membership and leadership resources to reflect
the rich diversity of the American population. AHIMA encourages the
celebration and promotion of human diversity through education,
mentoring, recognition, leadership, and other programs.*

American Health Information Management Association
233 North Michigan Avenue, Suite 2150
Chicago, Illinois 60601-5800

http://www.ahima.org

This book must be used with the 2006 edition of *ICD-9-CM* (code changes effective October 1, 2005).

Note to educators: *ICD-9-CM Diagnostic Coding and Reimbursement for Physician Services* is available with answers or without answers.

Additional Practice

AHIMA's publication, *Clinical Coding Workout: Practice Exercises for Skill Development* (AHIMA Prod. Nos. AC201504, with answers, and AC201604, without answers), is an excellent follow-up resource after the coder completes *ICD-9-CM Diagnostic Coding and Reimbursement for Physician Services*. Previously published under the title, *Coding in Context,* this exercise book is a perfect teaching tool for coders wanting to sharpen their ability to make critical coding decisions. The book contains beginning through advanced practice exercises, including case studies that help students and coders alike understand what they need to know when it comes to correct coding practices and procedures. The case studies in the book require users to make the kinds of decisions that coding professionals must make every day on the job.

Contents

About the Authors v

Preface vii

Chapter 1   Introduction to ICD-9-CM 1

Chapter 2   Supplementary Classification: V Codes. 33

Chapter 3   Late Effects 49

Chapter 4   Signs, Symptoms, and Ill-Defined Conditions. 55

Chapter 5   Infectious and Parasitic Diseases. 65

Chapter 6   Neoplasms 83

Chapter 7   Endocrine, Nutritional and Metabolic Diseases,
              and Immunity Disorders 97

Chapter 8   Mental Disorders 109

Chapter 9   Diseases of the Nervous System 119

Chapter 10   Diseases of the Blood and Blood-Forming Organs 127

Chapter 11   Diseases of the Circulatory System. 135

Chapter 12   Diseases of the Respiratory System. 155

Chapter 13   Diseases of the Digestive System 169

Chapter 14   Diseases of the Genitourinary System. 179

Chapter 15   Complications of Pregnancy, Childbirth, and the Puerperium 191

Chapter 16   Congenital Anomalies and Certain Conditions Originating
              in the Perinatal Period. 207

Chapter 17   Diseases of the Skin and Subcutaneous Tissue 219

Chapter 18   Diseases of the Musculoskeletal System and Connective Tissue 225

Chapter 19   Injury, Poisonings, and Adverse Effects. 235

Chapter 20   Complications of Surgical and Medical Care. 263

Chapter 21   Overview of Reimbursement and Coding Systems 273

Chapter 22   Challenges of Compliance and Ethical Coding 285

References and Bibliography 291

Appendix A   CMS-1500 Claim Form 293

Appendix B   Ethics in Coding. 297

Appendix C   AHIMA Practice Brief on Data Quality 307

Appendix D   AHIMA Position Statement on Data Quality. 313

Appendix E   ICD-9-CM Official Guidelines for Coding and Reporting 315

Appendix F   ICD-10-CM and ICD-10-PCS. 387

Index 407

About the Authors

Carol A. Venable, MPH, RHIA, FAHIMA, is a department head and a professor at the University of Louisiana at Lafayette, and Anita C. Hazelwood, MLS, RHIA, FAHIMA, is an associate professor at the same university. Their book, *ICD-10-CM Preview,* was first published by AHIMA in 2003 and was updated in 2004 with a new chapter on ICD-10-PCS.

Both authors have conducted numerous coding workshops at the local, state, and national levels. Moreover, they have published articles in *Educational Perspectives in Health Information Management,* in addition to serving on its editorial review board, and in the *Journal of AHIMA.*

Active volunteers of AHIMA, Ms. Venable and Ms. Hazelwood are members of the Assembly on Education and the Society for Clinical Coding and have served on the board of the Assembly on Education. Ms. Hazelwood also has served on the board of the Society for Clinical Coding.

Preface

The coding process requires a range of skills that combines knowledge and practice. *ICD-9-CM Diagnostic Coding and Reimbursement for Physician Services* was designed to provide a comprehensive text for students and physician-based coding personnel. It introduces the basic principles and conventions of ICD-9-CM coding, illustrates the application of coding principles with examples and exercises based on actual case documentation, and teaches students and/or physician-based coding personnel how to analyze clinical data for the purposes of coding and reimbursement.

Organization of the Book

Chapter 1, Introduction to ICD-9-CM, provides a general overview of coding and classification systems and presents the basic characteristics, conventions, and principles of ICD-9-CM. The chapter illustrates how to read and interpret documentation in the medical record and how to understand the basic steps and rules to follow for coding diagnoses. It also presents current, approved ICD-9-CM coding guidelines for assigning and sequencing accurate diagnosis codes.

Chapter 2, Supplementary Classification: V Codes, includes coding guidelines for situations when it is appropriate to use a V code. Some of the most commonly used V codes are reviewed.

Chapter 3, Late Effects, provides information on codes used to report late or residual effects of the acute phase of an injury or illness.

Chapter 4, Signs, Symptoms, and Ill-Defined Conditions, discusses the current, approved ICD-9-CM guidelines coders should follow when assigning and sequencing codes for diagnoses related to signs, symptoms, and ill-defined conditions.

Chapter 5, Infectious and Parasitic Diseases, presents general information on basic laboratory tests that physicians might order and reviews common microorganisms. Guidelines for coding infectious and parasitic conditions are covered.

Chapter 6, Neoplasms, describes the current, approved ICD-9-CM coding guidelines to follow when assigning and sequencing codes for diagnoses related to neoplasms. It also explains how to use the Neoplasm Table and the terms that apply to each of its columns.

Chapter 7, Endocrine, Nutritional and Metabolic Diseases, and Immunity Disorders, covers the most commonly diagnosed endocrine, nutritional, metabolic, and immunity disorders, such as diabetes mellitus, hypoglycemia, thyroid disorders, and cystic fibrosis.

Chapter 8, Mental Disorders, discusses the most common mental disorders and the correct way to assign codes for these types of diagnoses.

Chapter 9, Diseases of the Nervous System, describes the current, approved guidelines coders should follow when assigning and sequencing codes for diagnoses related to the nervous system.

Chapter 10, Diseases of the Blood and Blood-Forming Organs, presents coding rules related to diseases of the blood and blood-forming organs. Guidelines for assigning codes for anemia, coagulation defects, hemorrhagic conditions, and diseases of the white blood cells are included.

Chapter 11, Diseases of the Circulatory System, discusses the most common disorders of the circulatory system and the current, approved guidelines coders should follow when assigning and sequencing codes for these diagnoses.

Chapter 12, Diseases of the Respiratory System, explains the current, approved guidelines coders should follow when assigning and sequencing codes for diagnoses related to this system.

Chapter 13, Diseases of the Digestive System, discusses the major disorders of the digestive system and the approved guidelines coders should follow when assigning and sequencing codes related to this system.

Chapter 14, Diseases of the Genitourinary System, covers the most common disorders of the genitourinary system and provides the coding guidelines for assigning and sequencing codes for diagnoses related to this system.

Chapter 15, Complications of Pregnancy, Childbirth, and the Puerperium, clarifies the coding rules that apply to pregnancy and the postpartum period. It also discusses the guidelines for assigning codes from the various sections in chapter 11 of the ICD-9-CM codebook and reviews the V codes that are commonly used in physicians' coding.

Chapter 16, Congenital Anomalies and Certain Conditions Originating in the Perinatal Period, discusses the major anomalies and perinatal conditions that affect newborns. Definitions of congenital anomalies and perinatal conditions are reviewed. Some of the conditions covered include spina bifida, cleft lip, and perinatal infections.

Chapter 17, Diseases of the Skin and Subcutaneous Tissue, classifies diagnoses for disorders of the skin and subcutaneous tissue and provides guidelines for the proper coding and sequencing of diagnoses related to these conditions.

Chapter 18, Diseases of the Musculoskeletal System and Connective Tissue, provides information on the most common disorders related to the musculoskeletal system, such as arthritis.

Chapter 19, Injury, Poisonings, and Adverse Effects, covers a wide variety of injuries and also includes information on poisoning and adverse reactions to drugs. Coding guidelines for the reporting and sequencing of diagnoses are thoroughly reviewed.

Chapter 20, Complications of Surgical and Medical Care, provides an overview of complications of care that are not classified to other chapters in the ICD-9-CM codebook. A discussion of what constitutes postoperative complications is included.

Chapter 21, Overview of Reimbursement and Coding Systems, identifies various third-party payers and offers information on payment methodologies such as the Resource-based Relative Value System, or RBRVS. It also discusses the future of coding and coding systems and includes a glossary of reimbursement terms.

Chapter 22, Challenges of Compliance and Ethical Coding, delineates the issues of compliance and ethical coding and explains the coder's role in the process of reporting and reimbursement. It also gives examples of fraud and abuse and briefly overviews legislation that addresses these issues. Finally, the chapter presents guidelines for a physicians' compliance program.

The index and appendices at the back of the book make information readily accessible and provide additional resources for students and physician-based coders.

Chapter 1

Introduction to ICD-9-CM

Objectives

After completing this lesson, the student should be able to do the following:

- Explain the purpose of classification and coding systems

- Identify the basic characteristics, conventions, symbols, and principles of the ICD-9-CM classification system

- Understand the basic steps and rules to follow for the coding of diagnoses

- Apply knowledge of current, approved ICD-9-CM coding guidelines for the assignment and sequencing of codes for diagnoses

- Understand the appropriate use of the supplementary classifications of ICD-9-CM

Introduction

Healthcare data in the form of ICD-9-CM diagnostic codes are collected and reported for patients receiving medical care in all settings: inpatient, ambulatory care surgery, observation, outpatient, rehabilitation, skilled nursing, physician office, home health, and so on. The clinical health information is converted into coded data that are used for multiple purposes, including:

- Trending
- Planning
- Making comparisons
- Determining reimbursement
- Determining appropriate levels of service
- Justifying levels of service
- Measuring quality of care
- Measuring severity of illness
- Measuring intensity of service

The process of collecting and reporting these data is complex, and careful documentation is critical to accurate and complete data collection. The source document—the health record—must describe the encounter both qualitatively and quantitatively and must specify the reason for the visit (such as the condition, symptom, or diagnosis requiring attention) and the services provided.

Definition of Coding

In its simplest form, coding is the transformation of verbal descriptions into numbers. We are all familiar with this task because we use codes every day to carry out simple business and personal transactions. For example, a zip code transforms a geographical location into numbers. In the healthcare arena, specific codes describe diseases, injuries, and procedures. Whereas assigning zip codes is a rather simple task, assigning diagnostic and procedural codes is a detailed process that requires a thorough knowledge of medical terminology, anatomy, and pathophysiology.

The method of classifying diseases and procedures has evolved through the years into a sophisticated system that can track general and nonspecific conditions, such as abdominal pain, to specific diagnoses, such as acute cholecystitis with cholelithiasis. Hospitals have used coding systems to categorize diagnoses and procedures for many years. Since the 1980s, Medicare has required physicians to submit the appropriate diagnostic codes to identify the reason for a patient visit or encounter, such as a diagnosis (hypertension) or a symptom (chest pain).

Development of the Coding System

Healthcare providers such as physicians and hospitals index healthcare data by referring and adhering to a classification system published by the U.S. Department of Health and Human Services—the *International Classification of Diseases, 9th Revision, Clinical Modification*

(ICD-9-CM). As the title indicates, this coding system has been revised nine times, signifying that it has been in use for many years.

The notion of using classification systems can be traced back to the time of the ancient Greeks. In the seventeenth century, English statistician John Graunt developed the *London Bills of Mortality,* which was the first attempt to identify the proportion of children who died before reaching age six. In 1838, William Farr, registrar general of England, developed a system to classify deaths. And in 1893, a French physician, Jacques Bertillon, unveiled the *Bertillon Classification of Causes of Death* at the International Statistical Institute in Chicago.

Several countries adopted Bertillon's system; and in 1898, the American Public Health Association (APHA) recommended that the registrars of Canada, Mexico, and the United States also adopt it. In addition, APHA recommended revising the system every ten years to remain current with medical practice. The first international conference to revise the *International Classification of Causes of Death* was convened in 1900, and the system has been revised every ten years thereafter. At the time of the first conference, the classification system was contained in one book, which included an alphabetic index and a tabular list. As can be imagined, the book was quite small compared to current coding manuals.

Early revisions of the classification system involved only minor changes; however, the sixth revision brought drastic changes and the publication was expanded to two volumes. That revision included morbidity and mortality conditions, and its title was modified to reflect these changes—*Manual of International Statistical Classification of Diseases, Injuries and Causes of Death (ICD).* Prior to the sixth revision, responsibility for ICD revisions fell to the Mixed Commission, a group composed of representatives from the International Statistical Institute and the Health Organization of the League of Nations. In 1948, the World Health Organization (WHO), headquartered in Geneva, Switzerland, assumed responsibility for preparing and publishing the revisions to the ICD codebook. WHO sponsored the seventh and eighth revisions in 1957 and 1968, respectively.

The entire history of the ICD coding system emphasizes the determination of many people to provide an international classification system for compiling and presenting statistical data. Today, ICD is the most widely used statistical classification system in the world.

After WHO published the ninth revision of the ICD system in 1978, the United States modified it to meet the needs of American hospitals and called it *International Classification of Diseases, Ninth Revision, Clinical Modification (ICD-9-CM).* The ninth revision expanded the book to three volumes and introduced a fifth-digit subclassification.

A tenth revision of the ICD system has been developed at the international level. Currently, this revision is under review by the National Center for Health Statistics (NCHS), the Centers for Medicare and Medicaid Services (CMS), and other federal agencies in the United States for use in this country. No definitive date has been set for implementing the ICD-10 coding system in the United States.

Official Addenda to ICD-9-CM

ICD-9-CM represents the most current and comprehensive statistical classification system of its kind. Whereas ICD is updated approximately every ten years, ICD-9-CM is updated annually. Codes may be added, revised, or deleted. An *Official Authorized Addendum* documents these changes with their implementation effective October 1 of each year. CMS and NCHS publish the addenda with the approval of WHO. NCHS is responsible for maintaining the diagnosis classification in volumes 1 and 2; CMS is responsible for maintaining the procedure classification in volume 3. The American Health Information Management Association (AHIMA) and the American Hospital Association (AHA) give advice and assistance, as do health information management practitioners, physicians, and other users of ICD-9-CM.

To ensure accurate coding, all ICD-9-CM codebooks must be updated yearly with code revisions. In addition, all coding software (encoders) must be updated.

Coding Guidelines

To facilitate and standardize physician office coding, official coding guidelines were developed by CMS, AHA, AHIMA, and NCHS. Throughout this workbook, coding guidelines are presented for specific diseases and/or body systems. The most recent official coding guidelines for outpatient services, including physician offices, are provided in appendix E at the end of this workbook. A summary of these guidelines follows:

1. Use the appropriate code or codes from 001.0–V85.4 to identify diagnoses, symptoms, conditions, problems, complaints, or other reason(s) for the encounter or visit.

2. ICD-9-CM is composed of codes with three, four, or five digits. A three-digit code is used as the heading of a category of codes that may be further subdivided with fourth and/or fifth digits to provide greater specificity.

   Use a three-digit code only when it is not further subdivided and no fourth or fifth digits are available. Where fourth-digit subcategories and/or fifth-digit subclassifications are provided, they must be assigned. A code is invalid when it has not been coded to the full number of digits required for that code.

EXAMPLE:	250	Incorrect code assignment
	250.0	Incorrect code assignment
	250.01	Correct code assignment

   It is recognized that a specific diagnosis may not be known at the time of an initial office visit; however, this is not an acceptable reason for submitting a three-digit code when a four- or five-digit code is more appropriate.

3. First list the ICD-9-CM code for the diagnosis, condition, problem, or other reason for the encounter or visit shown in the health record to be chiefly responsible for the services provided; then list additional codes that describe any coexisting conditions.

   EXAMPLE: Patient was seen in the physician's office with a complaint of polyuria and polydipsia. During the visit, the patient's hypertension was evaluated and the prescription refilled. The first code listed may be either the polyuria or the polydipsia because this was the primary reason for the visit, followed by a code for the hypertension.

4. Do not code diagnoses documented as "probable," "suspected," "questionable," "rule out," or "working diagnosis." Rather, code the condition(s) to the highest degree of certainty for that encounter or visit, such as symptoms, signs, abnormal test results, or other reason for the visit.

   EXAMPLE: Patient was seen in the physician's office complaining of vomiting and nausea; rule out gastroenteritis. Because the gastroenteritis was not confirmed, only the vomiting and nausea should be coded.

5. Codes that describe symptoms and signs, as opposed to diagnoses, are acceptable for reporting purposes when a diagnosis has not been established or confirmed by the physician.

6. ICD-9-CM provides codes to deal with encounters for circumstances other than a disease or injury. The Supplementary Classification of Factors Influencing Health

Status and Contact with Health Services (V01.0–V85.4) is provided to deal with occasions when circumstances other than a disease or injury are recorded as diagnoses or problems.

7. Chronic diseases treated on an ongoing basis may be coded and reported as often as the patient receives treatment and care for the condition(s).

8. Code all documented conditions that coexist at the time of the encounter or visit and that require or affect patient care treatment or management. Do not code conditions that were treated previously and no longer exist. However, history codes (V10–V19) may be used as secondary codes when the historical condition or family history has an impact on current care or influences treatment.

9. For patients receiving diagnostic services only during an encounter or visit, sequence first the diagnosis, condition, problem, or other reason for the encounter or visit shown in the health record to be chiefly responsible for the outpatient services provided during the encounter or visit. Codes for other diagnoses (for example, chronic conditions) may be sequenced as additional diagnoses.

10. For patients receiving therapeutic services only during an encounter or visit, sequence first the diagnosis, condition, problem, or other reason for the encounter or visit shown in the health record to be chiefly responsible for the outpatient services provided during the encounter or visit. Codes for other diagnoses (for example, chronic conditions) may be sequenced as additional diagnoses. There is one exception: For patients receiving chemotherapy, radiation therapy, or rehabilitation, list first the appropriate V code that identifies the service and then the diagnosis or problem for which the service is being performed.

11. For patients receiving preoperative evaluations only, sequence a code from category V72.8, Other specified examinations, to describe the preoperative consultations. Assign a code for the condition to describe the reason for the surgery as an additional diagnosis. Code also any findings related to the preoperative evaluation.

12. For ambulatory surgery, code the diagnosis for which the surgery was performed. When the postoperative diagnosis is known to be different from the preoperative diagnosis at the time the diagnosis is confirmed, select the postoperative diagnosis for coding because it is the most definitive one.

13. For routine outpatient prenatal visits when no complications are present, codes V22.0, Supervision of normal first pregnancy, and V22.1, Supervision of other normal pregnancy, should be used as principal diagnoses. These codes should not be used in conjunction with chapter 11 codes.

Characteristics of ICD-9-CM

Since its October 1991 publication by the U.S. Department of Health and Human Services, the single, official ICD-9-CM codebook has consisted of three volumes:

- Volume 1: Tabular List of Diseases and Injuries

- Volume 2: Alphabetic Index to Diseases

- Volume 3: Tabular List of and Alphabetic Index to Procedures

The official version of ICD-9-CM is available only on CD-ROM from the U.S. Government Printing Office in Washington, DC. Because it has not been copyrighted and is in the public domain, many versions of the codebook are offered on the market. Although each version may offer special features, the ICD-9-CM codes themselves remain the same. The official version of ICD-9-CM is the codebook referred to throughout this book.

Although hospitals use all three volumes of ICD-9-CM for the billing of services, only volumes 1 and 2 are used for physician billing. CPT is used for coding outpatient procedures. Therefore, only volumes 1 and 2 are discussed in the subsequent chapters.

Because the ICD-9-CM system is reviewed annually, it is important to remember that all ICD-9-CM codebooks are kept current to reflect the revisions, deletions, and additions of codes implemented in the United States on October 1 of each year.

Volume 1: Tabular List of Diseases and Injuries

Volume 1 contains the following major subdivisions:

- Classification of Diseases and Injuries

- Supplementary Classifications (V Codes and E Codes)

- Appendices

Classification of Diseases and Injuries

The first major subdivision of volume 1, Classification of Diseases and Injuries, contains seventeen chapters that classify conditions according to etiology (cause of disease) or by a specific anatomical (body) system.

> **EXAMPLE:** Chapter 1, Infectious and Parasitic Diseases, represents classification by etiology or the cause of disease, but chapter 7, Diseases of the Circulatory System, represents classification by anatomical system.

The chapters in this subdivision are:

	Chapter Title	Categories
1.	Infectious and Parasitic Diseases	001–139
2.	Neoplasms	140–239
3.	Endocrine, Nutritional and Metabolic Diseases, and Immunity Disorders	240–279
4.	Diseases of the Blood and Blood-Forming Organs	280–289
5.	Mental Disorders	290–319
6.	Diseases of the Nervous System and Sense Organs	320–389
7.	Diseases of the Circulatory System	390–459
8.	Diseases of the Respiratory System	460–519
9.	Diseases of the Digestive System	520–579
10.	Diseases of the Genitourinary System	580–629
11.	Complications of Pregnancy, Childbirth, and the Puerperium	630–677
12.	Diseases of the Skin and Subcutaneous Tissue	680–709

13. Diseases of the Musculoskeletal System and Connective Tissue   710–739
14. Congenital Anomalies   740–759
15. Certain Conditions Originating in the Perinatal Period   760–779
16. Symptoms, Signs, and Ill-Defined Conditions   780–799
17. Injury and Poisoning   800–999

Each chapter is structured into the following subdivisions:

- Sections
- Categories
- Subcategories
- Subclassifications

Sections

A section consists of a group of three-digit categories that represents a single disease entity or a group of similar or closely related conditions, for example, Disorders of the Thyroid Gland (240–246).

Categories

An individual three-digit category represents a single disease entity or a group of similar or closely related conditions, for example, 520, Disorders of tooth development and eruption.

Subcategories

The fourth-digit subcategory provides more specificity or information regarding the etiology (cause), site, or manifestation (characteristic signs, symptoms, or secondary processes) of an illness. Fourth-digit subcategories are collapsible to the three-digit level. For example:

---

476 **Chronic laryngitis and laryngotracheitis**

    476.0 **Chronic laryngitis**
        Laryngitis:
          catarrhal
          hypertrophic
          sicca

    476.1 **Chronic laryngotracheitis**
        Laryngitis, (chronic) with tracheitis (chronic)
        Tracheitis, chronic, with laryngitis

Subclassifications

In some cases, fourth-digit subcategories have been expanded to the fifth-digit level to provide even greater specificity. Fifth-digit assignments and instructions can appear at different locations in the Tabular List. They can appear at the beginning of a chapter. For example:

13. DISEASES OF THE MUSCULOSKELETAL SYSTEM AND CONNECTIVE TISSUE (710–739)

The following fifth-digit subclassification is for use with categories 711–712, 715–716, 718–719, and 730:

0 **site unspecified**

1 **shoulder region**
  Acromioclavicular joint(s)
  Clavicle
  Glenohumeral joint(s)
  Scapula
  Sternoclavicular joint(s)

2 **upper arm**
  Elbow joint
  Humerus

3 **forearm**
  Radius
  Ulna
  Wrist joint

4 **hand**
  Carpus
  Metacarpus
  Phalanges [fingers]

5 **pelvic region and thigh**
  Buttock
  Femur
  Hip (joint)

6 **lower leg**
  Fibula
  Knee joint
  Patella
  Tibia

7 **ankle and foot**
  Ankle joint
  Digits [toes]
  Metatarsus
  Phalanges, foot
  Tarsus
  Other joints in foot

8 **other specified sites**
  Head
  Neck
  Ribs
  Skull
  Trunk
  Vertebral column

9 **multiple sites**

An instruction at the beginning of chapter 13, Diseases of the Musculoskeletal System and Connective Tissue, states that certain categories must be assigned a fifth digit to describe the affected body site. Fifth-digit assignments and instructions also may appear at the beginning of a section. For example:

MALIGNANT NEOPLASM OF LYMPHATIC
AND HEMATOPOIETIC TISSUE (200–208)

Excludes: *secondary neoplasm of:*
bone marrow (198.5)
spleen (197.8)
secondary and unspecified neoplasm of
lymph nodes (196.0–196.9)

The following fifth-digit subclassification is for use with categories 200–202:

0   **unspecified site, extranodal and solid organ sites**
1   **lymph nodes of head, face, and neck**
2   **intrathoracic lymph nodes**
3   **intra-abdominal lymph nodes**
4   **lymph nodes of axilla and upper limb**
5   **lymph nodes of inguinal region and lower limb**
6   **intrapelvic lymph nodes**
7   **spleen**
8   **lymph nodes of multiple sites**

The information at the beginning of section 200–208, Malignant Neoplasm of Lymphatic and Hematopoietic Tissue, notes that a fifth digit must be assigned to categories 200–202 to describe the site of the lymph nodes involved.

Fifth-digit assignments and instructions sometimes appear at the beginning of a three-digit category. For example:

250   **Diabetes mellitus**

Excludes: *gestational diabetes (648.8)*
hyperglycemia, NOS (790.6)
neonatal diabetes mellitus (775.1)
nonclinical diabetes (790.29)

The following fifth-digit subclassification is for use with category 250:

0   **type II or unspecified type, not stated as uncontrolled**

Fifth digit 0 is for use with type II patients, even if the patient requires insulin. Use additional code, if applicable, for associated long-term (current) insulin use V58.67

1   **type I [juvenile type], not stated as uncontrolled**

2   **type II or unspecified type, uncontrolled**

Fifth digit 2 is for use with type II patients, even if the patient requires insulin. Use additional code, if applicable, for associated long-term (current) insulin use V58.67

3   **type I [juvenile type], uncontrolled**

An instruction at the beginning of category 250, Diabetes mellitus, states that a fifth digit should be assigned to describe the type of diabetes mellitus.

Fifth-digit assignments and instructions also sometimes appear in a fourth-digit subcategory. For example:

786.5 Chest pain

> **786.50 Chest pain, unspecified**
> **786.51 Precordial pain**
> **786.52 Painful respiration**
>> Pain:
>>> anterior chest wall
>>> pleuritic
>> Pleurodynia
>>> *Excludes:* *epidemic pleurodynia (074.1)*
>
> **786.59 Other**
>> Discomfort ⎤
>> Pressure   ⎬ in chest
>> Tightness ⎦
>>> *Excludes:* *pain in breast (611.71)*

The fourth-digit subcategory of 786.5, Chest pain, is further subdivided to the fifth-digit level to describe specific types of chest pain.

The use of fifth digits is not optional. However, fifth digits are quite easy to overlook. To remember to assign them, it is helpful to highlight all the fourth-digit subcategories requiring a fifth-digit subclassification in volume 1 of the ICD-9-CM codebook. Many publishers include special symbols and/or color highlighting to identify codes requiring fourth and/or fifth digits.

Residual Subcategories

Residual subcategories are codes with titles of "other" and "unspecified." They were developed to classify conditions not assigned a separate subcategory to ensure that every disease always has a code. Residual subcategories titled "other" are easily distinguished because the fourth digit is often the number 8. Those codes describing "unspecified" conditions are usually assigned a fourth digit of 9. For example:

003.8 **Other specified salmonella infections**

003.9 **Salmonella infection, unspecified**

In the preceding examples, code 003.8 would include all other specified types of salmonella infections, excluding those listed in codes 003.0–003.29. However, code 003.9 is assigned when the physician documents a diagnosis of salmonella infection without further specification.

In a few instances, however, the fourth digit 9 is assigned for both "other" and "unspecified" because digits 0–8 have been used. For example:

478.9 Other and unspecified diseases of upper respiratory tract

> Abscess ⎤
>   ⎬ of trachea
> Cicatrix ⎦

Because codes 478.0–478.8 are used to describe specific upper respiratory tract diseases, code 478.9 includes both unspecified diseases and other diseases not classified in subcategories 478.0–478.8.

Supplementary Classifications (V Codes and E Codes)

Two supplementary classifications exist in addition to the main classification for diseases and injuries: Supplementary Classification of Factors Influencing Health Status and Contact with Health Services (V01–V84) and Supplementary Classification of External Causes of Injury and Poisoning (E800–E999). Unlike the numeric codes in the disease classification, the supplementary classifications contain alphanumeric codes. The codes in the Supplementary Classification of Factors Influencing Health Status and Contact with Health Services are known as V codes and consist of the letter V followed by two numeric digits, a decimal point, a fourth digit, and (where applicable) a fifth digit.

V64   **Persons encountering health services for specific procedures, not carried out**

     V64.0   **Vaccination not carried out**

         V64.00   **Vaccination not carried out, unspecified reason**

         V64.01   **Vaccination not carried out because of acute illness**

         V64.02   **Vaccination not carried out because of chronic illness or condition**

         V64.03   **Vaccination not carried out because of immune compromised state**

         V64.04   **Vaccination not carried out because of allergy to vaccine or component**

         V64.05   **Vaccination not carried out because of caregiver refusal**

         V64.06   **Vaccination not carried out because of patient refusal**

         V64.07   **Vaccination not carried out for religious reasons**

         V64.08   **Vaccination not carried out because patient had disease being vaccinated against**

         V64.09   **Vaccination not carried out for other reason**

     V64.1   **Surgical or other procedure not carried out because of contraindication**

     V64.2   **Surgical or other procedure not carried out because of patient's decision**

     V64.3   **Procedure not carried out for other reasons**

     V64.4   **Closed surgical procedure converted to open procedure**

         V64.41   **Laparoscopic surgical procedure converted to open procedure**

         V64.42   **Thoracoscopic surgical procedure converted to open procedure**

         V64.43   **Arthroscopic surgical procedure converted to open procedure**

The codes in the Supplementary Classification of External Causes of Injury and Poisoning are known as E codes and consist of the letter E followed by three numeric digits, a decimal point, and a fourth digit. For example:

E953   **Suicide and self-inflicted injury by hanging, strangulation, and suffocation**

      E953.0   **Hanging**

      E953.1   **Suffocation by plastic bag**

      E953.8   **Other specified means**

      E953.9   **Unspecified means**

Appendices

Volume 1 of ICD-9-CM has traditionally included five appendices. Changes as described below may cause publishers of paper codebooks to renumber the appendices in their October 2004 and subsequent publications.

Appendix A   Morphology of Neoplasms

This appendix includes a listing of all morphology types with the appropriate morphology, or M code. (Morphology codes are discussed in chapter 6 of this workbook.)

Appendix B   Glossary of Mental Disorders

In 2003 and prior years, the Glossary of Mental Disorders included definitions for the psychiatric terms found in chapter 5, Mental Disorders, of ICD-9-CM. However, this appendix was not maintained for many years and was considered to contain many inaccuracies. In response to a request from the American Psychiatric Association (APA), the Glossary of Mental Disorders has been removed from the official government (CD-ROM) version of ICD-9-CM, effective with the October 1, 2004 update. Coders should refer to the *Diagnostic and Statistical Manual of Mental Disorders, Fourth Edition, Text Revision (DSM-IV-TR),* published by the APA, for definitions of the mental disorders classified in chapter 5 of ICD-9-CM.

Appendix C   Classification of Drugs by AHFS List

The American Hospital Formulary Service (AHFS) list is published by the American Society of Hospital Pharmacists. The AHFS categorizes drugs to family-related groups. When coders must locate the category of a new drug or cannot find a new drug in the Table of Drugs and Chemicals, they turn to the AHFS as a helpful reference. The Table of Drugs and Chemicals lists the AHFS number under the main term "Drug." Appendix C includes a listing of the AHFS categories and the appropriate ICD-9-CM code.

Appendix D   Classification of Industrial Accidents according to Agency

Appendix D classifies industrial accidents according to agency, as adopted by the Tenth International Conference of Labor Statisticians on October 12, 1962.

Appendix E   List of Three-Digit Categories

Appendix E includes a listing of each three-digit category in ICD-9-CM, along with its appropriate title.

Appendix F   CC Exclusion List

Volume 2: Alphabetic Index to Diseases

Volume 2 is divided into three major sections:

- Index to Diseases and Injuries

- Table of Drugs and Chemicals

- Alphabetic Index to External Causes of Injury and Poisoning (E Codes)

Index to Diseases and Injuries

The Index to Diseases and Injuries includes the terminology for all the codes appearing in volume 1 of the ICD-9-CM codebook. It employs three types of indentations:

- Main terms

- Subterms

- Carryover lines

Main Terms

Printed in boldface type, the main terms are set flush with the left margin of each column for easy reference. Main terms may represent:

- Diseases (for example, influenza, bronchitis)

- Conditions (for example, fatigue, fracture, injury)

- Nouns (for example, disease, disturbance, syndrome)

- Adjectives (for example, double, large, kinking)

Main terms that are anatomical terms have cross-references to the condition. For example, bronchial asthma is found under the disease term "Asthma" rather than the site term "Bronchi, bronchial."

Many conditions can be found in more than one place in the index. For example:

- Complications of medical or surgical care are indexed under the name of the condition, as well as under the main term **"Complications."**

- Obstetrical conditions are found under the name of the condition and/or under entries such as **"Delivery," "Labor," "Pregnancy,"** and **"Puerperal"** (after delivery).

- Conditions that include the term *disease* or *syndrome* in their title or description may be found under the main terms **"Disease"** or **"Syndrome,"** as well as under the disease or syndrome's name. For example, chronic obstructive lung disease may be found in the Index to Diseases and Injuries under **"Obstruction, obstructed, obstructive,"** as well as under **"Disease, diseased."**

Subterms

Some main terms are followed by a list of indented subterms (modifiers) that affect the selection of an appropriate code for a given diagnosis. The subterms form individual line entries arranged in alphabetical order and printed in regular type beginning with a lowercase letter. Subterms are indented one standard indentation to the right under the main term. They describe essential differences in site, cause, or clinical type. More specific subterms are indented farther to the right, as needed; indented one standard indentation after the preceding subterm; and listed in alphabetical order.

Before a code can be selected, all subentries following the main term must be reviewed to determine which code is most appropriate. Note that the terms *with* and *without* are listed at the beginning of all the subterms, rather than in alphabetical order.

<table>
<tr><td>Incontinence 788.30</td><td>←   Main Term</td></tr>
<tr><td>without sensory awareness 788.34</td><td></td></tr>
<tr><td>anal sphincter 787.6</td><td>←   Site</td></tr>
<tr><td>continuous leakage 788.37</td><td></td></tr>
<tr><td>feces 787.6</td><td></td></tr>
<tr><td>   due to hysteria 300.11</td><td></td></tr>
<tr><td>   nonorganic origin 307.7</td><td></td></tr>
<tr><td>hysterical 300.11</td><td></td></tr>
<tr><td>mixed (male) (female) (urge</td><td></td></tr>
<tr><td>   and stress) 788.33</td><td></td></tr>
<tr><td>overflow 788.38</td><td></td></tr>
<tr><td>paradoxical 788.39</td><td></td></tr>
<tr><td>rectal 787.6</td><td></td></tr>
<tr><td>specified NEC 788.39</td><td></td></tr>
<tr><td>stress (female) 625.6</td><td>←   Cause</td></tr>
<tr><td>   male NEC 788.32</td><td></td></tr>
<tr><td>urethral sphincter 599.84</td><td></td></tr>
<tr><td>urge 788.31</td><td></td></tr>
<tr><td>   and stress (male) (female) 788.33</td><td></td></tr>
<tr><td>urine 788.30</td><td></td></tr>
<tr><td>   active 788.30</td><td>←   Clinical Type</td></tr>
<tr><td>   male 788.30</td><td></td></tr>
<tr><td>   stress 788.32</td><td></td></tr>
<tr><td>   and urge 788.33</td><td></td></tr>
<tr><td>   neurogenic 788.39</td><td></td></tr>
<tr><td>   nonorganic origin 307.6</td><td></td></tr>
<tr><td>   stress (female) 625.6</td><td></td></tr>
<tr><td>   male NEC 788.32</td><td></td></tr>
<tr><td>   urge 788.31</td><td></td></tr>
<tr><td>   and stress 788.33</td><td></td></tr>
</table>

Carryover Lines

Carryover lines are needed because there is a limit to the number of words that can fit on a single line of print in the Index to Diseases and Injuries. Carryover lines are indented two standard indent spaces from the preceding line. For example:

<table>
<tr><td>Rubella (German measles) 056.9</td></tr>
<tr><td>   complicating pregnancy, childbirth,</td></tr>
<tr><td>   or puerperium 647.5</td></tr>
</table>

Nonessential Modifiers

A series of terms in parentheses, called nonessential modifiers, sometimes directly follows a main term or a subterm. The presence or absence of nonessential modifiers in the diagnosis has no effect on the selection of the code listed for that main term or subterm. For example:

> **Pneumonia** (acute) (Alpenstich) (benign) (bilateral) (brain) (cerebral) (circumscribed) (congestive) (creeping) (delayed resolution) (double) (epidemic) (fever) (flash) (fulminant) (fungoid) (granulomatous) (hemorrhagic) (incipient) (infantile) (infectious) (infiltration) (insular) (intermittent) (latent) (lobe) (migratory) (newborn) (organized) (overwhelming) (primary) (progressive) (pseudolobar) (purulent) (resolved) (secondary) (senile) (septic) (suppurative) (terminal) (true) (unresolved) (vesicular) 486

EXAMPLE: Patient was diagnosed with congestive pneumonia. The appropriate code assignment is 486. ("Congestive" is a nonessential modifier.)

EXAMPLE: Patient was diagnosed with pneumonia. The appropriate code assignment is 486. (Nonessential modifier is not stated.)

Eponyms

Many disease names, as well as operations, carry the name of a person. Known as an eponym, the term is defined by *Stedman's Medical Dictionary* as: "The name of a disease, structure, operation, or procedure, usually derived from the name of the person who discovered or described it first" (Williams & Wilkins 2000, 589). The main terms for eponyms are located in the Alphabetic Index as follows:

1. Under the eponym itself; for example:

> **Alzheimer's**
>   disease or sclerosis 331.0

2. Under main terms such as disease, syndrome, and disorder; for example:

> **Disease . . .**
>   Alzheimer's—*see* Alzheimer's

3. A description of the disease or syndrome, usually enclosed in parentheses, follows the eponym. For example:

> **Chiari's**
>   disease or syndrome (hepatic vein thrombosis) 453.0

Terms in the Alphabetic Index Not Included in the Tabular List

Occasionally, a diagnostic or procedure term in the Alphabetic Index (volume 2) is not included in the Tabular List (Volume 1). In such situations, only similar terms are listed and the guidance of the index should be trusted.

EXAMPLE: The term *listlessness* is included in the Alphabetic Index with a code assignment of 780.79. However, in reviewing the Tabular List to verify the accuracy of the code, the following is noted:

780.79 **Other malaise and fatigue**

Asthenia NOS
Lethargy
Postviral (asthenic) syndrome
Tiredness

As shown in the example, *listlessness* does not appear in the Tabular List description, although similar terms do. In such cases, the coder should always trust the guidance of the index.

Index Tables

Two main entries in the Alphabetic Index, **"Hypertension, hypertensive"** and **"Neoplasm, neoplastic"** have subterms arranged in tables. Using tables for these terms simplifies access to complex combinations of subterms. The index tables are discussed in detail in chapters 6 and 11 of this workbook.

Table of Drugs and Chemicals

The Table of Drugs and Chemicals is an alphabetical listing of drugs and other chemical substances. Each substance is assigned a code according to a poisoning classification. The table also contains a listing of external causes of adverse effects of the different drugs and chemical substances.

Alphabetic Index to External Causes of Injury and Poisoning (E Codes)

The Alphabetic Index to External Causes of Injury and Poisoning lists the codes (E codes) that classify environmental events, circumstances, and other conditions as the cause of injury and other adverse effects. The index is organized with main terms that describe the environmental event, circumstance, or specific agent that caused the injury or adverse effect. E codes are discussed in detail in chapter 19 of this workbook.

Conventions in ICD-9-CM

To assign diagnostic codes accurately, a thorough understanding of ICD-9-CM conventions is necessary, including those for cross-references and instructional notations.

Cross-References

Cross-references in the Alphabetic Index are directions to look elsewhere in the codebook before a code is assigned. The following subsections discuss three types of cross-reference terms: *see, see also,* and *see category.*

See

The *see* cross-reference points to an alternative term. This mandatory instruction must be followed to ensure accurate assignment of ICD-9-CM codes. For example:

Hemorrhage ...
ulcer—*see* Ulcer, by site, with hemorrhage

In the preceding example, a code cannot be assigned until the instruction that has been provided is followed. The codes listed under the main term **"Ulcer"** must be reviewed.

Often, the *see* cross-reference is found under the anatomic site and directs the coder to the condition or disease affecting that site. For example:

Aorta, aortic—*see* condition

In the preceding example, the main term **"Aorta, aortic"** offers the instruction to "*see* condition." Therefore, the condition affecting the aorta, such as arteriosclerosis, should be sought out.

The *see* instruction also may be encountered when a condition is indexed under more than one main term. For example:

Metrorrhexis—*see* Rupture, uterus

In the preceding example, the direction is to "*see* Rupture, uterus" for a list of codes.

See Also

The second type of cross-reference direction is *see also.* This instruction requires a review of another main term in the index when all the needed information cannot be found under the first main term.

> **EXAMPLE:**   Patient's diagnosis is osteoarthritis, localized to the hip.

Osteoarthritis (*see also* Osteoarthrosis) 715.9
    distal interphalangeal 715.9
    hyperplastic 731.2
    interspinalis (*see also* Spondylosis) 721.90
    spine, spinal NEC (*see also* Spondylosis) 721.90
Osteoarthrosis (degenerative) (hypertrophic) (rheumatoid) 715.9

> *Note— Use the following fifth-digit*
> *subclassification with category 715:*
>
> *0   site unspecified*
> *1   shoulder region*
> *2   upper arm*
> *3   forearm*
> *4   hand*
> *5   pelvic region and thigh*
> *6   lower leg*
> *7   ankle and foot*
> *8   other specified sites except spine*
> *9   multiple sites*

    deformans alkaptonurica 270.2
    generalized 715.09
    juvenilis (Kohler's) 732.5
    localized 715.3
       idiopathic 715.1
       primary 715.1
       secondary 715.2
    multiple sites, not specified as generalized 715.89
    polyarticular 715.09
    spine (*see also* Spondylosis) 721.90
    temporomandibular joint 524.69

In the preceding example, when the main term **"Osteoarthritis"** is located in the index, the instruction states "*see also* Osteoarthrosis." But first the subterms under osteoarthritis need to be reviewed to find an entry titled "localized." If that subterm is found, the code provided after it is assigned. When the subterm is not found—as is the case in the preceding example— the next step is to turn to the main term **"Osteoarthrosis"** in the Alphabetic Index and review its subterms to find an entry of "localized." The entry is found, and code 715.3 is selected. The boxed note appearing under the main term **"Osteoarthrosis"** reminds the coder that a fifth digit is required. The final code assignment is 715.35.

See Category

The third type of cross-reference in the Alphabetic Index, *see category,* is used less often. This cross-reference term instructs the coder to consult a specific category in volume 1, the Tabular List. For example:

Delivery
    normal—*see category* 650

Instructional Notations

Three types of instructional notations are used in ICD-9-CM: inclusion notes, exclusion notes, and general notes.

Inclusion Notes

Inclusion (includes) notes are used throughout the Tabular List to further define or provide an example of a category or section. They can appear in the following areas: at the beginning of a chapter or section and directly below a category or subcategory code.

An inclusion note that appears at the beginning of a chapter or section applies to all the codes within that chapter (as in the first of the following examples) or section (as in the second example).

---

1. INFECTIOUS AND PARASITIC DISEASES (001–139)

Includes: diseases generally recognized as communicable or transmissible as well as a few diseases of unknown, but possibly infectious, origin

---

ISCHEMIC HEART DISEASE (410–414)

Includes: that with mention of hypertension

An inclusion note that falls directly below a category or subcategory code applies to all the codes within that range. For example:

---

461   Acute sinusitis

Includes: abscess
empyema
infection   } acute, of sinus (accessory) (nasal)
inflammation
suppuration

Because the inclusion note is not repeated, it is necessary to look back to the beginning of the subcategory, category, section, and chapter to ensure that important instructions are not missed.

Exclusion Notes

The exclusion (excludes) notes found in the Tabular List are readily visible on review because the word "excludes" is in italicized print with a box around it. Exclusion notes can appear at the beginning of a chapter, at the beginning of a section, and below a category, subcategory, or subclassification. Exclusion notes have three different meanings:

- The most common exclusion note indicates that the code under consideration cannot be assigned when the associated condition specified in the note is present. Rather, the code specified in the exclusion note is assigned to fully identify the condition. For example:

424.3**Pulmonary valve disorders**

Pulmonic: Pulmonic:
   incompetence NOS   regurgitation NOS
   insufficiency NOS   stenosis NOS

| *Excludes:* | *that specified as rheumatic (397.1)* |

The exclusion note under 424.3 indicates that code 397.1 should be assigned when the pulmonary valve disorder is specified as rheumatic.

- The second type of exclusion note indicates that the condition may have to be coded elsewhere. Depending on the etiology of the condition, either the code under review or the code suggested in the exclusion note should be assigned, but not both. For example:

603**Hydrocele**

Includes: hydrocele of spermatic cord, testis, or tunica vaginalis

| *Excludes:* | *congenital (778.6)* |

The exclusion note indicates that a code from category 603, Hydrocele, should not be assigned when the hydrocele is congenital. Instead, code 778.6, Congenital hydrocele, is assigned.

- The third type of exclusion note indicates that an additional code may be required to fully explain the condition. This note indicates conditions that are not included in the code under review. Should the condition specified in the exclusion note be present, the additional code should be assigned. For example:

4. DISEASES OF THE BLOOD AND BLOOD-FORMING ORGANS (280–289)

| *Excludes:* | *anemia complicating pregnancy or the puerperium (648.2)* |

The exclusion note indicates that two codes should be assigned to code an anemia occurring during pregnancy or the puerperium: code 648.2, Anemia in the mother classifiable elsewhere, but complicating pregnancy, childbirth, or the puerperium, which indicates that the anemia is occurring during pregnancy; and a code from chapter 4, Diseases of the Blood and Blood-Forming Organs, of the ICD-9-CM codebook to indicate the specific type of anemia.

The Tabular List usually instructs the coder to "use an additional code," therefore indicating that both codes are necessary.

Instructional Notes

Instructional notes appear in the Tabular List and the Alphabetic Index in all three volumes of the ICD-9-CM codebook.

Some notes carry an instruction to assign a fifth digit. For example:

---

831 **Dislocation of shoulder**

> *Excludes:* *sternoclavicular joint (839.61, 839.71)*
> *sternum (839.61, 839.71)*

The following fifth-digit subclassification is for use with category 831:

0 **shoulder, unspecified**
  Humerus NOS
1 **anterior dislocation of humerus**
2 **posterior dislocation of humerus**
3 **inferior dislocation of humerus**
4 **acromioclavicular (joint)**
  Clavicle
9 **other**
  Scapula

Other notes provide additional coding instructions and also define terms. For example in the Alphabetic Index:

Injury 959.9

> *Note—For abrasion, insect bite (nonvenomous), blister, or scratch, see Injury, superficial.*
>
> *For laceration, traumatic rupture, tear, or penetrating wound of internal organs, such as heart, lung, liver, kidney, pelvic organs, whether or not accompanied by open wound in the same region, see Injury, internal.*
>
> *For nerve injury, see Injury, nerve.*
>
> *For late effect of injuries, classifiable to 850–854, 860–869, 900–919, 950–959, see Late, effect, injury, by type.*

An example in the Tabular List is:

765.0 **Extreme Immaturity**

  Note: Usually implies a birthweight of less than 1,000 grams
  Use additional code for weeks of gestation (765.20–765.29).

The appearance of a note differs, depending on the volume of the ICD-9-CM codebook in which it is located. Alphabetic Index notes are boxed and set in italic type; Tabular List notes are located at various levels of the classification system and are not boxed.

Multiple Code Assignment

The use of more than one code to fully identify a given condition is often necessary in ICD-9-CM coding. In such cases, one code describes the cause, or etiology, of the condition and the other, the manifestation(s). Several instructional notations alert coders that the assignment of more than one code is required. Instructions for sequencing and coordinating multiple codes also should be followed.

Use Additional Code, If Desired

The instructional notation "use additional code, if desired" is found in volume 1 of the ICD-9-CM codebook. It indicates that use of an additional code may provide a more complete picture of the diagnosis or procedure. The phrase "if desired" should be ignored; the additional code must always be assigned when the health record provides supportive documentation. An instruction that appears at the beginning of a chapter applies to all the codes in that chapter. For example:

---

8. DISEASES OF THE RESPIRATORY SYSTEM (460–519)

Use additional code to identify infectious organism

Sometimes the instruction appears at the beginning of a section. For example:

INFLAMMATORY DISEASE OF FEMALE PELVIC ORGANS (614–616)

Use additional code to identify organism, such as Staphylococcus (041.1)
or Streptococcus (041.0)

Finally, the instruction sometimes also appears in a subcategory. For example:

530.2   Ulcer of esophagus

Ulcer of esophagus: Ulcer of esophagus due to ingestion of:
   fungal   aspirin
   peptic   chemicals
                                 medicines

Use additional E code to identify cause if induced
by chemical or drug

Code First Underlying Disease

The instruction "code first underlying disease" is found in volume 1 of the ICD-9-CM codebook for categories in which primary tabulation is not intended. The code, title, and instructions are set in italic type to serve as a red flag not to assign that code as a principal diagnosis. The note requires listing, first, the code for the underlying disease (etiology) and, second, the code for the manifestation. Although the note will suggest underlying diseases in most instances, it is not all-inclusive because the physician may identify other causes not included in that list. For example:

366.4 **Cataract associated with other disorders**

   366.41 *Diabetic cataract*

      Code first diabetes (250.5)

   366.42 *Tetanic cataract*

      Code first underlying disease, as:
        calcinosis (275.4)
        hypoparathyroidism (252.1)

   366.43 *Myotonic cataract*

      Code first underlying disorder (359.2)

   366.44 *Cataract associated with other syndromes*

      Code first underlying condition, as:
        craniofacial dysostosis (756.0)
        galactosemia (271.1)

   366.45 **Toxic cataract**
      Drug-induced cataract

      Use additional E code to identify drug or other toxic substance

   366.46 **Cataract associated with radiation and other physical influences**

      Use additional E code to identify cause

Connecting Words

Following are examples of subterms listed in the Alphabetic Index to Diseases and Injuries that indicate a relationship between the main term and an associated condition or etiology:

And	In
Associated with	Involving
Complicated (by)	Of
Due to	Secondary to
During	With
Following	With mention of
	Without

Diabetes, diabetic 250.00
   with
      coma (with ketoacidosis) 250.3
        hyperosmolar (nonketotic) 250.2

The connecting words *with* and *without* are sequenced before all other subterms, as in the preceding example. Other connecting words are listed in alphabetical order.

ICD-9-CM assumes a causal relationship between some combinations of conditions, even though the diagnostic statement might not make such a distinction.

    EXAMPLE: Mitral valve stenosis is assumed to be rheumatic in origin and is assigned code 394.0, Mitral stenosis, from the section titled "Chronic Rheumatic Heart Disease."

For cases in which conditions often occur together, ICD-9-CM developed combination codes to identify both the etiology and the manifestation.

> **EXAMPLE:** Streptococcal infection occurs often in the throat, resulting in streptococcal sore throat. Therefore, code 034.0, Streptococcal sore throat, incorporates both the underlying disease, the streptococcal infection, and the manifestation—the sore throat.

Abbreviations, Punctuation, and Symbols

ICD-9-CM uses a variety of symbols, punctuation, and abbreviations. These are discussed in the following subsections.

Abbreviations

Two abbreviations related to coding that are used in ICD-9-CM are NEC, for codes that are not elsewhere classifiable, and NOS, for codes not otherwise specified.

NEC: Not Elsewhere Classifiable

NEC serves two purposes. First, it can be used with ill-defined terms listed in the Tabular List to warn the coder that specified forms of the condition are classified differently. The codes given for such terms should be used only when more precise information is unavailable.

459.0   Hemorrhage, unspecified
     Rupture of blood vessel, not otherwise specified (NOS)
     Spontaneous hemorrhage, not elsewhere classified (NEC)

     | *Excludes:* | *hemorrhage:* |

          gastrointestinal NOS (578.9)
          in newborn NOS (772.9)
          secondary or recurrent following trauma (958.2)
          traumatic rupture of blood vessel (900.0–904.9)

The preceding example advises the coder to assign code 459.0 only when no other information is available. Furthermore, the exclusion note serves notice that other forms of hemorrhage are classified elsewhere, such as gastrointestinal hemorrhage, NOS (578.9).

Second, NEC can be used with terms for which a more specific code is unavailable, even though the diagnostic statement is specific.

008.67   Enteritis due to Enterovirus NEC
     Coxsackie virus
     Echovirus

     | *Excludes:* | *poliovirus (045.0–045.9)* |

In this example, code 008.67 would be reported even though a specific enterovirus, such as echovirus, has been identified, because ICD-9-CM does not provide a specific code for it.

NOS: Not Otherwise Specified

The equivalent of "unspecified," NOS (not otherwise specified) is used only in the Tabular List of Diseases and Injuries. Codes describing NOS conditions are assigned only when the diagnostic statement and/or the health record does not provide enough information to use more specific codes. For example:

382.9   **Unspecified otitis media**

Otitis media:
  NOS
  acute NOS
  chronic NOS

Code 382.9 is the appropriate code assignment because the diagnostic statement and/or the health record lack additional information, such as purulent or serous.

Punctuation

ICD-9-CM uses five punctuation marks with specialized meanings. It should be noted that some publishers of ICD-9-CM have elected not to use certain punctuation marks.

Parentheses ( )

Parentheses enclose supplementary words or explanatory information that may or may not be present in the statement of a diagnosis or procedure. They do not affect the code number assigned to the case. Terms in parentheses are considered nonessential modifiers, and all three volumes of ICD-9-CM use them. For example:

---

515   **Postinflammatory pulmonary fibrosis**

Cirrhosis of lung
Fibrosis of lung (atrophic)
  (confluent) (massive)
  (perialveolar)
  (peribronchial)   } chronic or unspecified
Induration of lung

In the preceding example, category 515 includes five nonessential modifiers: (atrophic), (confluent), (massive), (perialveolar), and (peribronchial). The presence or absence of these modifiers in the diagnostic statement has no bearing on the assignment of code 515.

Square Brackets [ ]

Square brackets are used to enclose synonyms, alternative wordings, abbreviations, and explanatory phrases. In effect, they are similar to parentheses in that they are not required as part of the diagnostic statement. Square brackets are used only in the Tabular List.

427.0   Paroxysmal supraventricular tachycardia

Paroxysmal tachycardia:
atrial [PAT]
atrioventricular [AV]
junctional
nodal

In the preceding example, paroxysmal atrial tachycardia (PAT) and atrioventricular (AV) are enclosed in brackets.

---

460   Acute nasopharyngitis [common cold]

Coryza (acute)	Rhinitis:
Nasal catarrh, acute	acute
Nasopharyngitis:	infective
NOS	
acute	
infective NOS	

In this example, a synonym for acute nasopharyngitis, the phrase "common cold," is enclosed in brackets.

Slanted Brackets [ ]

Slanted, or italicized, brackets are found only in the Alphabetic Index to Diseases and Injuries. They enclose a code number that must be used in conjunction with a code immediately preceding it. The code in the slanted brackets, then, is always sequenced second.

In the Alphabetic Index, the first code represents the underlying condition and the second code, enclosed in the italicized brackets, represents the manifestation. For example:

Retinitis (*see also* Chorioretinitis) 363.20
diabetic 250.5 *[362.01]*

The sequencing of the preceding example is as follows: 250.5x, Diabetes with ophthalmic manifestations, and *362.01, Background diabetic retinopathy.*

Colon :

The colon is used in the Tabular List after an incomplete term that needs one or more of the modifiers that follow so that it can be assigned to a given category or code. For example:

---

204   Lymphoid leukemia

Includes:	leukemia:		leukemia:
	lymphatic		lymphocytic
	lymphoblastic		lymphogenous

In the preceding example, the colon indicates that the type of leukemia must be lymphatic, lymphoblastic, lymphocytic, or lymphogenous in order to be assigned a code from category 204.

Brace }

The use of braces simplifies tabular entries and saves printing space by reducing repetitive wording. Braces connect a series of terms on the left or right with a statement on the other side of the brace. A term from the left must be associated with the term on the right before the code under consideration can be assigned. For example:

INTERNAL INJURY OF THORAX, ABDOMEN, AND PELVIS (860–869)

Includes: blast injuries
blunt trauma
bruise
concussion injuries
  (except cerebral)
crushing   } of internal organs
hematoma
laceration
puncture
tear
traumatic rupture

Without the brace, the narrative would take up more space and be difficult to read.

Symbols

The official ICD-9-CM codebook uses two symbols:

§   Section Mark

☐   Lozenge

Section Mark §

A section mark symbol precedes codes in the Tabular Lists of both procedures and diseases. It indicates the presence of a footnote at the bottom of the page or references an instructional note located earlier in the section. A section mark symbol preceding a category applies to all subdivisions in that category.

**§ 656   Other fetal and placental problems
           affecting management of mother**

The section mark symbol preceding category 656 indicates that a footnote with an instruction to assign fifth digits printed on a previous page can be found at the bottom of the page.

Some publishers have elected not to use the section mark symbol in their versions of the official coding manual, opting instead for some other symbol as an alert for special instructions.

Lozenge ☐

Found immediately preceding a four-digit code in volume 1, the lozenge symbol identifies the code as unique to the clinical modification of ICD-9 (or ICD-9-CM, the system used in the United States). However, this symbol does not correlate directly with ICD-9. Although researchers may find this information helpful, coders ignore it because it has no significance to their tasks.

---

§851   **Cerebral laceration and contusion**

☐ **851.0**   **Cortex (cerebral) contusion without mention of open intracranial wound**

☐ **851.1**   **Cortex (cerebral) contusion with open intracranial wound**

☐ **851.2**   **Cortex (cerebral) laceration without mention of open intracranial wound**

☐ **851.3**   **Cortex (cerebral) laceration with open intracranial wound**

☐ **851.4**   **Cerebellar or brain stem contusion without mention of open intracranial wound**

☐ **851.5**   **Cerebellar or brain stem contusion with open intracranial wound**

☐ **851.6**   **Cerebellar or brain stem laceration without mention of open intracranial wound**

☐ **851.7**   **Cerebellar or brain stem laceration with open intracranial wound**

☐ **851.8**   **Other and unspecified cerebral laceration and contusion, without mention of open intracranial wound**

☐ **851.9**   **Other and unspecified cerebral laceration and contusion, with open intracranial wound**

Use of the Health Record in the Coding Process

The coding process for each physician's office should be organized to address the following:

- Review of the health record

- Selection of codes significant for the current episode of care

- Criteria for the sequencing of diagnostic and procedural codes

- Interaction with physician(s) regarding documentation issues

- Generic coding guidelines

- System-specific coding guidelines for different body systems

- Reimbursement requirements

These elements of the process should be documented in a coding policy and procedure manual developed jointly by the health information office manager and the physician(s). In addition, the advice and support of any and all users of encoded medical data should be sought. The criteria should address the comprehensive, and sometimes unique, data needs of the office practice; local, state, and national reporting requirements; third-party reimbursement requirements; and professional standards of care as determined by the physician(s).

Coding policies and procedures should be continuously assessed and updated using the AHA's *Coding Clinic for ICD-9-CM.*

After a thorough review of the record has been completed, the coder must uniformly apply coding principles and official coding guidelines to report the appropriate diagnoses. In almost all instances, the coder can confidently identify the principal diagnosis after carefully reviewing the documentation. However, problems may be encountered in poorly or inconsistently documented records. In such instances, documentation deficiencies should be discussed with the physician(s).

Basic Steps in ICD-9-CM Coding

The following basic steps must be followed in ICD-9-CM coding:

1. Identify all main terms included in the diagnostic statement.

2. Locate each main term in the Alphabetic Index.

3. Refer to any subterms indented under the main term. The subterms form individual line entries and describe essential differences by site, etiology, or clinical type.

4. Follow cross-reference instructions when the needed code is not located under the first main term consulted.

5. Verify the code selected in the Tabular List.

6. Read and be guided by any instructional terms in the Tabular List.

7. Assign codes to their highest level of specificity:

    —Assign three-digit codes only when no four-digit codes appear within the category.

    —Assign a four-digit code only when no fifth-digit subclassification exists for that subcategory.

    —Assign a fifth digit for any subcategory where a fifth-digit subclassification is provided.

8. Continue coding the diagnostic statement until all the component elements are fully identified.

Chapter 1 Exercises

Multiple Choice

Select the correct answer:

1. Physicians use ICD-9-CM to describe:
   a. Diagnoses
   b. Procedures
   c. Services
   d. Supplies

2. Which of the following represents a subclassification?
   a. 692.9
   b. 185
   c. 414.01
   d. 486

Review the following diagnoses and underline the main term:

3. Tension headache

4. Irregular menstruation

5. Diverticula of cecum

6. Congestive heart failure

7. Ewing's sarcoma

Answer the following questions:

8. According to the inclusion note under category 056, what condition is included in codes 056.0 through 056.9?

9. According to the exclusion note under category 558, what conditions are assigned codes 009.2 and 009.3?

10. According to the note under code 766.0, how is an exceptionally large baby defined?

Review the following statements and assign the appropriate codes:

11. Localized osteoarthritis of right knee

12. Bleeding esophageal varices in liver cirrhosis

13. Urinary tract infection due to Escherichia coli

14. Bronchiolitis due to respiratory syncytial virus

15. Diabetic neuropathy

Chapter 1 Review Questions

Answer the following questions:

1. When is it permissible to use only a three-digit code in ICD-9-CM coding? *When no 4th or 5th digits are Available.*

2. In a physician's office setting, is it correct to code diagnoses documented as "probable," "suspected," "questionable," "rule out," or "working diagnosis"? *No*

3. What is the proper way to code chronic diseases? *As often as the patient receives treatment*

4. In the Alphabetic Index, how are conditions found that include the term *disease* or *syndrome* in their title or description? *Under "disease" or syndrome, or under the disease or syndrome name.*

5. What are nonessential modifiers, and how do they affect code selection? *They do not effect code selection.*

6. What are inclusion notes, and where are they found? *— They further define a category or section. Found at beginning of chapter or under category.*

7. What do slanted brackets indicate in the Alphabetic Index? *The code must be used in conjunction w/ preceding code and is always second.*

History of malignancies — use V. Codes.
Diabetes, Hypertension is Chronic

Chapter 2

Supplementary Classification: V Codes

Objectives

After completing this lesson, the student should be able to do the following:

- Understand the appropriate uses for codes in the supplementary classification, or V code, section of the ICD-9-CM codebook

- Apply knowledge of current, approved ICD-9-CM coding guidelines to assign and sequence accurate codes for diagnoses requiring V codes

- Identify the main terms in the Alphabetic Index where common problems or circumstances of admission are indexed

Introduction

Categories V01–V85 are included in the ICD-9-CM codebook in the chapter entitled Supplementary Classification of Factors Influencing Health Status and Contact with Health Services. Supplementary classification is useful for coding in the following situations:

- When a person who is currently well uses health services for a purpose such as acting as a donor or receiving prophylactic vaccination

> **EXAMPLE:** Physician office visit for prophylactic flu shot: V04.8, Need for prophylactic vaccination and inoculation against influenza

- When a circumstance or problem influences the patient's current illness or injury but is not in itself a current illness or injury

> **EXAMPLE:** Patient visits physician's office complaining of chest pain due to an undetermined cause. The patient is status post open-heart surgery for mitral valve replacement, six months ago: 786.50, Chest pain, unspecified; V43.3, Heart valve replaced by other means

As shown in the example, this V code is assigned as an additional code.

- When a person with a known disease or injury uses the healthcare system for specific treatment of that disease or injury

> **EXAMPLE:** Patient visits the clinic for chemotherapy for diagnosis of acute lymphocytic leukemia: V58.1, Encounter for chemotherapy; 204.00, Acute lymphocytic leukemia

The supplementary classification for health status is subdivided as follows:

Categories	Section Titles
V01–V06	Persons with Potential Health Hazards Related to Communicable Diseases
V07–V09	Persons with Need for Isolation, Other Potential Health Hazards, and Prophylactic Measures
V10–V19	Persons with Potential Health Hazards Related to Personal and Family History
V20–V29	Persons Encountering Health Services in Circumstances Related to Reproduction and Development
V30–V39	Liveborn Infants According to Type of Birth
V40–V49	Persons with a Condition Influencing Their Health Status
V50–V59	Persons Encountering Health Services for Specific Procedures and Aftercare
V60–V69	Persons Encountering Health Services in Other Circumstances
V70-V85	Persons without Reported Diagnosis Encountered during Examination and Investigation of Individuals and Populations

V codes sometimes are used in the inpatient hospital setting but more frequently are assigned in the outpatient setting, such as physicians' offices, clinics, or outpatient hospital departments. Moreover, third-party payers may reject some V codes in claims submitted for payment. A thorough understanding of which V codes are acceptable and/or payable will aid in prompt and appropriate payment.

Main Terms

V codes are indexed in the Alphabetic Index along with all of the other diseases, conditions, symptoms, and so on. However, coders must familiarize themselves with the main terms where common problems or circumstances are indexed. They should look for terms that describe the reason for the encounter or admission.

> **EXAMPLE:** Patient is seen for closure of a colostomy: V55.3, Attention to colostomy

The statement in the above example requires a V code because the patient was admitted for attention to an artificial opening.

The following main terms included in the Alphabetic Index lead to V codes:

Admission (encounter)	History (personal) of
Aftercare	Maintenance
Attention to	Maladjustment
Boarder	Newborn
Care (of)	Observation
Carrier (suspected) of	Outcome of delivery
Checking	Pregnancy
Contact	Problem
Contraception, contraceptive	Prophylactic
Convalescence	Replacement by artificial or mechanical device
Counseling	or prosthesis of
Dependence	Resistance, resistant
Dialysis	Screening
Donor	Status
Examination	Supervision (of)
Exposure	Test(s)
Fitting (of)	Therapy
Follow-up	Transplant(ed)
Health	Unavailability of medical facilities
Healthy	Vaccination

The main terms listed in the Alphabetic Index are highlighted in boldface type.

Categories V01–V06

Categories V01–V06, Persons with Potential Health Hazards Related to Communicable Diseases, include codes that describe patients who have come in contact with, or been exposed to, a communicable disease, and who are in need of prophylactic vaccination and inoculation against a disease. The codes in these categories are referenced in the Alphabetic Index under **"Contact," "Exposure," "Prophylactic,"** and **"Vaccination."**

> **EXAMPLE:** Exposure to rubella: V01.4, Contact with or exposure to rubella

> **EXAMPLE:** Vaccination against diphtheria: V03.5, Need for prophylactic vaccination and inoculation against diphtheria alone

Reporting "exposure to" codes may justify the need for services provided to both symptomatic and asymptomatic patients with negative test results.

Categories V07–V09

Within categories V07–V09, Persons with Need for Isolation, Other Potential Health Hazards, and Prophylactic Measures, category V09 is used as an additional code for infectious conditions classified elsewhere to indicate the presence of drug resistance of the infectious organism. The codes in this category are to be used when the documentation in the health record indicates that the patient's infectious condition is resistant to the medication therapy administered. These codes are indexed in the Alphabetic Index under "**Resistance, resistant** (to)."

> **EXAMPLE:** Staphylococcus aureus infection resistant to penicillin medication: 041.11, Staphylococcus aureus; V09.0, Infection with micro-organisms resistant to penicillins

Categories V10–V19

Categories V10–V19, Persons with Potential Hazards Related to Personal and Family History, include codes for personal or family history of malignant neoplasms. In addition, these categories include codes for personal history of other diseases, allergy to medicines and other agents, and other history presenting hazards to health, as well as family history of other diseases. Typically, the codes in these categories are assigned as additional diagnoses to fully describe the reason for a visit or procedure and are indexed in the Alphabetic Index under "**History** (personal) of."

> **EXAMPLE:** Patient has had an allergic reaction to penicillin in the past: V14.0, Personal history of allergy to penicillin

> **EXAMPLE:** Patient's mother was diabetic: V18.0, Family history of diabetes mellitus

> **EXAMPLE:** Patient is known to have been noncompliant with treatment in the past: V15.81, Personal history of noncompliance with medical treatment

Categories V20–V29

Categories V20–V29, Persons Encountering Health Services in Circumstances Related to Reproduction and Development, include codes that describe supervision of normal and high-risk pregnancy, supervision or care of an infant, postpartum care, contraceptive management and surveillance, sterilization, procreative management, outcome of delivery, and antenatal screening. Code V20.2 is assigned for routine health checks or care of a healthy infant or child, which often is documented as "well-baby care."

Premature babies with a low birth weight are often prone to lifetime problems associated with the low birth weight. Subcategory V21.3, Low birth weight status, is used to identify patients who have a current condition attributable to low birth weight. Fifth digits specify the birth weight. This subcategory would not be used when the patient still has a condition that is classifiable to codes 760–779.

Category V22

Category V22 includes codes for supervision of a normal pregnancy. Generally, codes V22.0, Supervision of normal first pregnancy, and V22.1, Supervision of other normal pregnancy, are used in the outpatient setting. These codes are referenced in the Alphabetic Index under "**Pregnancy,** supervision (of) (for)." Code V22.2, Incidental pregnancy, is assigned as an additional code when a pregnant patient is seen for a reason that is unrelated to the pregnancy and does not affect the management of the pregnancy or the pregnancy itself. Further, to use this code, the physician must state that the condition is not affecting the pregnancy. Code V22.2 is indexed in the Alphabetic Index under **"Pregnancy."**

EXAMPLE:	Patient seen in emergency services with a sprained wrist and also is 30 weeks pregnant: 842.00, Sprains and strains of unspecified site of wrist; V22.2, Pregnant state, incidental
EXAMPLE:	Routine office visit for patient who is three months pregnant; this is her first pregnancy: V22.0, Supervision of normal first pregnancy

Category V23

Category V23 provides information on conditions that may add risk to a present pregnancy. The codes in this category are indexed in the Alphabetic Index under "**Pregnancy,** supervision (of) (for)" or "**Pregnancy,** management affected by." Code V23.7 may be assigned to patients who have had little or no prenatal care. For the information to be valuable, healthcare providers must define insufficient prenatal care and consistently capture this code.

EXAMPLE:	Pregnancy, 19 weeks' gestation with history of infertility: V23.0, Pregnancy with history of infertility
EXAMPLE:	Pregnancy, 23 weeks' gestation with history of preterm labor; V23.41, Pregnancy with history of preterm labor

Category V24

Category V24 is appropriate for use in the physician's office or clinic setting for uncomplicated follow-up care during the postpartum period (six weeks following delivery). When a postpartum complication is found, however, the appropriate diagnosis code should be assigned rather than a code from category V24. The codes in this category are referenced in the Alphabetic Index under "**Postpartum,** observation."

EXAMPLE:	Visit to physician for routine postpartum exam; no complications noted: V24.2, Routine postpartum follow-up
EXAMPLE:	Patient delivered at home and admitted to hospital with postpartum hemorrhage: 666.14, Other immediate postpartum hemorrhage

Category V25

Category V25 includes codes that describe contraceptive management, such as general contraceptive counseling and advice, insertion of intrauterine contraceptive device, menstrual extraction, encounter for emergency contraceptive counseling and prescription, and surveillance of previously prescribed contraceptive methods. Codes from this category are indexed in the Alphabetic Index under **"Contraception, contraceptive."**

Category V26

Category V26, Procreative management, describes healthcare services related to producing an offspring. The codes in this category can be used to describe services related to genetic testing and infertility. Healthcare encounters for reversal of a previous tubal ligation or vasectomy, artificial insemination, investigation and testing, and genetic counseling and testing are included in this category. Codes to describe a person's sterilization status also are included for both men and women.

> **EXAMPLE:** Female patient undergoes fertility testing by fallopian insufflation, V26.21

> **EXAMPLE:** Male patient is admitted for a vasoplasty after previous sterilization two years ago, V26.0

Category V27

Category V27, Outcome of delivery, contains codes that should be assigned on the mother's health record to indicate whether the outcome of delivery was single or multiple and liveborn or stillborn. The codes in this category are referenced in the Alphabetic Index under **"Outcome of delivery."**

> **EXAMPLE:** Spontaneous delivery of full-term live infant: 650, Normal delivery; V27.0, Outcome of delivery, single liveborn

Category V29

Category V29, Observation and evaluation of newborns for suspected condition not found, includes codes that are available for situations in which a newborn (defined as an infant during the first 28 days of life) is suspected of having a particular condition but exhibits no signs or symptoms and the suspected condition is ruled out after examination and observation. The codes in this category are located in the Alphabetic Index under **"Observation** (for), suspected, condition, newborn." A code from this category typically is reserved to be the principal or primary diagnosis code submitted on the claim form when the V30 code no longer applies.

> **EXAMPLE:** A 10-day-old infant is seen by a physician who is concerned that the baby may be affected by the mother's cocaine addiction. Drug screens were negative and the baby is fine: V29.8, Observation for other specified suspected condition

Categories V30–V39

A code from categories V30–V39, Liveborn Infants According to Type of Birth, is used to identify each type of birth and is always the first code listed on a newborn's health record. The categories describe single or multiple liveborns, and single or multiple stillborns. Codes for these categories are located in the Alphabetic Index under **"Newborn."** Any disease or birth injury also should be coded as additional diagnoses, when applicable.

Instructions for fourth and fifth digits are given at the beginning of this section of categories, as follows:

.0 Born in hospital (requires a fifth digit)
.1 Born before admission to hospital
.2 Born outside hospital and not hospitalized

The fourth digit .0 is assigned when a baby is born in the hospital. The following fifth-digit subclassification is used with the fourth digit .0:

0 delivered without mention of cesarean delivery
1 delivered by cesarean delivery

> **EXAMPLE:** Exceptionally large liveborn male infant delivered in hospital via low cervical cesarean section: V30.01, Single liveborn, delivered in hospital by cesarean delivery; 766.0, Exceptionally large baby

The fourth digit .1 is assigned when a baby is admitted to the hospital immediately after birth. The V codes in these categories are not assigned to newborns transferred from other hospitals.

> **EXAMPLE:** Infant admitted to hospital after birth at home: V30.1, Single liveborn, delivered before admission to hospital

> **EXAMPLE:** Infant with tetralogy of Fallot, a congenital heart defect, transferred to hospital B from hospital A. Hospital B would assign the following: 745.2, Tetralogy of Fallot

The fourth digit .2 is assigned to the V code when a baby is born outside the hospital and is not hospitalized. Therefore, this fourth digit should not be used in the acute care setting.

> **EXAMPLE:** Single liveborn infant, examined at home after birth; physical examination is essentially normal; infant will remain at home. Home visit is coded: V30.2, Single liveborn, born outside hospital and not hospitalized

Categories V40–V49

The note at the beginning of categories V40–V49, Persons with a Condition Influencing Their Health Status, indicates that "these categories are intended for use when these conditions are recorded as 'diagnoses' or 'problems.'" Often the codes in these categories further explain, and perhaps justify, the service or test being performed. They typically are assigned as additional diagnoses.

Category V42

Category V42, Organ or tissue replaced by transplant, is used to report homologous or heterologous (animal or human) organ transplants. The codes in this category are indexed in the Alphabetic Index under "**Status** (post), transplant."

> **EXAMPLE:** Status post heart transplant (human donor): V42.1, Heart replaced by transplant

Category V43

Category V43, Organ or tissue replaced by other means, is used to code replacement of an organ with an artificial device, a mechanical device, or a prosthesis. The codes in this category are indexed in the Alphabetic Index under "**Status** (post), organ replacement, by artificial or mechanical device or prosthesis of."

> **EXAMPLE:** Status post hip replacement with a prosthetic device: V43.64, Hip joint replaced by other means

Category V44

Category V44 is subdivided to identify the presence of an artificial opening such as tracheostomy (V44.0), gastrostomy (V44.1), ileostomy (V44.2), colostomy (V44.3), and cystostomy (V44.50–V44.59). These codes are indexed in the Alphabetic Index under "**Status** (post)."

> **EXAMPLE:** Status post colostomy: V44.3, Colostomy status

The exclusion statement at the beginning of category V44 should be noted. It serves as an instruction to use a different code (V55.0–V55.9) when the encounter or admission is for attention to, or management of, the artificial opening.

Category V45

Category V45 describes a variety of postsurgical states such as cardiac pacemaker in situ (V45.01), renal dialysis status (V45.1), presence of cerebrospinal fluid drainage device (V45.2), acquired absence of organ (V45.7x), and aortocoronary bypass status (V45.81). Codes in this category are located in the Alphabetic Index under "**Status** (post)."

> **EXAMPLE:** Patient is seen by the physician with diagnosis of coronary artery disease; patient is also status post CABG procedure three years ago: 414.00, Coronary artery disease; V45.81, Status post aortocoronary bypass procedure

Subcategory code V45.7 was created to indicate the status of an acquired absence of an organ in contrast to a congenital absence. This status is useful in describing the reason for the visit when a patient is seen for reconstructive surgery. The code is intended for use in patient care where the absence of an organ affects treatment. Fifth digits describe the absence of the breast, intestine, kidney, lung, stomach, eye, urinary sites, genital organs, or other organs. Subcategory code V45.84 indicates post status dental restoration such as crowns and fillings.

Category V46

Category V46, Other dependence on machines, includes codes that are assigned to cases of patients who have become dependent on respirators, aspirators, and other devices. The codes in this category are indexed in the Alphabetic Index under "**Dependence, on.**"

> **EXAMPLE:** Patient in acute respiratory failure dependent on respirator: 518.81, Acute respiratory failure; V46.11, Dependence on respirator, status

EXAMPLE: Severely disabled patient with emphysema is dependent on supplemental oxygen; 492.8, Emphysema; V46.2, Supplemental oxygen

Code V46.12 is used for encounters where patients are admitted for respirator dependence during power failure. Code V46.13 is used to report an encounter for weaning from mechanical failure of the respirator, and code V46.14 is used to indicate mechanical failure of the respirator.

Category V49

Within category V49, Other conditions influencing health status, code V49.81 is used to describe asymptomatic postmenopausal status for patients who present for services or testing related to this condition. For example, an asymptomatic woman may seek testing for bone density. In the absence of any conditions, syndromes, or postmenopausal disorders, code V49.81 is used.

Code V49.82 is used to indicate the presence of dental sealant, and V49.84 is used to specify bed confinement status.

Categories V50–V59

The following note appears at the beginning of categories V50–V59, Persons Encountering Health Services for Specific Procedures and Aftercare: "Categories V51–V58 are intended for use to indicate a reason for care in patients who may have already been treated for some disease or injury not now present, or who are receiving care to consolidate the treatment, to deal with residual states, or to prevent recurrence." The section is subdivided to describe the type of service provided. Codes in categories V50–V59 are indexed in the Alphabetic Index under "**Admission** (encounter), for," "**Aftercare,**" and "**Attention to.**" Typically, codes from these categories are sequenced first.

For encounters specifically for prophylactic removal of breasts, ovaries, or another organ due to a genetic susceptibility to cancer or a family history of cancer, the principal or first-listed code should be a code from subcategory V50.4, Prophylactic organ removal, followed by the appropriate genetic susceptibility code and the appropriate family history code.

If the patient has a malignancy of one site and is having prophylactic removal of another site to prevent either a new primary malignancy or metastatic disease, a code for the malignancy should also be assigned in addition to a code from subcategory V50.4. A V50.4 code should not be assigned if the patient is having organ removal for treatment of a malignancy, such as the removal of the testes for the treatment of prostate cancer.

Categories V52–V53

Categories V52–V53 include codes that describe the fitting and adjustment of prosthetic devices and implants, such as:

- V52.4, Fitting and adjustment of breast prosthesis and implant
- V53.2, Fitting and adjustment of hearing aid
- V53.31, Fitting and adjustment of cardiac pacemaker
- V53.7, Fitting and adjustment of orthopedic device
- V53.91, Fitting and adjustment of insulin pump
- V53.99, Fitting and adjustment, other device

Category V54

Category V54 is used for orthopedic aftercare and is further subdivided to describe the removal of an internal fixation device and other orthopedic aftercare. Code V54.0x is reported to describe a visit for removal of an internal fixation device, an encounter for lengthening/adjustment of growth rod, or other aftercare for internal fixation device, and subcategory code V54.8x is reported for other orthopedic aftercare, such as aftercare following joint replacement or cast removal. Subcategory V54.1 is used to report aftercare for continuing treatment of healing traumatic fractures. Fifth digits indicate the site of the fracture. Subcategory V54.2 is used to report aftercare for healing pathologic fractures with fifth digits indicating the site of the fracture.

> **EXAMPLE:** Removal of screw from healed fracture of arm: V54.01, Aftercare involving internal fixation device

Category V55

Unlike category V44, Artificial opening status, category V55 describes attention to the artificial opening, which may include any of the following:

- Closure
- Passage of sounds or bougies
- Reforming
- Removal or replacement of catheter
- Toilet or cleansing
- Adjustment or repositioning of catheter

> **EXAMPLE:** Replacement of cystostomy tube: V55.5, Attention to cystostomy

Category V56

Category V56 includes codes that describe encounters for dialysis, dialysis catheter care, and adequacy testing for hemodialysis and peritoneal dialysis. The instruction to "use additional code to identify the associated condition," such as renal failure, at the beginning of this category should be noted. The codes in this category are located in the Alphabetic Index under "Dialysis."

> **EXAMPLE:** Visit for renal dialysis for patient with end-stage renal disease: V56.0, Encounter for extracorporeal dialysis; 585.6, End-stage renal disease

Category V57

Category V57 includes codes that describe admissions or encounters for physical therapy, speech therapy, or occupational therapy. When a patient is admitted for a rehabilitation procedure, the first code listed is the V code, followed by the disease or condition requiring rehabilitation. Codes in this category are indexed in the Alphabetic Index under "Therapy."

> **EXAMPLE:** Encounter for physical therapy for hemiplegia due to CVA that occurred eight months ago: V57.1, Care involving other physical therapy; 438.20, Late effect of cerebrovascular disease, hemiplegia affecting unspecified side

Category V58

Category V58, Encounter for other and unspecified procedures and aftercare, includes codes that describe admissions or encounters for radiotherapy, chemotherapy, blood transfusion, attention to surgical dressings and sutures, therapeutic drug monitoring, other aftercare following specified surgery, and so on. An excludes note following code V58.4 reminds the coder that orthopedic aftercare (V54.0–V54.9) is excluded from this subcategory.

> **EXAMPLE:** Patient seen in the physician's office for removal of sutures from healed open wound of the forearm: V58.3, Attention to surgical dressings and sutures

Category code V58.6, Long-term (current) drug use, classifies a patient who is on long-term drug therapy such as anticoagulants (V58.61), antibiotics (V58.62), antiplatelets/antithrombotics (V58.63), non-steroidal anti-inflammatories (V58.64), steroids (V58.65), aspirin (V58.66), and insulin (V58.67).

Categories V60–V69

Categories V60–V69, Persons Encountering Health Services in Other Circumstances, include a variety of codes that identify other circumstances in which patients would encounter healthcare services.

Category V64 is used to report encounters for health services that are ultimately not carried out. Subcategory code V64.0 is used when a vaccination is not carried out for some reason, with fifth digits indicating the specific reason the vaccination was not done. Other codes in this category include:

V64.1	Surgical or other procedure not carried out because of contraindication
V64.2	Surgical or other procedure not carried out because of patient's decision
V64.3	Procedure not carried out for other reasons
V64.4	Closed surgical procedure converted to open procedure
	V64.41 Laparoscopic surgical procedure converted to open procedure
	V64.42 Thoracoscopic surgical procedure converted to open procedure
	V64.43 Arthroscopic surgical procedure converted to open procedure

Category V65

Category V65 is used to report encounters when a person is seeking consultation without complaint or sickness. Codes in V65 are used to report encounters for dietary surveillance; for counseling, including prebirth counseling for expectant mothers; for insulin pump training; and for patients with feared complaints in whom no diagnosis is made. V65.19 is used when another person is consulting on behalf of the patient. Code V65.11 is used when expectant mothers visit pediatricians for prebirth interviews.

Category V66

The codes in category V66, Convalescence and palliative care, are used primarily for patients during convalescence, often in a long-term care facility or hospice, after surgery, radiotherapy, or chemotherapy. This category is further subdivided to describe the reason for the convalescence.

The convalescence codes are indexed in the Alphabetic Index under "**Convalescence** (following)" and "**Admission** (encounter), for, convalescence following."

> **EXAMPLE:** Seventy-year-old patient admitted to a long-term care facility for convalescence following repair of hip fracture: V66.4, Convalescence following treatment of fracture

Category V67

The codes in category V67 are used to describe follow-up examinations. A note below the category title indicates that this category includes surveillance only following completed treatment. Thus, a code from this category would not be assigned for patients undergoing treatment, such as chemotherapy, for a particular condition. Instead, the appropriate code for the condition or treatment would be assigned from categories 001–999 or other V codes, as applicable. Category V67 is further subdivided to describe the completed treatment, such as surgery, radiotherapy, and chemotherapy. Codes in this category are indexed in the Alphabetic Index under "**Follow-up** (examination) (routine) (following)" and "**Admission** (encounter), for, follow-up examination (routine) (following)."

> **EXAMPLE:** Patient admitted for follow-up cystoscopy to rule out recurrence of malignant neoplasm of the urinary bladder; patient underwent a transurethral resection of the bladder a year ago and has been cancer free to date; cystoscopy revealed no recurrence: V67.09, Follow-up examination following other surgery; V10.51, History of malignant neoplasm of the urinary bladder

> **EXAMPLE:** Patient admitted for follow-up colonoscopy to rule out recurrent adenoma of the colon; patient underwent removal of adenoma three years ago; colonoscopy was positive for recurrence and adenoma was removed: 211.3, Benign neoplasm of colon

Categories V70–V85

Categories V70–V85, Persons without Reported Diagnosis Encountered during Examination and Investigation of Individuals and Populations, include codes that describe different types of medical examinations and special screenings.

Category V70

Category V70 includes several codes for general medical examinations. These codes are appropriate for routine visits, especially for preventive care when no complaints are present. In most cases, when a specific condition, sign, or diagnosis is presented and being evaluated, that code should be reported rather than a V code. Specifically:

- V70.0, Routine general medical examination at a healthcare facility

- V70.1, General psychiatric examination, requested by the authority

- V70.2, General psychiatric examination, other and unspecified

- V70.3, Other medical examination for administrative purposes

- V70.4, Examination for medicolegal reasons
- V70.5, Health examination of defined subpopulations
- V70.6, Health examination in population surveys
- V70.7, Examination of participant in clinical trial
- V70.8, Other specified general medical examinations
- V70.9, Unspecified general medical examination

Category code V70 excludes preprocedural general physical exams.

Category V71

Category V71, Observation and evaluation of suspected conditions, not found, includes codes that are assigned for encounters or admissions to evaluate the patient's condition when some evidence suggests the existence of an abnormal condition, but no supporting evidence for the suspected condition is found and no treatment is currently required. Codes in this category are located in the Alphabetic Index under "**Admission** (encounter), for, observation (without need for further medical care)" and "**Observation** (for)."

> **EXAMPLE:** Patient is admitted to the hospital for observation after an automobile accident because serious head trauma is suspected; all diagnostic tests are negative for head injury: V71.4, Observation following other accident

Category V72

Category V72, Special investigations and examinations, includes codes to describe ancillary services provided to a patient, such as radiological, laboratory, and preoperative examinations. The codes in this category are indexed in the Alphabetic Index under "**Admission** (encounter), for, examination" and "**Examination.**" When a patient receives only diagnostic services during a visit, the diagnosis, condition, problem, or other reason identified as the chief circumstance for the outpatient encounter should be sequenced first. Other diagnoses also should be coded, when appropriate.

> **EXAMPLE:** Patient visits the radiology department for chest x-ray:
> V72.5, Radiology examination, NEC

Because the patient has no other complaints documented, only the V code is appropriate.

> **EXAMPLE:** Patient visits the radiology department for chest x-ray to rule out pneumonia; patient complains of cough and fever: 786.2, Cough; 780.6, Fever

Because the patient presents with a complaint of fever and cough, either of these symptoms should be listed first, rather than the V code. The pneumonia is not coded because it was not established during the encounter.

> **EXAMPLE:** Patient visits the laboratory department for routine blood work:
> V72.6, Laboratory examination

Because the patient has no other complaints documented, only the V code is appropriate.

> **EXAMPLE:** Patient visits the laboratory department with complaints of polydipsia; a blood glucose test is performed to rule out diabetes: 783.5, Polydipsia

The symptom code for polydipsia is listed first. Because the diabetes has not been established during this encounter, it is not coded.

Code V72.31 is used to code a routine gynecological examination, while V72.32 is used when a repeat Pap smear is done following an initial abnormal smear.

Pregnancy test, unconfirmed, and pregnancy test, negative, are classified to V72.40 and V72.41, respectively.

Visits that require only preoperative evaluations are sequenced as follows:

1. Code from category V72.8x, Other specified examinations, to identify the preoperative consultation or visit

2. Code to describe the condition for which the surgery is being performed

3. Code to describe any conditions found during the preoperative evaluation

Categories V73–V85

Categories V73–V85 include codes to identify screening examinations for specific conditions and disorders that are currently inactive. Codes in categories V73–V84 are referenced in the Alphabetic Index under "**Screening** (for)."

> **EXAMPLE:** Patient visits the laboratory department for a diabetes blood test screening: V72.6, Laboratory examination; V77.1, Special screening for diabetes mellitus

When a code from category V72 is assigned, an additional code from categories V73–V84 also may be assigned to identify any special screening test performed. Category V85 identifies the body mass index for various age categories of adults.

Chapter 2 Exercises

Review the following statements and assign the appropriate codes:

1. Status post unilateral kidney transplant, human donor

   V42.0

2. Encounter for removal of cast

   V54.89

3. Encounter for chemotherapy for patient with Hodgkin's lymphoma

   V58.11   201.90

4. Reprogramming of cardiac pacemaker

   V53.41

Chapter 2 Exercises (Continued)

5. Replacement of tracheostomy tube

   _V55.0_

6. Encounter for speech therapy for patient with dysphasia secondary to an old CVA

   _V57.3 , 787.2_

7. Encounter for fitting of artificial leg

   _V52.1_

8. Office visit for gynecological examination, including Papanicolaou smear

   _V72.31_

9. Visit to radiology department for barium swallow

   _V72.5_

10. Follow-up examination of colon adenocarcinoma resected one year ago, no recurrence found

    _V58.42 , 153.9_

11. Admission to long-term care facility for convalescence following partial surgical resection, malignant neoplasm of brain

    _V66.0 , 191.9_

12. Routine general medical examination

    _V70.0_

13. Examination of eyes

    _V72.0_

14. Infant to clinic for developmental handicap screening

    _V79.9_

15. Encounter for laboratory test, patient complains of fatigue

    _780.79_   _sign only - No V-code_

16. Unconfirmed pregnancy test

    _V72.40_

17. Tetanus vaccination

    _V03.7_

18. Visit to the emergency department after falling 10 feet at work; no injuries noted

    _V71.3_

19. Patient presenting for a screening mammogram has a strong family history of breast cancer and is at high risk for cancer

    _V76.11   V16.3_

Chapter 2 Review Questions

Answer the following questions:

1. When is code V22.2, Incidental pregnancy, used?

2. How long is the postpartum period according to ICD-9-CM?

3. When is a code from V29 assigned on a baby's chart?

4. What code should be used when a postmenopausal asymptomatic woman presents for a bone density study?

5. When a patient has an encounter for dialysis, a code from category V56 is used. What additional code or codes are required?

6. When is it appropriate to use a code from category V71, Observation and evaluation of suspected condition?

7. What code(s) is used when a patient is seen for a chest x-ray due to a lingering cough?

Chapter 3

Late Effects

Objectives

After completing this lesson, the student should be able to do the following:

- Apply knowledge of current, approved ICD-9-CM coding guidelines to assign and sequence codes for diagnoses related to the late effects of disease and injury

- Differentiate between "late effect" and "residual" and be able to recognize terms and phrases that indicate a late effect

- Identify the time limit that applies to the occurrence of residual conditions

Introduction

ICD-9-CM coding provides diagnostic codes for disease processes related to all of the systems of the body. It also provides codes for the late effects of disease and injuries. A physician of any medical specialty can use any ICD-9-CM code.

Definition of Late Effects

Most illnesses or injuries completely resolve after medical treatment, but in some instances some type of healthcare problem remains. The temporary or permanent condition that follows the acute phase of an illness or injury is called a residual or late effect. Documentation in the health record may include the following terms and phrases to indicate a late effect:

- Residuals of
- Old
- Sequela of
- Late
- Due to a previous illness or injury
- Following a previous illness or injury

> **EXAMPLES:**   Hemiplegia following old cerebral thrombosis
> Scarring following third-degree burn
> Traumatic arthritis following fracture

The hemiplegia, scarring, and traumatic arthritis represent residuals of a previous illness or injury. The cerebral thrombosis, third-degree burn, and fracture represent the causes of the residuals.

Passage of Time and Residual Effects

A diagnosis sometimes reflects the fact that enough time has passed since the occurrence of an acute illness or injury that a residual effect is now present. For example, a fracture in a young person should heal in four to six weeks; in an older person, healing should take six to twelve weeks. When healing does not occur, the physician may state that the patient has a nonunion fracture, which is a condition that requires a late effect code.

There is no time limit within which the designation of a residual effect must be made. A late effect may be apparent early, as in a cerebrovascular accident, or it may occur months or even years later, as in the case of a previous injury such as a fracture (*Coding Clinic*, March–April 1986).

Coding of Late Effects

ICD-9-CM contains the following limited number of late effect codes to identify the cause of the late effect:

137   Late effects of tuberculosis
138   Late effects of acute poliomyelitis
139   Late effects of other infectious and parasitic diseases
268.1   Rickets, late effects
326   Late effects of intracranial abscess or pyogenic infection
438   Late effects of cerebrovascular disease
677   Late effect of complication of pregnancy, childbirth, and the puerperium
905   Late effects of musculoskeletal and connective tissue injuries
906   Late effects of injuries to skin and subcutaneous tissues
907   Late effects of injuries to the nervous system
908   Late effects of other and unspecified injuries
909   Late effects of other and unspecified external causes
997.6   Amputation stump complication

Late effects of specific diseases are discussed in the chapters on specific diseases in the ICD-9-CM codebook. For example, late effects of cerebrovascular disease, category 438, are included in the chapter on diseases of the circulatory system.

The code for the cause of the late effect can be located in the Alphabetic Index under "**Late,** effect(s) of."

Late—*see also* condition
    effect(s) (of)—*see also* condition
    cerebrovascular disease (conditions classifiable to 430–437) 438.9
      with
        alterations of sensations 438.6
        aphasia 438.11
        apraxia 438.81
        ataxia 438.84
        cognitive deficits 438.0
        disturbances of vision 438.7
        dysphagia 438.82
        dysphasia 438.12
        facial droop 438.83
        facial weakness 438.83
        hemiplegia/heriparesis
          affecting
            dominant side 438.21
            nondominant side 438.22
            unspecified side 438.20

Coding Guideline

The residual condition or nature of the late effect is sequenced first, followed by the cause of the late effect.

> **EXAMPLE:**   Scar of the right hand secondary to a laceration sustained two years ago: 709.2, Scar conditions and fibrosis of skin; 906.1, Late effect of open wound of extremities, without mention of tendon injury

Coding Guideline Exceptions

Exceptions to the preceding coding guideline are as follows:

- When the late effect code has been expanded at the fourth- and fifth-digit levels to include the manifestations.

  EXAMPLE: Dysphasia secondary to old cerebrovascular accident sustained one year ago: 438.12, Late effect of cerebrovascular disease, speech and language deficits, dysphasia

- When the health record does not identify the specific residual effect, only the late effect should be coded.

  EXAMPLE: Documentation in the health record states "late effect of polio": 138, Late effects of acute poliomyelitis

- When the Alphabetic Index indicates a different sequence, the directions of the index should be followed.

  EXAMPLE: Scoliosis due to poliomyelitis during childhood

  The following entries appear in the Alphabetic Index:

Scoliosis (acquired) (postural) 737.30
   congenital 754.2
   due to or associated with . . .
      poliomyelitis 138 *[737.43]*

- The index directs the coder to sequence, first, the late effect code (138), followed by the residual *[737.43]*, which is in italicized print and thus should not be reported as the principal diagnosis or first-listed code.

---

138   Late effects of acute poliomyelitis
737.43   *Scoliosis associated with other conditions*

- When ICD-9-CM does not provide a code to describe the cause of the late effect, only a code for the residual should be assigned. Conditions that are stated to be due to previous surgery are not considered late effects. Depending on the circumstances, a "history of" or surgical complication code may be reported.

Chapter 3 Exercises

Review the following statements and cases and assign the appropriate codes:

1. Epileptic seizures due to previous encephalitis

2. Malunion fracture of humerus due to old fracture

3. Residuals of old gunshot wound of leg

4. Paraplegia from previous laceration of spinal cord

5. Keloid of arm due to old crushing injury

6. Traumatic arthritis following fracture of left ankle

7. Scarring due to third-degree burn of left leg

8. Mild mental retardation due to viral encephalitis

9. Scar of skin of right leg secondary to open wound sustained eight months ago caused by accidental cut with knife

10. Dr. Smith, an orthopedic surgeon, sees a 20-year-old female suffering from painful swelling of the semilunar cartilage of the right knee due to a past sports injury. During the visit, she also states that her wrist seems to be pulling inward toward her body and that, at times, she is barely able to straighten it. After a thorough examination and further questioning, Dr. Smith discovers that a year earlier the patient suffered second-degree burns to that wrist resulting from a grease fire in a skillet.

    Impression: Contracture of the wrist due to past second-degree burns of the wrist; painful swelling of semilunar cartilage of the right knee

    Code(s):

11. A physician is called to emergency services to see a 46-year-old male who is having post-traumatic convulsions. A couple of years earlier, the patient suffered a skull fracture in a railway accident. Since the accident, he has experienced occasional dizziness and headaches that have always gone away until he began having the convulsions.

    Discharge diagnosis: Posttraumatic convulsions following a skull fracture two years ago

    Code(s):

Review Questions

Answer the following questions:

1. What is the difference between a late effect and a residual condition?

2. What is the time limit on when a residual condition can occur?

3. How is the code for the cause of a late effect located?

4. What is the coding guideline regarding the sequencing of a residual condition and a late effect?

5. What should be coded when the health record does not identify the specific residual effect, only the late effect?

6. What terms or phrases recorded in the health record indicate a late effect?

Chapter 4

Signs, Symptoms, and Ill-Defined Conditions

Objectives

After completing this lesson, the student should be able to do the following:

- Apply knowledge of current, approved ICD-9-CM coding guidelines to assign and sequence accurate codes for diagnoses related to signs, symptoms, and ill-defined conditions

- Differentiate between a sign and a symptom

- Identify those conditions that are integral to a disease process and those that are not

- Recognize the most common signs and symptoms

Introduction

Chapter 16 of the ICD-9-CM codebook, Signs, Symptoms, and Ill-Defined Conditions, is divided into the following sections. The codes in these sections, like all ICD-9-CM codes, may be used by physicians of any medical specialty or by general practitioners:

Categories	Section Titles
780–789	Symptoms
790–796	Nonspecific Abnormal Findings
797–799	Ill-defined and Unknown Causes of Morbidity and Mortality

A sign is objective evidence of a disease observed by a physician. A symptom is any subjective evidence of disease reported by the patient to the physician. It should be noted that the symptoms associated with a given organ system are classified to that particular chapter in the codebook. Examples include metabolic acidosis (276.2), gastrointestinal hemorrhage (578.9), and dehydration (276.51). Symptoms associated with many other body/organ systems or those of unknown causes are classified to chapter 16. Examples include nausea and vomiting (787.01), cough (786.2), chest pain (786.50), respiratory arrest (799.1), and anorexia (783.0).

Categories 780–789

Categories 780–789, Symptoms, include a variety of symptoms, many of which are appropriately reported as additional diagnoses. The signs and symptoms described in these categories are used when the following occur:

- Cases exist for which no more specific diagnosis can be made even after all the facts bearing on the cases have been investigated.

- Signs or symptoms existing at the time of the initial encounter prove to be transient and their causes cannot be determined.

- Provisional diagnoses remain for a patient who fails to return for further investigation or care.

- Cases are referred elsewhere for investigation or treatment before the diagnosis is made.

- A more precise diagnosis is unavailable for any other reason.

- Certain symptoms represent important problems in medical care, and it might be desirable to classify them in addition to a known cause.

- A symptom that was treated in an outpatient setting did not have the workup necessary to determine a definitive diagnosis.

The following coding guidelines apply for categories 780–789:

1. Conditions that are integral to the disease process should not be assigned as additional codes.

> **EXAMPLE:** Nausea and vomiting with gastroenteritis: 558.9, Other and unspecified noninfectious gastroenteritis and colitis

Only the code for gastroenteritis (558.9) is assigned. The code for nausea and vomiting (787.01) is not assigned because these symptoms are associated with gastroenteritis.

2. Conditions that are not an integral part of a disease process should be coded separately when present.

> **EXAMPLE:** Patient with metastasis to the brain is admitted in comatose state:
> 198.3, Secondary malignant neoplasm of brain and spinal cord;
> 780.01, Coma

The code for the coma (780.01) should be added as an additional diagnosis because coma is a significant condition that is not routinely associated with brain metastasis.

Symptoms and signs are used frequently to describe reasons for service in outpatient settings. Outpatient visits do not always allow for the type of study that is needed to determine a diagnosis. Often the purpose of the outpatient visit is to relieve the symptom rather than to determine or treat the underlying condition. Coders must code the outpatient's condition to the highest level of certainty. The highest level of certainty is often an abnormal sign or symptom code that is assigned as the reason for the outpatient visit.

Categories 790–796

Categories 790–796, Nonspecific Abnormal Findings, include codes for nonspecific abnormal findings on laboratory, x-ray, pathologic, and other diagnostic tests. In the outpatient setting, these codes may provide further explanation of the service provided, such as an elevated blood pressure reading (796.2) that requires further monitoring and workup.

The following guidelines apply when nonspecific abnormal findings in the inpatient setting are coded:

- Abnormal findings from laboratory, x-ray, pathologic, and other diagnostic results are not coded and reported unless the physician indicates their clinical significance. When the findings are outside the normal range and the physician has ordered other tests to evaluate the condition or has prescribed treatment, it is appropriate to ask the physician whether the diagnosis code(s) for the abnormal findings should be added.

- Exclusion notes in the section on nonspecific findings direct coders to search elsewhere in the ICD-9-CM codebook when documentation in the health record states the presence of a specific condition. Codes for these specific conditions are located in the Alphabetic Index under **"Findings, abnormal, without diagnosis."**

Often abnormal findings are the reason for additional testing to be performed on patients in the outpatient setting. For example, elevated prostate specific antigen (PSA) (code 790.93) may be a reason for continued testing or monitoring of a patient. The code does not provide a specific diagnosis but, rather, indicates an abnormal finding for a specific organ. Abnormal findings that are documented in the record may or may not be appropriate to code. When the coder notes an abnormal laboratory finding that appears to have triggered additional testing or therapy, he or she should ask the physician whether the abnormal finding is a clinically significant condition.

On other occasions, the coder will notice abnormal findings on radiological studies that may well be incidental to the patient's current condition. For example, an elderly patient with congestive heart failure is given a chest x-ray. A finding of degenerative arthritis is noted in the radiologist's conclusion, but no apparent treatment or further evaluation has occurred. It is unlikely that the arthritis should be coded.

The radiologist's findings can be used to identify the specific site of a fracture when the physician's diagnosis statement is nonspecific. For example, the attending physician writes "Fracture, left tibia." However, the radiologist describes the injury as a fracture of the shaft of the tibia. The coder may code 823.20, Fracture, tibia, shaft, based on the specific findings by the radiologist .

The radiologist's findings also may be used to clarify an outpatient's diagnosis or reason for services. For example, a patient comes to the hospital for an outpatient x-ray. The physician's order for the x-ray is "possible kidney stones." The radiologist's statement on the radiology report is "bilateral nephrolithiasis." Based on the fact that the radiologist is a physician, it is appropriate to code the calculus of the kidney, 592.0, as the patient's diagnosis (*Coding Clinic,* 2nd Quarter 2000).

Categories 797–799

Categories 797–799, Ill-Defined and Unknown Causes of Morbidity and Mortality, include conditions for which further specification is not provided in the health record or for which the underlying cause is unknown. These codes should not be used when a more definitive diagnosis is available.

> **EXAMPLE:** 799.01 Asphyxia
> 799.1 Respiratory arrest
> 799.2 Nervousness

In the preceding example, without further specification as to the underlying cause, the codes from chapter 16 are assigned. However, when the cause of the respiratory arrest is documented as congestive heart failure, that condition should be coded and not the arrest.

Common Signs and Symptoms

As previously discussed, when symptoms are routinely associated with a particular condition, only that condition is reported. However, when the symptom is not routinely associated with a specific condition, two separate codes may be assigned.

Some of the most common signs and symptoms are:

Syncope (780.2): Syncope is a fainting spell that usually follows a feeling of lightheadedness and may be prevented either by lying down or by sitting with the head between the knees. It may be caused by many different factors, including emotional stress, pooling of blood in the legs, heavy sweating, or a sudden change in room temperature or body position. Code 780.2 may be assigned when the diagnostic statement indicates blackout, fainting, near syncope, presyncope, collapse, or vasovagal attack.

Convulsions or seizures (780.31–780.39): Convulsions or seizures are characterized by a sudden, violent, and uncontrollable contraction of a group of muscles. Convulsions and seizures designated as febrile are assigned code 780.31; all other nonspecific seizures or convulsions are assigned code 780.39.

Dizziness and giddiness (780.4): This condition is a feeling of faintness or an inability to keep normal balance in a standing or a seated position. It sometimes is linked to mental confusion, nausea, and weakness. Code 780.4 also may be assigned when the diagnostic statement indicates lightheadedness, vertigo, or giddiness.

Early satiety (780.94): Early satiety is common in many conditions, such as hormone problems or a brain tumor. It is not the same as anorexia. Early satiety occurs in persons who have hunger and are eating but feel full.

Facial weakness (781.94): Code 781.94 is used when facial weakness is not a late effect of a CVA.

Disturbance of skin sensation (782.0): This condition describes the loss of skin sensation, often associated with tingling. Code 782.0 is assigned when the documentation states anesthesia of the skin, burning or prickling sensation of the skin, hyperesthesia or hypoesthesia of the skin, numbness, paresthesia, or tingling of the skin.

Abnormal weight loss or underweight (783.21 and 783.22): A relatively recent weight loss is reported with code 783.21, while the condition of weighing less than a person's standard weight for height is reported with code 783.22. The coder is instructed to also identify the Body Mass Index (V85.0) if it is known.

Lack of expected normal physiological development in childhood (783.4): Fifth-digit codes in this category describe three distinctive conditions relating to developmental problems. Failure to thrive, 783.41, is assigned when infants or children lose weight or fail to gain weight in accordance with standardized growth charts. Delayed milestones, 783.42, describes a child who fails to achieve developmental milestone(s) within the expected age windows. Short stature, 783.43, is a diagnosis for a slower-than-normal rate of maturation.

Epistaxis (784.7): Epistaxis is a nosebleed caused by irritation of the soft inner lining of the nose, violent sneezing, or fragile arteries in the nose. Additionally, it may be caused by long-term infection, injury, high blood pressure, leukemia, or lack of vitamin K. Epistaxis may result from tiny blood vessels breaking in the wall between the nostrils (nasal septum). It often occurs in children. In adults, it is more common among men than women and may be severe in elderly persons. Epistaxis may cause respiratory distress, dizziness, and nausea, and blood loss may lead to fainting.

Palpitations (785.1): Palpitations are characterized by a pounding or racing of the heart and are linked to normal emotional responses or with some heart disorders. Some people may complain of a pounding heart and show no sign of heart disease. Others, who have serious heart disorders, may not detect palpitations. When the palpitations occur as a result of an established condition, such as atrial fibrillation (427.31), the palpitation code is not reported.

Enlargement of lymph nodes (785.6): Enlargement of lymph nodes also is referred to as lymphadenopathy or swollen glands. Code 785.6 is reported when a definitive diagnosis has not been established. When the documentation indicates a diagnosis of acute or chronic lymphadenitis, the following codes are assigned: 683, Acute lymphadenitis, and 289.1, Chronic lymphadenitis.

Symptoms involving respiratory system and other chest symptoms (786): This category describes a classification of a variety of conditions, including:

786.01	Hyperventilation
786.02	Orthopnea
786.03	Apnea
786.04	Cheyne-Stokes respiration
786.05	Shortness of breath
786.06	Tachypnea
786.07	Wheezing

786.09	Other dyspnea and respiratory abnormalities
786.1	Stridor
786.2	Cough
786.3	Hemoptysis
786.4	Abnormal sputum
786.50	Unspecified chest pain
786.51	Precordial pain
786.52	Painful respiration/pleurodynia
786.59	Other specified chest pain, including chest discomfort, tightness, or pressure
786.6	Swelling, mass, or lump in chest
786.7	Abnormal chest sounds
786.8	Hiccough
786.9	Other symptoms involving respiratory system and chest

Hyperventilation (786.01): Hyperventilation is characterized by a breathing rate that is greater than that necessary for the exchange of oxygen and carbon dioxide. Its causes include asthma or early emphysema; increased metabolism because of exercise, fever, hyperthyroidism, or infections; damage to the central nervous system, as in cerebral thrombosis; encephalitis, head injuries, or meningitis; certain hormones and drugs; difficulties with mechanical respirators; and mental factors such as anxiety and pain.

Nausea and vomiting (787.0): This category refers to a common stomach upset. Fifth digits indicate whether both conditions were present, as follows:

787.01	Nausea with vomiting
787.02	Nausea alone
787.03	Vomiting alone

However, when the condition is documented as vomiting of blood (hematemesis), code 578.0 should be assigned.

Heartburn (787.1): Heartburn is a painful burning sensation in the throat (esophagus) just below the breastbone. Typically, heartburn is caused by stomach contents flowing back into the esophagus, but it also may be caused by too much acid in the stomach or by a peptic ulcer.

Dysphagia (787.2): Dysphagia is difficulty in swallowing, commonly linked to blockage or motor disorders of the esophagus. Patients with blockages such as esophageal tumors or lower esophageal rings are unable to swallow solids but can tolerate liquids. Other conditions included in this category are achalasia, aphagia, or corkscrew esophagus.

Diarrhea (787.91): Usually, diarrhea is a symptom of some other disorder or of a more severe disease, in which case it should not be coded separately. It may be accompanied by vomiting and various other symptoms that should be coded when present.

Retention of urine (788.2): This is the abnormal accumulation of urine in the bladder due to the inability to urinate. This code excludes urinary retention due to hyperplasia of the prostate.

Incontinence of urine (788.3x): This is the inability to completely control urination with involuntary passage of urine. Fifth digits indicate specific types such as urge, stress, mixed, post-void dribbling, nocturnal enuresis, and overflow.

Urgency of urination (788.63): This is a common symptom of feeling an intense need to urinate.

Abdominal pain (789.0): Fifth digits identify the specific parts of the abdomen affected, as follows:

789.00	Abdominal pain, unspecified site
789.01	Abdominal pain, right upper quadrant
789.02	Abdominal pain, left upper quadrant
789.03	Abdominal pain, right lower quadrant
789.04	Abdominal pain, left lower quadrant
789.05	Abdominal pain, periumbilic
789.06	Abdominal pain, epigastric
789.07	Abdominal pain, generalized
789.09	Abdominal pain of other specified site or multiple sites

Chapter 4 Exercises

Review the following statements and cases and assign the appropriate codes:

1. Right lower quadrant abdominal pain with nausea, vomiting, and diarrhea

2. Abnormal mammogram

3. Ten-month-old infant with excessive crying, fever, and runny nose; final diagnoses: acute rhinitis and acute left otitis media

4. Abnormal glandular Pap smear of the cervix

5. Sudden infant death syndrome

6. Sleep apnea with insomnia

7. Shortness of breath, cause undetermined

8. Septicemia and septic shock

9. Pneumonia with cough

10. Elevated blood pressure reading; hypertension not confirmed

(Continued on next page)

Chapter 4 Exercises (Continued)

11. Stress urinary incontinence in male patient

788.32

12. Seizures; epilepsy, ruled out

13. Abdominal mass with jaundice

789.30 , 782.4

14. Abnormal glucose tolerance test

790.29 → 790.22 because it is a TEST

15. Elevated PSA

790.93

16. Failure to thrive in 2-year-old child

783.41

17. A male patient was admitted because of severe midsternal chest pain also involving both arms. Several cardiac procedures were performed (heart catheterization, arteriography, and angiography), but they revealed no coronary artery disease. The patient's pain improved, and he was discharged in no apparent distress.

Discharge diagnosis: Chest pain with no coronary artery disease

Code(s):

786.50, 786.51 because it's midsternal

18. A 43-year-old female patient was seen in emergency services with generalized abdominal pain that was moderate to severe in intensity. Blood work showed an elevated white blood count. The diagnosis at the time the patient was seen was thought to be possible acute cholecystitis. Several tests were run (IVP, cholecystogram, and gallbladder ultrasound), all of which came back within normal limits. Within a couple of days, the patient became pain free, her white count returned to normal, and she asked to leave the hospital because she was feeling better.

Discharge diagnoses: Abdominal pain; leukocytosis

Code(s):

789.07, 288.8

19. A 63-year-old type II diabetic female was admitted because of elevated liver function studies and known cholelithiasis. A hepatitis profile was done and found to be normal. Her blood sugar was constantly monitored and remained in the normal range throughout her hospital stay. Upon discharge, the physician was unsure whether the elevated liver function studies were due to her cholelithiasis or her diabetic condition.

Discharge diagnoses: Abnormal liver function studies secondary to either cholelithiasis or diabetes mellitus

Code(s):

790.6 (794.8) ✓ correct because its liver function study

250.00 – diabetes
574.20 – cholelithiasis

See page 381 section E for why you code both Hypertension and Cholelithiasis

pag 381 letter E

Review Questions

Answer the following questions:

1. What is the difference between a sign and a symptom?

2. Should abnormal laboratory findings that have triggered additional testing or therapy always be coded?

3. When is it appropriate to assign codes from categories 797–799, Ill-Defined and Unknown Causes of Morbidity and Mortality?

4. Are conditions that are integral to the disease process assigned as additional codes?

5. On an outpatient basis, what is coded when only a sign or symptom is known?

6. When laboratory, x-ray, pathologic, and other diagnostic results are outside the normal range and the physician has either ordered additional tests to evaluate the condition or even prescribed treatment, should a coder assign a code for these abnormal findings?

1. Sign - observed by the physician
   Symptom - reported by the patient

2. No, unless the physician indicates clinical significance

3. When further specification is not provided in the health record.

4. No

5. The code for the abnormal sign or symptom — to highest certainty

6. The coder should ask the physician if the should code for abnormal findings — No.

Chapter 5

Infectious and Parasitic Diseases

Objectives

After completing this lesson, the student should be able to do the following:

- Apply knowledge of current, approved ICD-9-CM coding guidelines to assign and sequence accurate codes for infectious and parasitic diseases

- Generally understand the basic laboratory tests performed to assist physicians in the diagnosis and treatment of infectious diseases

- Identify the general categories of microorganisms that cause infections

- List V codes appropriate to infectious and parasitic diseases

Introduction

Chapter 1 of the ICD-9-CM codebook includes diseases recognized as communicable or transmissible and some diseases of unknown, but possibly infectious, origin. The infectious and parasitic diseases incorporated within chapter 1 are classified by body site and organism. Noncommunicable diseases are classified by site to other chapters in the codebook. Physicians of all specialties use these codes to identify infections that affect any body system. The infectious and parasitic diseases chapter is further subdivided into the following broad sections:

Categories	Section Titles
001–009	Intestinal Infectious Diseases
010–018	Tuberculosis
020–027	Zoonotic Bacterial Diseases
030–041	Other Bacterial Diseases
042	Human Immunodeficiency Virus [HIV] Infection
045–049	Poliomyelitis and Other Non-Arthropod-Borne Viral Diseases of Central Nervous System
050–057	Viral Diseases Accompanied by Exanthem
060–066	Arthropod-Borne Viral Diseases
070–079	Other Diseases Due to Virus and Chlamydiae
080–088	Rickettsioses and Other Arthropod-Borne Diseases
090–099	Syphilis and Other Venereal Diseases
100–104	Other Spirochetal Diseases
110–118	Mycoses
120–129	Helminthiases
130–136	Other Infectious and Parasitic Diseases
137–139	Late Effects of Infectious and Parasitic Diseases

Laboratory Tests Used in the Diagnosis and Treatment of Infectious Diseases

Before reviewing specific categories in this chapter, it will be helpful to have a general understanding of some of the basic laboratory tests that can assist the physician in the diagnosis and treatment of infectious diseases.

Smear and Stain Examinations

The Gram stain technique is named for Dr. Christian Gram, who first described it in 1884. This technique can assist a physician in making a diagnosis by providing clues to the agent causing an infection, thus helping the physician determine the appropriate antibiotic to prescribe while waiting for culture results. Gram-positive organisms stain purple; Gram-negative organisms shed the stain and appear red. Some examples of Gram-positive and Gram-negative organisms include the following:

Gram-Positive Organisms	Gram-Negative Organisms
Staphylococcus	Neisseria
Streptococcus	Branhamella (Moraxella)
Bacillus	Campylobacter
Clostridium	Enterobacteriaceae
Lactobacillus	Salmonella Proteus
Actinomyces	Klebsiella Serratia
Listeria	Yersinia Shigella
Corynebacterium	Morganella Citrobacter
Peptococcus	Vibrio
Peptostreptococcus	Aeromonas
	Proteus
	Serratia
	Shigella
	Citrobacter

When a good sputum specimen is obtained, the Gram stain is a rapid, simple, and inexpensive technique for diagnosing bacterial pneumonia.

In addition to separating bacteria into Gram-positive and Gram-negative groups, the Gram-staining process also indicates the shape of the bacterium. Bacteria may appear as rods or cocci. Examples of how the shape is used to classify bacteria include the following:

Shape	Organism
Cocci in chains	Streptococci
Cocci in clusters	Staphylococci
Straight rods	Salmonella
Brick-shaped rods	Clostridium perfringens

Acid-fast stains are used when bacteria do not stain easily with the Gram stain. Examples of acid-fast stains are Ziehl-Neelsen stain, Fluorochrome stain, and Kinyoun stain.

Other staining methods and the types of organisms that are examined by microscope include the following:

Name of Stain	Organism(s) Examined
Tzanck stain	Herpes simplex and varicella-zoster skin lesions
Silver stain	Treponema, fungi, P. carinii, Legionella, rickettsiae
Periodic Acid-Schiff	Fungi
Acridine orange	Bacteria, fungi, trichomonads
Methylene blue	Fecal leukocytes
Giemsa and Wright	Malaria, Helicobacter pylori

Cultures

In culturing specimens, the rate of growth, atmospheric needs (such as aerobic or anaerobic), and nutritional requirements of the bacterium are clues to its identification. Media commonly used in culturing are liquid (broths) and gel (agar). The grouping of bacterium growth on a culture is referred to as a colony. Additional clues for bacteria identification include odor, pigment production, and shape, size, and consistency of the colony.

Serologic Studies

Serologic studies are used to provide a specific diagnosis when attempts to identify an infectious agent are unsuccessful or impractical, or when culture techniques or facilities are unavailable. Often therapeutic decisions are made before the serologic test results can be made available. Infectious diseases commonly diagnosed by serologic testing include syphilis, rubella, Mycoplasma pneumoniae, Lyme disease, and infectious mononucleosis.

Microorganisms That Cause Infections

Coders need to know the general categories of microorganisms that cause infections. Microorganisms that infect humans and induce disease include bacteria, parasites, fungi, and viruses. In terms of medicine, microbial diseases are classified according to the affected organ or system. For example, the bacterium Staphylococcus aureus can cause disease of the skin, bones, and respiratory tract. The coxsackie virus B5 can induce symptoms involving the central nervous system, serous membranes, and skeletal and cardiac musculature.

Bacteria

Bacteria are one-celled, microscopic organisms that multiply by cell division. For millions of years, they were the dominant forms of life on earth. Today, they are found in virtually all environments. Some bacteria are vital to the functioning of ecosystems; others cause infections and diseases in humans and animals.

Streptococcus pyogenes (Group A) is an inhabitant of the upper respiratory tract and is spread by droplets or direct contact, especially in overcrowded conditions. When infection occurs in the upper respiratory tract, the result is acute exudative pharyngitis, with or without tonsillitis, peritonsillar abscess, or suppurative lymphadenitis. Other manifestations of S. pyogenes are impetigo, chronic renal failure, rheumatic fever, and carditis.

Streptococcus pneumoniae (Group C) is a common organism found in the mouth of 10 to 40 percent of healthy people. Often referred to as pneumococcus, this organism causes lobar pneumonia in adults and sinusitis and otitis media in children. Group C streptococcus also is the most common cause of meningitis in the elderly. A vaccine is available for these high-risk people. Other organisms include Group D streptococcus, which sometimes is seen in patients with gastrointestinal neoplasms, and Group G streptococcus, which causes a variety of infections including bursitis, pleuropulmonary infections, and skin and soft-tissue infections.

Staphylococcus aureus organisms may cause infections involving the skin and subcutaneous tissues, the eye, or the ear. These organisms also cause diseases such as pneumonia, endocarditis, osteomyelitis, food poisoning, and toxic shock syndrome. This organism can be transmitted by direct spread or through the bloodstream.

Clostridium difficile normally inhabits the bowel. In recent years, it has been recognized as a cause of pseudomembranous colitis. Diarrhea and fever are symptoms of intestinal infection caused by this organism.

Mycoplasma is a genus of bacteria, of which the three most common species that produce disease in humans are M. pneumoniae, M. hominis, and Ureaplasma urealyticum. The latter two organisms are together referred to as genital mycoplasmas because of their connection with the genital tract. M. pneumoniae can cause other respiratory diseases such as pneumonia, pharyngitis, laryngitis, bronchiolitis, and bronchitis.

The Enterobacteriaceae is a large group of bacteria characterized by the shape of Gram-negative rods. Infections that primarily affect the gastrointestinal tract are caused by the bacterium Escherichia coli (E. coli).

Bacillus includes many bacteria, but only a few cause disease in humans. Bacillus anthracis and Bacillus cereus are causes of anthrax and food poisoning, respectively.

Clostridium perfringens is an organism that normally inhabits the human intestines. This organism can cause cellulitis and food poisoning.

Chlamydia trachomatis bacteria cause an infection that affects the conjunctiva, the urethra, and the cervical canal. Conjunctival infections are spread by contaminated hands. A neonate born to an infected mother may contract an infection by passing through the infected birth canal. Genital chlamydia trachomatis infections are spread by sexual contact.

Table 5.1 describes the locations of infections caused by common pathogens.

Table 5.1.   Infection sites with common pathogens

Location of Infection	Common Pathogen
Urinary tract infections	E. coli, Klebsiella, Proteus, Pseudomonas sp., Enterococci

Intravenous catheter phlebitis and/or sepsis:
   Peripheral catheter
 	
   Hyperalimentation line
	Staphylococcus aureus, S. epidermidis, Klebsiella, Enterobacter, Pseudomonas sp., Candida sp., S. aureus, S. epidermidis, Enterococci

Arteriovenous shunt	S. aureus, S. epidermidis
Septic bursitis	S. aureus
Septic arthritis	S. aureus, Gram-negative organisms in high-risk patients,* H. influenzae in children, Group B streptococci in neonates
Biliary tract	E. coli, Klebsiella sp., Enterococci, Bacteroides fragilis in elderly patients
Intra-abdominal abscess, peritonitis	E. coli, B. fragilis, Klebsiella sp., Enterococci
Burn wounds	Early: S. aureus, Streptococci Later: Gram-negative bacilli, fungi
Cellulitis, wound, and soft tissue infections or large bowel perforation	S. aureus, Streptococci, Clostridium sp.
Pelvic abscess, postabortion or postpartum	Anaerobic streptococci, B. fragilis, Clostridium sp., E. coli, Enterococci
Acute osteomyelitis	S. aureus, H. influenzae in children, Group B streptococci in neonates, Gram-negative organisms in high-risk patients*

*High-risk patients include the elderly, IV drug abusers, diabetics, and debilitated or immunocompromised patients.

Parasites

A parasite is an organism that lives in or on another living organism. The Sporozoea is a class of microscopic parasites that can cause many human and animal diseases, including malaria. Worms also are classified as parasites, including the tapeworm, fluke, roundworm, pinworm, hookworm, and whipworm.

Fungi

Fungi also can cause infectious diseases, including poisonings, allergies, cutaneous or mucous membrane infections, and subcutaneous and invasive infections. However, most fungal infections do not spread from person to person.

One fungal infection, Candidiasis infection, is so common that the disease has received several other names, such as moniliasis, thrush, and mycotic vulvovaginitis. Essentially, the Candida albicans species causes this fungus disease. The disease may be localized to the mouth, throat, skin, scalp, vagina, fingers, nails, bronchi, lungs, or GI tract.

The following conditions can lead to opportunistic infection by the pathogen Candida:

- Extreme youth (thrush or diaper rash)
- Physiologic change (pregnancy with vaginitis, postsurgical status)
- Administration of steroids
- Prolonged administration of antibiotics
- General debility (diabetes, malignancy, AIDS)

Viruses

A virus is a minute infectious microorganism that is much smaller than a bacterium and replicates only within a living host cell.

Following is a list of commonly known viral infections:

Adenoviridae (adenoviruses)	Measles
Arbovirus (encephalitis)	Mumps
Aseptic meningitis	Papilloma viruses
Cytomegalovirus (CMV)	Paralytic poliomyelitis
Epstein-Barr virus	Respiratory syncytial virus
Hepatitis viruses	Rubella
Herpes simplex virus	Varicella zoster
Human immunodeficiency virus	Zoonoses (rabies)
Influenza virus types A and B	

More information on common viral infections is presented later in this chapter.

In coding infectious and parasitic diseases, the entire health record must be reviewed to identify the following:

- Body site (such as lungs, liver, skin, or vagina)
- Severity of the disease (acute versus chronic)

- Specific organism or parasite (such as Candida, bacteria, or virus)

- Etiology of the infection (such as food poisoning)

- Associated signs, symptoms, or manifestations (such as jaundice or Kaposi's sarcoma)

Combination Codes and Multiple Coding

Chapter 1 of the ICD-9-CM codebook includes many combination codes to identify both the condition and the causative organism.

> **EXAMPLE:** 112.0 Candidiasis of mouth
> 006.1 Chronic intestinal amebiasis without mention of abscess
> 130.1 Conjunctivitis due to toxoplasmosis

Multiple coding is often necessary to completely describe an infectious condition or disease.

Categories 041 and 079

Typically, both categories 041 and 079 are assigned as additional diagnoses to describe the causative organism in diseases that are classified elsewhere in ICD-9-CM. Category code 041, Bacterial infection in conditions classified elsewhere and of unspecified site, is assigned when the organism is a bacterium. Category code 079, Viral and chlamydial infection in conditions classified elsewhere and of unspecified site, is assigned when the organism is a virus or chlamydia. In both categories, the codes may be located using the main term **"Infection"** in the Alphabetic Index to Diseases.

Category 041 is further subdivided to identify specific bacteria such as streptococcus, staphylococcus, pneumococcus, and so forth.

> **EXAMPLE:** Urinary tract infection due to E. coli
> 599.0 Urinary tract infection, site not specified
> 041.4 Escherichia coli (E. coli)

Category 079 is further subdivided to identify specific viruses, such as adenovirus; ECHO virus; Coxsackie virus; retrovirus; human T-cell lymphotrophic virus, types I and II; human immunodeficiency virus, type 2; and so forth.

> **EXAMPLE:** Acute viral osteomyelitis of the hip
> 730.05 Acute osteomyelitis, pelvic region and thigh
> 079.99 Unspecified viral infection

Infection with Drug-Resistant Microorganisms

The note given for this category in the ICD-9-CM codebook states that the codes in category V09 are intended for use as additional codes for infectious conditions classified elsewhere to indicate the presence of drug resistance in the infectious organism. Code assignment should not be based on the laboratory or sensitivity reports alone. The physician statement should be the source for learning whether an infectious organism is drug resistant. When referring to drug resistance, physicians make common statements such as multidrug-resistant tuberculosis and methicillin-resistant Staphylococcus aureus.

A category V09 code is intended for use as an additional code(s) to either the disease caused by the infectious organism or the complication or comorbid condition.

Common Infectious Diseases

This section looks at various infectious diseases for which codes may need to be assigned. Each disease is described along with the coding used to report it.

Tuberculosis

Tuberculosis (010–018) is an acute or chronic infection caused by Mycobacterium tuberculosis. Infection commonly occurs in the lungs, although it can occur in other sites, such as the meninges. In the primary infection of pulmonary tuberculosis, symptoms include fatigue, weakness, anorexia, weight loss, night sweats, and low-grade fever. Secondary infections are characterized by productive cough, hemoptysis, chest pain, and anorexia.

The diagnostic workup for tuberculosis includes the following:

- Purified protein derivative (PPD)

- Sputum culture (results may take three to six weeks)

- Acid-fast bacilli of sputum

- Chest x-ray

The fifth-digit subclassification for use with categories 010–018 identifies the method used to establish the diagnosis of tuberculosis. For example, the fifth digit 0 is assigned when the method is unknown or not documented; fifth digit 2 is assigned when a bacteriological or histological examination was performed, but the results were unavailable in the health record at the time of coding. Nonspecific reaction to tuberculin skin test without documentation of active tuberculosis is reported to code 795.5. A positive PPD also is classified to 795.5.

Streptococcal Sore Throat

Streptococcal sore throat (strep throat) is defined as an infection of the throat due to beta-hemolytic Streptococci. It is characterized by a sudden onset of fever, malaise, headache, and nausea. The throat appears edematous and red, and exudate may or may not be present. When such symptoms are present, a throat culture is indicated. ICD-9-CM classifies strep throat to code 034.0, which also includes the following diagnoses:

- Septic sore throat

- Septic angina

- Streptococcal angina

- Streptococcal laryngitis

- Streptococcal pharyngitis

- Streptococcal tonsillitis

No additional code is necessary to identify the organism (Streptococcus) because it is already included in the title of code 034.0.

Septicemia

Septicemia (038) is the entry of bacteria into the bloodstream. Symptoms include spiking fever, chills, and skin eruptions in the form of petechiae or purpura. Although blood cultures are usually positive, a negative culture does not exclude the diagnosis of septicemia in patients with clinical evidence of the condition. Clinical evidence may include the symptoms just listed, as well as hyperventilation with respiratory alkalosis, changes in the mental status of the patient, and thrombocytopenia (*Coding Clinic,* 2nd Quarter 2000).

ICD-9-CM classifies septicemia by the underlying organism involved. Bacterial septicemia is classified to category 038, which is further subdivided to identify the specific bacterium, such as staphylococcus. Without further specification, septicemia is reported with code 038.9. Septicemia due to Candida albicans is reported with code 112.5. A note at code category 038 (Septicemia) directs the coder to use an additional code for systemic inflammatory response syndrome (SIRS) (995.91–995.92).

When the diagnosis of septicemia with shock or of general sepsis with septic shock is documented in the health record, septicemia should be coded and listed first, followed by the SIRS code (995.92) and then followed by the appropriate code for septic shock (785.52). The official coding guidelines should be referenced for detailed information on septicemia, sepsis, SIRS, and shock.

Meningitis

Bacterial meningitis, category 320, is an inflammation of the meninges, which is a trio of membranes that surrounds the spinal cord and brain. Signs of infection are fever, chills, and malaise; increased cranial pressure exhibited as headache; and vomiting. When the meningitis is due to organisms other than bacteria, a code from category 321, Meningitis due to other organisms, is assigned. Meningococcal meningitis is coded with 036.0.

Other Bacterial Diseases

Bacterial infections that cannot be coded elsewhere should be assigned code 040.89, Other specified bacterial diseases. Subcategory code 040.8 also includes tropical pyomyositis (040.81) and toxic shock syndrome (040.82).

Childhood Communicable Diseases

Chickenpox (052), or varicella, is a common acute and highly contagious infection caused by the herpes virus Varicella-zoster. Category 052 is further subdivided to identify the presence or absence of complications.

Measles (055) is one of the most common illnesses known. Symptoms present with fever, followed by a rash. Category 055 is further subdivided to identify the presence or absence of complications.

Rubella (056), or German measles, is an acute, mildly contagious viral disease that produces a rash for approximately three days, along with lymphadenopathy. It is transmitted through contact with blood, urine, stools, or nasopharyngeal secretions. Category 056 is further subdivided to identify complications. When rubella is documented as congenital (present at birth), code 771.0 should be assigned.

Herpes

Herpes zoster (053), or shingles, is a severe infection caused by the Varicella-zoster virus. It presents with painful skin blisters that follow the posterior roots of the spinal nerves or the fifth cranial nerve. Category 053 is further subdivided to identify the presence or absence of complications.

Herpes simplex (054) is a recurrent viral infection caused by herpes virus hominis. Herpes type I is transmitted by oral and respiratory secretions and affects skin and mucous membranes. It commonly produces fever blisters and cold sores. Herpes type II affects primarily the genital area and is transmitted by sexual contact. Category 054 is further subdivided to identify specific complications. When herpes simplex is congenital (present at birth), code 771.2 should be assigned.

Viral Hepatitis

Viral hepatitis (070) is an inflammation of the liver caused by a virus. Signs and symptoms of hepatitis include jaundice, nausea, aversion to smoking, and abdominal pain on liver palpitation. Serum levels such as SGOT, SGPT, and serum bilirubin will be elevated. The five forms of hepatitis include the following:

- Type A (HAV) is highly contagious and usually transmitted by a fecal–oral route.

- Type B (HBV) is transmitted by direct exchange of contaminated blood, human secretions, and feces.

- Type C (HCV) is usually transmitted through transfused blood from asymptomatic donors.

- Type D (HDV-delta) is found only in patients with an acute or chronic episode of hepatitis B.

- Type E (HEV) is transmitted enterally.

Category 070 is further subdivided to identify the specific type and whether hepatic coma is present. A fifth-digit subclassification is required for subcategories 070.2–070.7.

Nonviral hepatitis is classified under diseases of the digestive system and reported with codes from chapter 9 of the ICD-9-CM codebook.

Candidiasis

Candidiasis (112) is an infection caused by the Candida species moniliasis. It usually is a mild, superficial fungal infection commonly occurring in the nails, skin, mucous membranes, vagina, esophagus, and gastrointestinal tract. Occasionally, the fungi can enter the bloodstream and invade major organs such as the kidneys, lungs, or brain. Category 112 is further subdivided to identify the specific site affected. Neonatal Candida monilia infection is excluded from this category; it is assigned to 771.7.

Sexually Transmitted Diseases

Sexually transmitted diseases (STDs), or venereal diseases, are contagious conditions usually spread through sexual intercourse or genital contact. Syphilis is classified to categories 090–097, which include types specified as congenital, juvenile, latent, or symptomatic (those affecting specific body systems, such as the cardiovascular or neurologic systems). Gonorrhea is classified to category 098, which is further subdivided to identify the specific sites affected and the severity (acute versus chronic).

Chlamydial venereal diseases are classified to subcategory 099.5, with the fifth digits used to identify the specific sites affected. When further specification as to cause and site is lacking, venereal disease is classified to code 099.9.

Infectious Gastroenteritis

Infectious gastroenteritis can be caused by a variety of organisms, including bacteria, viruses, and parasites. It is characterized by severe nausea, vomiting, anorexia, abdominal cramps, fever, malaise, muscular aches, prostration, hypokalemia, acidosis, metabolic alkalosis, and hyponatremia.

Several categories exist within ICD-9-CM to classify infectious gastroenteritis, including the following:

- Subcategory 003.0, Salmonella gastroenteritis, which includes Salmonella food poisoning with gastroenteritis (Salmonella food poisoning not further specified as with gastroenteritis is reported with code 003.9)

- Category 005, Other food poisoning (bacterial), which is further subdivided to identify specific organisms or types, such as Staphylococcal (005.0), botulism (005.1), and Clostridium perfringens (005.2)

- Category 008, Intestinal infections due to other organisms, which is further subdivided to identify specific causes, such as Escherichia coli (008.0x), Aerobacter aerogenes (008.2), and Clostridium difficile (008.45)

Gastroenteritis not specified as infectious is assigned code 558.9. Other codes demonstrating noninfectious gastroenteritis include:

558.1   Gastroenteritis and colitis due to radiation
558.2   Toxic gastroenteritis and colitis
558.3   Allergic gastroenteritis and colitis

Under code 558.3, there is a note to "use additional code" to identify type of food allergy (V15.01–V15.05).

Bacteremia

Bacteremia (790.7), the presence of bacteria in the blood, is demonstrated by a positive blood culture. A patient with positive blood culture may or may not have symptoms and may have only a low-grade fever. Whenever a diagnosis of urosepsis is encountered, the coder should query the physician as to whether it is intended to mean generalized sepsis caused by leakage of urine into the vascular circulation or urine contaminated by bacteria. Septicemia due to a nonbacterial microorganism is coded as an infection caused by the particular organism. For example, Candidal septicemia is assigned code 112.5, Disseminated (systemic) candidiasis, because this is a fungal infection. Bacteremia in a newborn during the perinatal period is assigned code 771.83, while septicemia (sepsis) in a newborn (during the perinatal period) is assigned code 771.81.

Human Immunodeficiency Virus Disease

Two types of human immunodeficiency virus (HIV) are known to exist: HIV-1 and HIV-2. HIV-1 is widespread throughout the world and causes acquired immune deficiency syndrome (AIDS). Found primarily in West Africa, HIV-2 causes a different type of illness. Infection with HIV can initiate a process of gradual and accelerating destruction of the body's immune system. To ensure uniform reporting of AIDS cases, the Centers for Disease Control (CDC) has developed specific definition criteria that must be met prior to establishing a diagnosis of AIDS.

HIV Classification

Code assignment for HIV depends on whether the patient is symptomatic or asymptomatic. The codes used include the following:

- 042, Human immunodeficiency virus [HIV] disease: Patients with HIV-related illness should be coded to 042. Category 042 includes AIDS, AIDS-like syndrome, AIDS-related complex, and symptomatic HIV infection.

- V08, Asymptomatic human immunodeficiency virus [HIV] infection: Patients with physician-documented asymptomatic HIV infection who have never had an HIV-related illness should be coded to V08.

- 795.71, Nonspecific serologic evidence of human immunodeficiency virus [HIV]: Code 795.71 should be used for patients (including infants) with inconclusive HIV test results.

Health records with diagnostic statements of "suspected," "likely," "possible," or "questionable" HIV infection should be returned to the physician for clarification before coding.

Patients who are seen for an HIV-related illness should be assigned a minimum of two codes in the following order:

1. Code 042 to identify the HIV disease

2. Additional codes to identify other diagnoses, such as Kaposi's sarcoma

> **EXAMPLE:** Disseminated candidiasis secondary to AIDS
> 042   Human immunodeficiency virus [HIV] disease
> 112.5   Disseminated candidiasis
>
> **EXAMPLE:** Acute lymphadenitis with HIV infection
> 042   Human immunodeficiency virus [HIV] disease
> 683   Acute lymphadenitis

During pregnancy, childbirth, or the puerperium, a patient admitted because of an HIV-related illness should receive a principal diagnosis of 647.6x, Other specified infectious and parasitic diseases in the mother classifiable elsewhere, but complicating the pregnancy, childbirth, or the puerperium, followed by 042 and the code(s) for the HIV-related illness(es). **Note:** This is an exception to the sequencing rule previously discussed.

> **EXAMPLE:** Delivery of a liveborn male in mother with AIDS
> 647.61, Other specified infectious and parasitic diseases in the mother classifiable elsewhere, but complicating the pregnancy, childbirth, or the puerperium
> 042, Human immunodeficiency virus [HIV] disease
> V27.0, Outcome of delivery, single liveborn

> **EXAMPLE:** Patient is admitted for evaluation and treatment of pneumonia; workup reveals Pneumocystis carinii pneumonia. Patient is also 25 weeks pregnant and has AIDS.
> 647.63, Other specified infectious and parasitic diseases in the mother classifiable elsewhere, but complicating the pregnancy, childbirth, or the puerperium
> 042, Human immunodeficiency virus [HIV] disease
> 136.3, Pneumocystosis

When a patient with symptomatic HIV disease, or AIDS, is admitted for an unrelated condition, such as a traumatic injury, the code for the unrelated condition should be the principal diagnosis. An additional diagnosis would include code 042, as well as all other manifestations or conditions associated with the HIV disease.

> **EXAMPLE:** Patient was seen by the physician who diagnosed acute appendicitis. Patient also has AIDS.
> 540.9, Acute appendicitis
> 042, Human immunodeficiency virus [HIV] disease

Code V08, Asymptomatic HIV infection, is reported when the diagnosis is listed as HIV positive, known HIV, HIV test positive, or similar terminology. Furthermore, the health record must *not* include any documentation describing the presence of symptoms related to HIV disease. Code V08 should not be reported when the term *AIDS* is used or when the patient is treated for any HIV-related illness or is described as having any condition(s) resulting from the HIV infection. Rather, code 042 should be reported in these circumstances.

Code 795.71, Inconclusive serologic test for human immunodeficiency virus [HIV], is reported for patients with inconclusive HIV serology, but with no definitive diagnosis or manifestations of the illness.

Patients with any known prior diagnosis of an HIV-related illness should be assigned code 042. After having developed an HIV-related illness, the patient should *always* be assigned code 042 at every subsequent encounter. Patients previously diagnosed with any HIV illness (042) should *never* be assigned code 795.71 or V08.

Testing for HIV

Patients requesting testing for HIV should be assigned code V73.89, Screening for other specified viral disease. In addition, code V69.8, Other problems related to lifestyle, may be assigned to identify patients who are in a known high-risk group for HIV. Code V65.44, HIV counseling, also may be assigned when these services are provided during the encounter.

When the results of the test are positive and the patient is asymptomatic, code V08, Asymptomatic HIV infection, should be assigned. When the results are positive and the patient is symptomatic with an HIV-related illness, such as Kaposi's sarcoma, code 042, HIV disease, should be assigned.

Late Effects of Infectious and Parasitic Diseases

The following three categories (137–139) are identified for use in describing late effects of infectious and parasitic diseases:

Category 137 Late effects of tuberculosis
Category 138 Late effects of acute poliomyelitis
Category 139 Late effects of other infectious and parasitic diseases

Late effects are located in the Alphabetic Index under "**Late,** effect(s) (of)." In sequencing, the first code listed is the residual (retardation, hemiplegia, and so forth) followed by the late effect code (137.0, 137.2, 138, and so forth) identifying the underlying cause, unless otherwise directed by the Alphabetic Index.

> **EXAMPLE:** Mental retardation due to old viral encephalitis
> 319 Unspecified mental retardation
> 139.0 Late effects of viral encephalitis

V Codes

Several V code categories apply to infectious and parasitic diseases. Some of these are particularly relevant to the outpatient setting. They include the following:

V01	Contact with or exposure to communicable diseases
V02	Carrier or suspected carrier of infectious diseases
V03	Need for prophylactic vaccination and inoculation against bacterial diseases
V04	Need for prophylactic vaccination and inoculation against certain viral diseases
V05	Need for other prophylactic vaccination and inoculation against single diseases
V06	Need for prophylactic vaccination and inoculation against combinations of diseases
V07	Need for isolation and other prophylactic measures
V12.0x	Personal history of infectious and parasitic diseases
V46.2	Other dependence on machines, supplemental oxygen
V73	Special screening examination for viral and chlamydial diseases
V74	Special screening examination for bacterial and spirochetal diseases
V75	Special screening examination for other infectious diseases

Chapter 5 Exercises

Review the following statements and cases and assign the appropriate codes:

1. AIDS with Kaposi's sarcoma of skin of lower leg

2. Urinary tract infection due to Escherichia coli

3. Aseptic meningitis

4. Viral hepatitis, type A

5. Measles with no complications

6. Gastroenteritis due to Salmonella

7. Rotavirus enteritis

8. Asymptomatic HIV infection

9. Septicemia due to streptococcus

10. Acute poliomyelitis

11. Left lower extremity paralysis; late effect of poliomyelitis

12. Candidiasis infection of the mouth

13. Tinea pedis

14. Anthrax pneumonia

15. Encephalitis due to typhus

16. Chronic urinary tract infection due to Monilia with microorganisms resistant to cephalosporin

(Continued on next page)

Chapter 5 Exercises (Continued)

17. Outpatient visit #1: Patient was seen in the physician's office for Pneumocystis carinii. He is HIV positive.

____

Outpatient visit #2 (same patient): Patient is HIV positive and comes in for a complete physical examination. Patient is currently symptom free.

____

18. Inpatient admission—History and physical findings: This 33-year-old male gives a history of fever with chills on and off for the past two weeks, headaches, myalgias, history of URI, sore throat, and sinusitis two weeks ago. He took antibiotics with no improvement. Still has fever up to 102° F and chills. No history of hemoptysis, hematemesis, or melena. No history or diagnosis of diabetes mellitus, hypertension, or cardiovascular problems. No history of weight loss. Main complaints are fever, chills, headaches, and myalgias for the past two weeks. Chest x-ray was obtained as outpatient, but no diagnosis was entertained.

Significant lab, x-ray, and consult findings: CBC showed white blood cell count 10.7, hemoglobin 13.7, crit 40.9, segments 32, lymphs 52, atypical lymphocytes 11. Hepatitis profile showed hepatitis-B core antibody positive. Urinalysis within normal limits. Blood, urine, and throat cultures were negative. Stool cultures were negative. Chest x-ray was normal.

Course in hospital: Initially, the patient was placed on IV fluids and IV antibiotics and treated symptomatically and supportively. After hepatitis-B core antibody came back, IV antibiotics were discontinued and treated supportively. The patient became afebrile, felt better, and was discharged home on 3/13.

Discharge diagnosis: Hepatitis B.

Code(s):

____

19. History and physical findings: This 71-year-old male is a nursing home resident as a result of a cerebrovascular accident two years ago. On the day of admission, he was noted to be clammy with tachypnea, to have decreased level of responsiveness, and to show increased fever. He was seen in emergency services, where evaluation revealed the presence of probable urinary tract infection and sepsis. His WBC count was 23,000, with decreased hemoglobin and hematocrit. He was admitted for treatment of urinary sepsis. Physical examination revealed an elderly male who is aphasic secondary to CVA. The patient has a right hemiplegia from previous CVA. The heart has a regular rhythm, the lungs are clear, and the abdomen is soft.

Significant lab, x-ray, and consult findings: Initial white blood cell count was 23,700; final blood count was 9,000. Urinalysis showed white cells too numerous to count. The urine culture had greater than 100,000 colonies of E. coli and Group D strep. The chest x-ray showed known thoracic aortic aneurysm that was unchanged. No acute abnormalities were noted. EKG showed sinus tachycardia.

Course in hospital: Initially, the patient was started empirically on Primaxin. He underwent fluid rehydration, and his electrolytes were followed closely. Electrolytes improved through his hospital stay. He was continued on IV Primaxin until the date of discharge, when he was changed to Cipro by tube. All of the bacteria grown in the urine were sensitive to the Cipro. The chest x-ray showed no change from previous admissions, and he was followed closely with additional oxygen as needed. The patient has a history of chronic obstructive lung disease and is dependent on oxygen at the nursing home. At this time, he has reached maximal hospital benefit and is switched to oral antibiotics. He is to continue on tube feedings, which he is tolerating quite well. The patient was discharged back to the nursing home.

Discharge diagnoses: Urinary sepsis; COPD; post cerebrovascular accident with residual

Code(s):

Review Questions

Answer the following questions:

1. When would a code from category V09, Infection with drug-resistant microorganisms, be used?

2. What do the fifth digits indicate with categories 010–018?

3. How is septicemia with septic shock coded?

4. What code is used when a patient is HIV positive, but asymptomatic?

5. What code is used to identify AIDS in a pregnant woman?

6. How are late effects of infectious and parasitic diseases coded?

7. Is congenital rubella coded differently from rubella occurring after birth?

Chapter 6

Neoplasms

Objectives

After completing this lesson, the student should be able to do the following:

- Apply knowledge of current, approved ICD-9-CM coding guidelines to assign and sequence accurate codes for diagnoses related to neoplasms

- Understand the definitions that describe the behavior of neoplasms

- Discuss the use and construction of morphology (M) codes

- Interpret the guidelines for the use of V codes in the neoplasm chapter

- Understand how to use the neoplasm table in the Alphabetic Index to Diseases

- Know how to correctly code neoplasms that are described as metastatic

Introduction

The term *neoplasm* refers to any new or abnormal growth. Chapter 2 in the Tabular List in volume 1 of the ICD-9-CM codebook classifies *all* neoplasms. Generally, these conditions are treated by referral to an oncologist. The following categories and section titles are included:

Categories	Section Titles
140–149	Malignant Neoplasm of Lip, Oral Cavity and Pharynx
150–159	Malignant Neoplasm of Digestive Organs and Peritoneum
160–165	Malignant Neoplasm of Respiratory and Intrathoracic Organs
170–176	Malignant Neoplasm of Bone, Connective Tissue, Skin, and Breast
179–189	Malignant Neoplasm of Genitourinary Organs
190–199	Malignant Neoplasm of Other and Unspecified Sites
200–208	Malignant Neoplasms, Stated or Presumed to Be Primary, of Lymphatic and Hematopoietic Tissue
210–229	Benign Neoplasms
230–234	Carcinoma in Situ
235–238	Neoplasms of Uncertain Behavior
239	Neoplasms of Unspecified Nature

In ICD-9-CM coding, neoplasms are classified according to the following three criteria:

- Behavior of the neoplasm, such as malignant or benign

- Morphology type, such as leukemia, melanoma, or adenocarcinoma

- Anatomical site involved, such as lung, brain, or stomach

Behavior of the Neoplasm

Definitions that describe the behavior of neoplasms include:

- **Malignant:** Malignant neoplasms are collectively referred to as cancers. A malignant neoplasm can invade and destroy adjacent structures, as well as spread to distant sites to cause death.

- **Primary:** A primary site is the site where a neoplasm originated.

- **Secondary:** A secondary site is the site(s) to which the neoplasm has spread via:

  —Direct extension, in which the primary neoplasm infiltrates and invades adjacent structures

  —Metastasis to local lymph vessels by tumor cell infiltration

  —Invasion of local blood vessels

  —Implantation in which tumor cells shed into body cavities

- **In situ:** In an in situ neoplasm, the tumor cells undergo malignant changes but are still confined to the point of origin without invasion of surrounding normal tissue. The following terms also describe in situ malignancies:

  —Noninfiltrating

  —Noninvasive

  —Intraepithelial

  —Preinvasive carcinoma.

- **Benign:** In benign neoplasms, growth does not invade adjacent structures or spread to distant sites but may displace or exert pressure on adjacent structures.

- **Uncertain behavior:** Neoplasms of uncertain behavior are tumors that a pathologist cannot determine to be either benign or malignant because features of both are present.

- **Unspecified nature:** Neoplasms of unspecified nature include tumors in which neither behavior nor histological type is specified in the diagnosis.

Neoplasm Table

As mentioned previously, the Alphabetic Index to Diseases contains two tables. One of them is the neoplasm table, which is indexed under the main term **"Neoplasm."**

The neoplasm table contains seven columns. The first column lists the anatomical sites in alphabetical order. The next six columns identify the behavior of the neoplasm. The first three of these six columns include codes for malignant neoplasms and are further classified as primary, secondary, and carcinoma (Ca) in situ. The fourth column identifies codes for benign neoplasms. The last two columns include codes for neoplasms of uncertain behavior and of unspecified type.

When many sites are indented under a main term, the listing for that term may run several pages long. Accurate coding requires the coder to search through all of the subterms under the main heading.

Morphology Codes

Morphology codes (M codes) consist of five digits: the first four digits identify the histological type of the neoplasm; the fifth digit indicates the behavior. A complete listing of morphology codes can be found in appendix A of volume 1 of the ICD-9-CM codebook. M codes are used primarily by cancer or tumor registries in hospitals to identify the specific histology and behavior of neoplasms.

The one-digit behavior codes that are appended to the four-digit histological codes include the following:

/0   Benign

/1   Uncertain whether benign or malignant
     Borderline malignancy

/2   Carcinoma in situ
     Intraepithelial
     Noninfiltrating
     Noninvasive

/3   Malignant, primary site

/6   Malignant, metastatic site
     Secondary site

/9   Malignant, uncertain whether primary or metastatic site

Morphology codes appear next to each neoplastic term in the Alphabetic Index.

> **EXAMPLE:**   **Adenocarcinoma** (M8140/3)—*see also* Neoplasm, by site, malignant

In the preceding example, M8140 identifies the histological type as adenocarcinoma and the digit /3 indicates the malignant behavior as a primary site.

Although the behavior code listed in ICD-9-CM is appropriate to the histological type of neoplasm, the behavior type should be changed to fit the diagnostic statement.

> **EXAMPLE:**   Patient was admitted to the hospital with a diagnosis of adeno-carcinoma of the lung with metastasis to the bone.
>
> M8140/3   Adenocarcinoma (lung)
> M8140/6   Metastatic adenocarcinoma (bone)

Facilities would not use the behavior digit /9 with morphology codes because all malignant neoplasms are coded as primary or secondary, based on the documentation in the health record.

Occasionally, a difficulty arises in assigning a morphologic number when a diagnosis contains two qualifying adjectives with different morphology codes. In such cases, the higher number should be selected.

> **EXAMPLE:**   Patient was admitted to the hospital with a diagnosis of malignant intraductal lobular carcinoma of the breast.
>
> The following two morphology codes are available:
>
> M8500/2   Intraductal
> M8520/3   Lobular
>
> Because the higher number is M8520/3, this code is assigned.

V Codes

V codes provide a method for reporting encounters for chemotherapy, radiation therapy, and follow-up visits, as well as a way to indicate a history of primary malignancy or a family history of cancer.

Coding Guidelines for V Codes

Coders should consider the following guidelines when using V codes:

- When the treatment is directed at the malignancy, designate the malignancy as the principal diagnosis. When the purpose of the encounter is for radiation therapy or radiotherapy (V58.0) or for chemotherapy (V58.1), sequence the malignancy as an additional diagnosis and include the V code as the first-listed diagnosis.

> **EXAMPLE:** Patient with right UOQ breast carcinoma was seen for radiation therapy.
>
> The following codes are reported:
>
> V58.0   Encounter for radiotherapy
>
> 174.4   Malignant neoplasm of upper, outer quadrant of breast

- When a patient is admitted for the purpose of radiotherapy or chemotherapy and develops a complication, such as uncontrolled nausea and vomiting or dehydration, the principal diagnosis is the admission for radiotherapy (V58.0) or the admission for the chemotherapy (V58.1). Additional codes would include the cancer and the complication(s).

> **EXAMPLE:** Patient was admitted for chemotherapy for acute lymphocytic leukemia. During the hospitalization, the patient developed severe nausea and vomiting treated with medications.
>
> The following codes are reported:
>
> V58.1   Encounter for chemotherapy
>
> 204.00   Acute lymphocytic leukemia
>
> 787.01   Nausea with vomiting

- When the primary malignancy has been previously excised or eradicated from its site, and there is no adjunct treatment directed to that site and no evidence of any remaining malignancy at the primary site, the appropriate code from category V10 should be used to indicate the former site of the primary malignancy. Any mention of extension, invasion, or metastasis to a nearby structure or organ or to a distant site is coded as a secondary malignant neoplasm to that site and may be the first-listed diagnosis in the absence of the primary site.

- When a patient is seen for a follow-up exam and there is no evidence of recurrence or metastasis, a code from category V67, Follow-up examination, should be used. A code from V10, Personal history of malignant neoplasm, should be used as an additional code.

The instructional notes listed under each subcategory of V10 refer to specific code ranges for primary malignancy categories (140–195 and 200–208) and carcinoma in situ categories (230–234). Secondary malignancies are excluded from the V10 codes.

Instructions in the Alphabetic Index for Coding Neoplasms

The main terms and subentries in the Alphabetic Index to Diseases assist the coder in locating the morphological type of neoplasms. When a specific code or site is not listed in the index, cross-references direct the coder to the neoplasm table. The following steps should be followed in coding neoplasms:

1. Locate the morphology of the tumor in the Alphabetic Index. In most cases, the coder is directed to the neoplasm table. In other cases, he or she is provided with a code under the morphology type.

Adenocarcinoma of the colon
    Adenocarcinoma (M8140/3)—*see also* Neoplasm, by site, malignant

---

> Acute lymphocytic leukemia
> **Leukemia, leukemic** (congenital) (M9800/3) 208.9
> lymphocytic (M9820/3) 204.9
> acute (M9821/3) 204.0

2. Follow the instructions under the main term in the Alphabetic Index. Instructions in the Alphabetic Index should be followed when determining which column to use in the neoplasm table.

> **Adenomyoma** (M8932/0)—*see also*
> Neoplasm, by site, benign

The instructions can be overridden when the documentation in the health record specifies a different behavior.

> **EXAMPLE:**   Malignant adenoma of colon
>
> 153.9   Malignant neoplasm of colon, unspecified

Although the Alphabetic Index says to "*see also* Neoplasm, by site, benign," the coder should assign code 153.9, Malignant neoplasm of colon, unspecified, rather than code 211.3, Benign neoplasm of the colon.

When a diagnostic statement indicates which column of the neoplasm table to reference but does not identify the specific type of tumor, the neoplasm table should be consulted directly.

> **EXAMPLE:**   Carcinoma in situ of cervix
>
> 233.1   Carcinoma in situ of cervix uteri

After consulting the neoplasm table, code 233.1 from the "in situ" column is selected.

Instructions in the Tabular List for Coding Neoplasms

Specific instructions for coding neoplasms appear in the Tabular List as well as in the Alphabetic Index. The following information applies to the coding of neoplasms:

1. Code functional activity associated with a neoplasm. Some categories in the neoplasm chapter in the Tabular List offer the instructional notation "Use additional code, if desired" as advice to also code any functional activity associated with a particular neoplasm, such as increased or decreased hormone production due to the presence of a tumor.

> **183**   **Malignant neoplasm of ovary and other uterine adnexa**
>
> | *Excludes:* | *Douglas' cul-de-sac (158.8)* |
>
> **183.0**   **Ovary**
> Use additional code to identify any functional activity

EXAMPLE: Patient was admitted to the hospital with carcinoma of the ovary and menometrorrhagia due to hyperestrogenism.

    183.0   Malignant neoplasm of ovary
    256.0   Hyperestrogenism
    626.2   Excessive or frequent menstruation

2. Note variations in categories 150 and 201. Two categories in the malignant section depart from the usual principles of classification: 150, Malignant neoplasms of the esophagus; and 201, Hodgkin's disease. In both cases, the fourth-digit subdivisions are not mutually exclusive.

---

150   **Malignant neoplasm of esophagus**
    150.0   Cervical esophagus
    150.1   Thoracic esophagus
    150.2   Abdominal esophagus
    150.3   Upper third of esophagus
    150.4   Middle third of esophagus
    150.5   Lower third of esophagus

In the preceding example, the anatomy of the esophagus is classified in two ways because no uniform agreement exists on the use of these terms. Some physicians prefer the terms *upper, middle,* and *lower* to describe the site of the esophagus; others prefer the terms *cervical, thoracic,* and *abdominal.* The code that correlates with documentation in the health record should be assigned.

---

201   **Hodgkin's disease**
    201.0x   Hodgkin's paragranuloma
    201.1x   Hodgkin's granuloma
    201.2x   Hodgkin's sarcoma
    201.4x   Lymphocytic-histiocytic predominance
    201.5x   Nodular sclerosis
    201.6x   Mixed cellularity
    201.7x   Lymphocytic depletion
    201.9x   Hodgkin's disease, unspecified

In the preceding example, a dual axis reflects the different terminology used by pathologists. One pathologist may use Hodgkin's paragranuloma; another may indicate the type of involvement as Hodgkin's lymphoma of mixed cellularity. Again, no uniform agreement exists on the use of these terms, so the terminology in the health record should be the guide in assigning a code.

Anatomical Site Involved

ICD-9-CM provides guidelines for coding the anatomical site of a neoplasm to the highest degree of specificity. These guidelines are discussed in the following subsections.

Classification of Malignant Neoplasms

Malignant neoplasms are separated into primary sites (140–195) and secondary or metastatic sites (196–198), with further subdivisions by anatomic site.

Neoplasms of the lymphatic and hematopoietic system are *always* coded to categories 200–208, regardless of whether the neoplasm is stated as primary or secondary. Neoplasms of the lymphatic and hematopoietic system, such as leukemias and lymphomas, are considered widespread and systemic in nature and, as such, do not metastasize. Therefore, they are *not* coded to category 196, Secondary and unspecified malignant neoplasms of lymph nodes, which includes codes identifying secondary or metastatic neoplasms of the lymphatic system. In coding lymphomas (200–203), extranodal sites, such as the brain or stomach, are identified with a fifth digit 0.

Determination of the Primary Site

The primary site is defined as the origin of the tumor. Physicians usually identify the origin of the tumor in the diagnostic statement. In some cases, however, the physician cannot identify the primary site. For these situations, ICD-9-CM provides an entry in the neoplasm table titled "unknown site or unspecified," which is assigned to code 199.1. Code 199.1 can be assigned whether or not the site is primary or secondary (metastatic) in nature.

Category 195

Category 195, Malignant neoplasms of other and ill-defined sites, is available for use only when a more specific site cannot be identified. This category includes malignant neoplasms of contiguous sites, not elsewhere classified, whose point of origin cannot be determined.

> **EXAMPLE:**   Carcinoma of the neck
>
> 195.0   Malignant neoplasm of head, face, and neck

Definition of the Asterisk (*)

At the beginning of the neoplasm table, a boxed note defines the use of the asterisk (*). When the asterisk follows a specific site in the neoplasm table, the following rules apply:

- When the neoplasm is identified as a squamous cell carcinoma or an epidermoid carcinoma, that condition should be classified as a malignant neoplasm of the skin.

  > **EXAMPLE:**   Squamous cell carcinoma of the ankle
  >
  > 173.7   Malignant neoplasm of skin of lower limb, including hip (ankle)

  The asterisk following the term *ankle* in the neoplasm table indicates that it would be incorrect in this case to assign code 195.5, Malignant neoplasm of lower limb, because the neoplasm is a squamous cell carcinoma. Instead, the malignant column for the entry "skin . . . ankle" in the neoplasm table should be referenced to assign the correct code: 173.7.

- When the neoplasm is identified as a papilloma of any type, that condition should be classified as a benign neoplasm of the skin.

  > **EXAMPLE:**   Papilloma of the arm
  >
  > 216.6   Benign neoplasm of skin of upper limb, including shoulder (arm)

The asterisk following the term *arm* in the neoplasm table indicates that it would be incorrect to assign code 229.8, Benign neoplasm of other specified sites, if the neoplasm is a papilloma. The benign column for the entry "skin, . . . arm" in the neoplasm table should be referenced to assign the correct code: 216.6.

Coding of Contiguous Sites

In some cases, the origin of the tumor (primary site) may involve two adjacent sites. Therefore, neoplasms with overlapping site boundaries are classified to the fourth-digit subcategory 8, titled "Other."

> **EXAMPLE:**   A malignant lesion of the jejunum and ileum

---

152   **Malignant neoplasm of small intestine, including duodenum**

    152.8   **Other specified sites of small intestine**

        Duodenojejunal junction
        Malignant neoplasm of contiguous
          or overlapping sites of small
          intestine whose point of origin
          cannot be determined

Code 152.8 is obtained by referencing the entry "intestine, . . . small . . . contiguous sites" in the neoplasm table.

Classification of Primary Sites

As defined earlier in this lesson, a primary site refers to the site where the tumor originated. This section discusses some of the complexities involved in determining whether to code a neoplasm as a primary or a secondary site.

Surgical Removal Followed by Adjunct Therapy

When surgical removal of a primary site malignancy is followed by adjunct chemotherapy or radiotherapy, the malignancy code (from categories 140–198 or 200–208) is assigned as long as the chemotherapy or radiotherapy is actively administered. Even though the neoplasm has been removed surgically, the patient is still receiving therapy for that condition and the active code for the malignant neoplasm must be assigned, rather than a code describing "history of carcinoma."

> **EXAMPLE:**   Office visit for chemotherapy; patient has adenocarcinoma of the breast with mastectomy performed one month ago: V58.1, Encounter for chemotherapy; 174.9, Malignant neoplasm of breast

After the chemotherapy/radiation therapy is complete, a code for category V10 may be reported, rather than an active malignancy code.

> **EXAMPLE:**   Astrocytoma of the brain surgically removed one year ago; chemotherapy was completed three months ago: V10.85, Personal history of malignant neoplasm of the brain

Visits in which the patient receives only chemotherapy or radiation therapy are sequenced as follows:

- When the encounter is solely for chemotherapy, code V58.1 is sequenced first, followed by the appropriate ICD-9-CM code to identify the malignant neoplasm.

- When the encounter is solely for radiation therapy, code V58.0 is sequenced first, followed by the appropriate ICD-9-CM code to identify the malignant neoplasm.

- When the encounter is for radium implant or insertion or for treatment by radioactive iodine, code V58.0 is not used. The code for the malignant neoplasm is reported.

Surgical Removal Followed by Recurrence

When a primary malignant neoplasm previously removed by surgery or eradicated by radiotherapy or chemotherapy recurs, the primary malignant code for that site is assigned, unless the Alphabetic Index directs otherwise.

> **EXAMPLE:**   Recurrence of carcinoma of inner aspect lower lip
>
> 140.4   Malignant neoplasm of lower lip, inner aspect

The Alphabetic Index refers to the neoplasm table, where code 140.4 is found for neoplasm of the inner aspect of the lower lip.

"Metastatic from" in Diagnostic Statements

When cancer is described as "metastatic from a specific site," it is interpreted as a primary neoplasm of that site.

> **EXAMPLE:**   Carcinoma in cervical lymph nodes metastatic from lower esophagus
>
> 150.5   Malignant neoplasm of lower third of esophagus
> 196.0   Secondary malignant neoplasm of lymph nodes of head, face, and neck

The lower esophagus is the primary site (150.5); the secondary site is the cervical lymph nodes (196.0).

Classification of Secondary Sites

The patient's health record is the best source of information on differentiating between a primary and a secondary site. Some of the principal terms used in diagnostic statements that refer to secondary malignant neoplasms are described below.

"Metastatic to" and "Direct Extension to"

The terms *metastatic to* and *direct extension to* are used in classifying secondary malignant neoplasms in ICD-9-CM. For example, cancer described as "metastatic to a specific site" is interpreted as a secondary neoplasm of that site.

> **EXAMPLE:**   Metastatic carcinoma of the colon to the lung
>
> 153.9   Malignant neoplasm of colon, unspecifie
> 197.0   Secondary malignant neoplasm of lung

The colon (153.9) is the primary site, and the lung (197.0) is the secondary site.

"Spread to" and "Extension to"

When expressed in terms of malignant neoplasm with "spread to" or "extension to," diagnoses should be coded as primary sites with metastases.

> **EXAMPLE:** Adenocarcinoma of the stomach with spread to the peritoneum
>
> 151.9   Malignant neoplasm of stomach, unspecified
> 197.6   Secondary malignant neoplasm of retroperitoneum and peritoneum

The stomach (151.9) is the primary site. The peritoneum (197.6) is the secondary site.

Metastatic of One Site

When only one site is stated in the diagnostic statement and it is identified as metastatic, the coder determines whether the site should be coded as primary or secondary (assuming the health record does not provide additional information to assist in assigning a code).

> **EXAMPLE:** Metastatic serous papillary ovarian carcinoma

In the preceding example, the diagnostic statement identifies the carcinoma as metastatic. Before the code can be assigned, however, the following steps must be taken:

1. In the Alphabetic Index, locate the morphology type of the neoplasm as described in the diagnostic statement.

   > **EXAMPLE:** In the preceding example, the morphology type is carcinoma with subterms "serous" and "papillary."

2. Review subterms for the specific site as identified in the diagnostic statement. When the specific site is identified, assign that code. When the specific site is not included as a subterm, assign the code for primary of an unspecified site.

   > **EXAMPLE:** In the preceding example, the specific site, ovary, is not identified in the Alphabetic Index; however, a code is provided for unspecified site.

Carcinoma (M8010/3) . . .
    serous (M8441/3)
        papillary (M8460/3)
            specified site—*see* Neoplasm, by
          site, malignant
        unspecified site 183.0

Code 183.0, Malignant neoplasm of ovary, is assigned to indicate the primary malignant site.

3. When the code obtained in step 2 is 199.0 or 199.1, the directions in step 5 must be followed.

4. Now that the primary site of the carcinoma has been identified, a code must be assigned to describe the metastatic or secondary site. A review of the diagnostic statement finds no other site identified. Therefore, the neoplasm table must be used to determine the metastatic code. Because the metastatic site is unspecified, review the

neoplasm table for a subterm of "unknown site or unspecified." From the second column, "malignant, secondary," select the code 199.1.

5. When the morphology is not stated, or the code obtained in step 2 is 199.0 or 199.1, the site described as metastatic in the diagnostic statement should be coded as a primary malignant neoplasm unless it is included in the following list of exceptions, in which case it must be coded as a secondary neoplasm of that site:

Bone	Brain
Diaphragm	Heart
Liver	Lymph nodes
Mediastinum	Meninges
Peritoneum	Pleura
Retroperitoneum	Spinal cord

Sites classifiable to 195.0–195.8

> **EXAMPLE:** Metastatic carcinoma of the bronchus. The morphology is carcinoma. After locating **"Carcinoma,"** the first step is to look for a subterm of unspecified site. In reviewing the entries, no subterm is found for unspecified site. However, "*see also* Neoplasm, by site, malignant" appears after the main term.

6. The next step is to turn to the neoplasm table and look for a subterm of unspecified site. A code is selected from the "malignant, primary" column—199.1. However, step 5 informs coders to assign the site listed in the diagnostic statement as the primary site when code 199.1 is identified. The next step is to review the exception list to determine whether bronchus is included. Because bronchus is not included in the list, it is assigned as the primary site and identified by code 162.9, Malignant neoplasm of bronchus and lung, unspecified. To assign a code for the secondary site, unknown in this example, use the "malignant, secondary" column of the neoplasm table to locate the subterm "unknown site or unspecified"—199.1.

Chapter 6 Exercises

Review the following statements and cases and assign the appropriate codes. Assign M codes to these cases for practice.

1. Glioma of the parietal lobe of the brain

    ____

2. Adenocarcinoma of prostate

    ____

3. Carcinoma in situ of vocal cord

    ____

4. Epidermoid carcinoma of the middle third of the esophagus

    ____

5. Galactorrhea due to pituitary adenoma

    ____

6. Benign melanoma of skin of shoulder

    ____

Chapter 6 Exercises (Continued)

7. Adrenal adenoma with primary hyperaldosteronism

8. Acute myeloid leukemia in remission

9. Hodgkin's granuloma of intra-abdominal lymph nodes and spleen

10. Recurrence of papillary carcinoma of bladder, low-grade transitional cell

11. Burkitt's lymphoma in multiple lymph nodes and spleen

12. Carcinoma of the brain from the lower lobe of the lungs

13. A 54-year-old female was taken to emergency services following episodes of shortness of breath and lethargy. She was treated mainly for her breathing difficulties. When a CT scan of the lungs was done to evaluate her breathing problem, it was noted that she had a mass in the right upper lobe of the lung. MRIs also were done at that time of the bone, brain, and kidneys, all of which came back positive for metastatic deposits. A biopsy of the lung mass was done, and pathology was consistent with oat cell carcinoma. Radiation and chemotherapy were recommended.

    Discharge diagnosis: Oat cell carcinoma of the right upper lobe of the lung with metastasis to the bone (shoulder and hip), brain stem, and kidneys

    Code(s):

14. Inpatient encounter: An 87-year-old male was transferred from a local nursing home with complaints of partial hemiparesis. Immediately upon arrival, a CT scan of the brain was done that showed a mass in the left temporal lobe. The mass was biopsied and determined to be a glioblastoma. Radiation therapy was thought to be the best method of handling this tumor due to the patient's age and overall condition. He will return in a couple of weeks for his first treatment.

    Discharge diagnosis: Glioblastoma multiforme, left temporal lobe

    Code(s):

    Outpatient encounter: The elderly male patient was seen in the outpatient department for administration of his first radiation treatment for glioblastoma multiforme, which was diagnosed only recently.

    Diagnosis: Radiotherapy for management of glioblastoma multiforme in the left temporal lobe

    Code(s):

15. A 53-year-old male was diagnosed with carcinoma of the lower portion of the esophagus one month ago. To date, he has received one chemotherapy treatment and, since the treatment, has been quite nauseated and not felt much like eating or drinking. He presents to the physician today for evaluation.

    Impression: Dehydration; carcinoma of the lower third of the esophagus

    Code(s):

Review Questions

Answer the following questions:

1. What is the difference between a primary and a secondary neoplastic site?

2. How are the morphology (M) codes primarily used?

3. Which encounters in this chapter are appropriately assigned a V code?

4. What is the proper sequence of codes when a patient is seen for chemotherapy and then develops a complication?

5. When a patient is seen for a follow-up exam and there is no evidence of recurrence or metastasis, what code(s) should be used?

6. What codes are used for neoplasms of the lymphatic and hematopoietic system?

7. How are neoplasms with overlapping site boundaries coded?

8. How is the recurrence of a primary malignant neoplasm removed by surgery or radio-therapy or chemotherapy coded?

Chapter 7

Endocrine, Nutritional and Metabolic Diseases, and Immunity Disorders

Objectives

After completing this lesson, the student should be able to do the following:

- Apply knowledge of current, approved ICD-9-CM coding guidelines to assign and sequence accurate codes for diagnoses related to endocrine, nutritional, and metabolic diseases, and immunity disorders

- Identify the types of diabetes mellitus and the complications and manifestations associated with the various types

- Delineate the major types of thyroid disorders and immunity disorders

- List V codes appropriate to endocrine, nutritional, and metabolic diseases, and immunity disorders

Introduction

Chapter 3 of the ICD-9-CM codebook provides codes for endocrine, nutritional, and metabolic disorders, and immunity disorders. Typically, these types of disorders are treated by endocrinologists, allergists, immunologists, and physicians specializing in internal medicine or general practice.

The endocrine system involves glands that are located throughout the body. These glands secrete hormones into the bloodstream. Some of the major endocrine glands are the thyroid, adrenals, ovaries, and testicles. The best known of the endocrine disorders is diabetes mellitus.

Vitamin and mineral disorders such as rickets and various vitamin deficiencies are included in chapter 3. Immunology codes identify conditions of the immune system caused by the action of antibodies. Gout, dehydration, obesity, and cystic fibrosis are some of the conditions classified to chapter 3.

Chapter 3 is subdivided into the following sections:

Categories	Section Titles
240–246	Disorders of Thyroid Gland
250–259	Diseases of Other Endocrine Glands
260–269	Nutritional Deficiencies
270–279	Other Metabolic and Immunity Disorders

Diabetes Mellitus

Diabetes mellitus, or DM, is a metabolic disease in which insulin production by the pancreas is damaged. DM may be due to both hereditary and nonhereditary factors, such as obesity, surgical removal of the pancreas, and the action of certain drugs. When the pancreas does not produce insulin, glucose (sugar) is not broken down so that it can be used and stored by the body cells. The result is too much sugar in the blood (hyperglycemia), which in turn spills into the urine (glycosuria). Saturation of the blood and urine with glucose draws water out of the body causing dehydration and thirst. Other symptoms of DM include excessive hunger, marked weakness, and weight loss.

The following laboratory findings indicate a diagnosis of diabetes mellitus:

- Results of blood sugar analysis after glucose tolerance test: one hour after a meal—160 mg/100 ml; two hours after a meal—120 mg/100 ml (normal is 115–130 mg/100 ml blood one hour after a meal)

- Glycosuria evident in urine specimen

DM affects 6 percent of the total U.S. population and is the leading cause of new cases of blindness. One of every three patients on dialysis has end-stage renal disease secondary to diabetic nephropathy. Between 50 and 75 percent of cases of lower extremity amputations take place in people with diabetes.

Treatment consists of insulin regulation by either insulin injection or oral antidiabetic agents and/or a controlled diet.

Complications and Manifestations

ICD-9-CM classifies diabetes mellitus to category 250, which is further subdivided to identify the presence or absence of complications and/or manifestations of the diabetes:

<table>
<tr><td>250</td><td colspan="2">Diabetes mellitus</td></tr>
<tr><td></td><td>250.0</td><td>Diabetes mellitus, without mention of complication</td></tr>
<tr><td></td><td>250.1</td><td>Diabetes with ketoacidosis</td></tr>
<tr><td></td><td>250.2</td><td>Diabetes with hyperosmolarity</td></tr>
<tr><td></td><td>250.3</td><td>Diabetes with other coma</td></tr>
<tr><td></td><td>250.4</td><td>Diabetes with renal manifestations</td></tr>
<tr><td></td><td>250.5</td><td>Diabetes with ophthalmic manifestations</td></tr>
<tr><td></td><td>250.6</td><td>Diabetes with neurological manifestations</td></tr>
<tr><td></td><td>250.7</td><td>Diabetes with peripheral circulatory disorders</td></tr>
<tr><td></td><td>250.8</td><td>Diabetes with other specified manifestations</td></tr>
<tr><td></td><td>250.9</td><td>Diabetes with unspecified complication</td></tr>
</table>

The following fifth digits identify the type of diabetes (type I or type II) and the current state (controlled versus uncontrolled) of the condition:

0   Type II or unspecified type, not stated as uncontrolled

Fifth digit 0 is for use for type II, adult-onset diabetic patients, even when the patient requires insulin.

There is also a note to "Use additional code, if applicable, for associated long-term (current) insulin use V58.67."

Type II diabetes is the most common type, affecting 90 percent of the diabetic population. It is usually diagnosed in older adults, but it can occur in teenagers and young adults. Risk factors include obesity and heredity. The cause is unknown.

An important characteristic of type II diabetes mellitus is the lack of ketone bodies in the urine, which means type II diabetics have some effective insulin. These patients generally do not require insulin therapy to sustain life. However, insulin therapy may be required in some cases to correct symptomatic or persistent hyperglycemia. Usually, these cases are managed by weight reduction in the obese, diabetic diets, and/or oral hypoglycemic agents. These patients seldom develop ketoacidosis and, instead, are prone to the development of a hyperosmolar state and dehydration.

1   Type I [juvenile type], not stated as uncontrolled

Type I diabetes occurs when there is an absolute lack of insulin production. This occurs most often in children and young adults, although type I diabetes can develop at any age. The cause of type I diabetes is unknown.

Insulin therapy is required to maintain normal blood glucose levels. There may be brief symptom-free intervals (often referred to as honeymoon periods) during which insulin-dependent patients do not require insulin therapy. In type I patients, there is a tendency to develop diabetic ketoacidosis (DKA). Nonketosis-prone diabetics also may develop DKA, but this is rare.

When coding the case of a patient who receives insulin during a hospitalization, the coder should not assume that the patient is a type I diabetic. It is not unusual for type II diabetics to need the administration of insulin for a short time to regulate their diabetes; however, this does not imply that such patients are now insulin dependent. Documentation in the health record must support assignment of a type I diabetes.

Fifth digits 2 and 3 classify type I and type II diabetics with uncontrolled blood sugars. Diabetes mellitus should not be considered out of control unless the physician identifies it as such in the diagnostic statement and/or body of the record. When evidence in the record appears to indicate an uncontrolled state, the physician should be queried.

Code V58.67 can be used to identify long-term use of insulin for type II diabetics.

Two types of complications may occur with diabetes mellitus. One is the acute metabolic complication that is part of the diabetes itself and does not require an additional code. The other is the chronic effect that occurs in another body system due to the diabetes and that requires a code from the 250.4x–250.8x series with an additional code for the manifestation.

Acute Metabolic Complications

A number of acute metabolic complications may occur with diabetes mellitus. Many of these are discussed in the following subsections.

Diabetes with Ketoacidosis (250.1x)

Diabetic ketoacidosis (DKA) is assigned to code 250.11 unless the DM is identified specifically as type II. In those cases, it is coded as 250.10. DKA occasionally occurs in a type II diabetic patient suffering from an infection, myocardial infarction, trauma, or other serious illness.

DKA is caused by the lack of effective insulin or carbohydrate, protein, and fat metabolism. Symptoms include polyuria, weakness, lethargy, myalgia, headache, nausea, vomiting, abdominal pain, and hyperventilation. Typical findings are glycosuria 4+ (urinary glucose), strong ketonuria (urinary ketones), hyperglycemia (blood glucose), ketonemia (blood ketones), acidosis (low arterial blood pH), and low plasma bicarbonate.

Diabetes with Hyperosmolarity (250.2x)

Diabetes with hyperosmolarity is a form of hyperglycemic coma involving an altered state of consciousness (not necessarily an unconscious state) without significant ketosis, but with hyperosmolarity (increase in the concentration of the blood) and dehydration. Another term for this state is hyperosmolar nonketotic syndrome (HNKS).

HNKS usually occurs in type II (250.20) and is commonly associated with the following conditions: infections, acute pancreatitis, pancreatic carcinoma, thyrotoxicosis, subdural hematoma, and uremia. This code assignment includes patients who have an altered state of consciousness, altered sensorium, or other acute neurological deficits related to the hyperosmolar state.

Diabetes with Unspecified Complication (250.9x)

The diabetes with unspecified complication category includes those metabolic complications of diabetes mellitus that cannot be assigned elsewhere.

Late Effect Complications

Diabetes mellitus with complicating conditions in the 250.4x–250.8x series is coded, first, to the appropriate diabetic code and, second, with an additional code to identify the specific complicating condition. Conditions qualified as diabetic or due to diabetes are coded in this manner even though the index may not indicate dual coding. However, conditions listed with a diagnosis of DM or in a diabetic patient are not necessarily complications of the diabetes.

Thus, the condition should be coded as such only when the physician identifies it as a diabetic complication.

> **EXAMPLE:** Proliferative diabetic retinopathy due to type I diabetes mellitus
>
> 250.51   Diabetes with ophthalmic manifestations
> 362.02   Proliferative diabetic retinopathy

The diabetes code must be sequenced first, followed by the code for the retinopathy.

When a patient develops several complications due to diabetes, more than one code from subcategories 250.4x–250.8x may be assigned to describe the condition completely.

> **EXAMPLE:** Diabetic polyneuropathy and peripheral angiopathy due to type I diabetes mellitus
>
> 250.61   Diabetes with neurological manifestations, type I
> 357.2   Polyneuropathy in diabetes
> 250.71   Diabetes with peripheral circulatory disorders, type I
> 443.81   Peripheral angiopathy in diseases classified elsewhere

Diabetes with Renal Manifestations (250.4x)

Diabetic nephropathy NOS (not otherwise specified) is coded as 250.4x, Diabetes with renal manifestations, and 583.81, Nephritis and nephropathy, not specified as acute or chronic, in diseases classified elsewhere. Diabetic nephrosis and diabetic nephrotic syndrome are coded as 250.4x and 581.81, Nephrotic syndrome in diseases classified elsewhere.

When the renal condition has progressed to end-stage renal disease, only two codes are required: one for the diabetes (250.4x) and one for the end-stage renal disease (585.6). It is unnecessary to code the intermediate kidney condition (*Coding Clinic,* 3rd Quarter 1991).

Diabetes with Ophthalmic Manifestations (250.5x)

A true diabetic cataract, or snowflake cataract, is rare and occurs mainly in type I diabetes mellitus: codes 250.51, Diabetes mellitus with ophthalmic manifestations, type I; and 366.41, Diabetic cataract. Senile cataracts in persons with DM are not classified as manifestations of the diabetes. Typical senile cataracts (366.10) occur earlier and more frequently in diabetics but are not diabetic cataracts. Code the diabetes and the senile cataract(s) as separate entities (250.0x and 366.10).

Diabetes with Neurological Manifestations (250.6x)

Peripheral, cranial, and/or autonomic neuropathy is a chronic manifestation of diabetes mellitus. The codes for peripheral or cranial neuropathy are 250.6x, Diabetes with neurological manifestations, and 357.2, Polyneuropathy in diabetes; and for autonomic neuropathy, 250.6x and 337.1, Peripheral autonomic neuropathy in disorders classified elsewhere.

Diabetes with Peripheral Circulatory Disorders (250.7x)

Arteriosclerosis occurs earlier and more extensively in diabetics than in nondiabetics. For example, peripheral vascular disease causing intermittent claudication is coded 250.7x, and 443.81, Peripheral angiopathy in diseases classified elsewhere.

Diabetic atherosclerosis with gangrene is coded to 250.7x, Diabetes with peripheral circulatory disorders, and 440.24, Atherosclerosis of arteries of the extremities with gangrene.

Diabetes with Other Specified Manifestations (250.8x)

Other specified manifestations of diabetes mellitus would include, for example, diabetic osteomyelitis, which is coded as 250.8x and 730.8x. Other infections involving bone in diseases are classified elsewhere.

Diabetic Foot Ulcers

The underlying cause of foot ulcers in a diabetic patient may be diabetic neuropathy (250.6x), peripheral vascular disease (250.7x), or superimposed infection. In the latter case, the ulcers are not coded as a diabetic complication; that is, code the diabetes (250.0x), the infection or causative organism (when applicable), and the foot ulcer (707.1x).

Diabetic foot ulcers that result from diabetic neuropathy, with insults to the feet due to loss of sensation and from peripheral vascular disease, are coded, first, to the appropriate diabetes code (250.6x or 250.7x) and, second, to the code for ulcer of the lower extremity (707.1x).

When information is unavailable as to whether the ulcer is due to peripheral vascular disease or polyneuropathy, code 250.8x, Diabetes with other specified manifestations, should be assigned. It must be emphasized, however, that *not all* ulcers in diabetic patients are diabetic ulcers; when there is a question as to linkage, the coder should consult the physician.

Organic Impotence

When impotence is due to peripheral vascular disease, it should be coded first as 250.7x; when it is due to peripheral neuropathy, it should be coded first as 250.6x. When information on whether the impotence is due to diabetic peripheral vascular disease or diabetic peripheral neuropathy is unavailable, code 250.8x should be assigned. The code for diabetes is followed by 607.84, Impotence of organic origin.

Additional Coding for Diabetes Mellitus

When patients are seen in the ambulatory setting for workup of possible DM, the codes describing the presenting symptoms, such as polydipsia (783.5) or polyuria (788.42), are assigned when the diabetes is not confirmed.

Abnormal Glucose

Code 790.2, Abnormal glucose, is used to classify situations in which an individual does not have diabetes mellitus but does exhibit an abnormal glucose level. Fifth digits differentiate between impaired fasting glucose (code 790.21) and an impaired glucose tolerance test (code 790.22). Code 790.29 is used for other abnormal glucose.

Diabetes Mellitus Complicating Pregnancy

Code 648.0x is used for pregnant women with preexisting DM whose diabetes in some way complicates the pregnant state, is aggravated by the pregnancy, or is a main reason for obstetrical care. A secondary code is used to identify the specific type of diabetes.

Code 648.8x, Abnormal glucose tolerance (gestational diabetes), refers to abnormal glucose tolerance that appears during pregnancy in previously nondiabetic women and resolves during the postpartum period. These patients are placed on a diabetic diet and may require insulin therapy to maintain normal blood glucose levels. Further, they may be at risk for subsequent development of type II diabetes mellitus in later years.

Diabetes Mellitus in Newborns of a Diabetic Mother

Code 775.0, Syndrome of "infant of a diabetic mother," should be assigned when the newborn infant of a diabetic mother or gestational diabetic mother manifests features of this condition.

Neonatal diabetes mellitus (775.1) refers to a transient diabetic state, usually hyperglycemia, occurring in the newborn infant of a diabetic mother. It may be referred to as pseudodiabetes and may require a short course of insulin therapy.

Secondary Diabetes Mellitus

Secondary diabetes mellitus usually results from some type of medical or surgical treatment, such as removal of the pancreas. The underlying condition that caused the diabetes should be coded with an additional code, from category 251, used to identify the diabetes (*Coding Clinic, 3rd Quarter 1991*).

Hypoglycemia

Hypoglycemia is defined by a blood sugar level below 50 to 60 mg/dL. It can be caused by an imbalance in the amount of insulin taken, food eaten, and activity. The 251 subcategory codes are intended for application to patients *without* diabetes mellitus.

The difference between codes 251.0 and 251.2 is the degree of hypoglycemia. Code 251.0 classifies nondiabetic hypoglycemic coma or shock due to excessive administration of insulin or oral hypoglycemic drugs. Code 251.2 classifies hypoglycemic reaction without mention of coma or shock in nondiabetic patients (*Coding Clinic,* March–April 1985).

Thyroid Disorders

Hypothyroidism is characterized by a low-serum thyroid hormone resulting from hypothalamic, pituitary, or thyroid insufficiency. Early features of hypothyroidism include fatigue, forgetfulness, sensitivity to cold, unexplained weight gain, and constipation. With progression, the characteristic myxedematous symptoms appear: decreasing mental stability; dry, flaky, inelastic skin; puffy face, hands, and feet; hoarseness; periorbital edema; upper eyelid droop; dry, sparse hair; and thick, brittle nails. Cardiovascular involvement may lead to decreased cardiac output. Progression to myxedema coma is gradual.

In ICD-9-CM, hypothyroidism is classified to category 244, Acquired hypothyroidism, and includes separate codes for specific types, such as postsurgical hypothyroidism (244.0). When the hypothyroidism is congenital in nature, code 243 is reported.

Hyperthyroidism is a metabolic imbalance that results from thyroid hormone overproduction. The most common form of hyperthyroidism is Graves' disease, which increases thyroxine production, enlarges the thyroid gland (goiter), and causes multiple system changes. The classic symptoms of Graves' disease are goiter, nervousness, heat intolerance, weight loss despite increased appetite, sweating, diarrhea, tremor, and palpitations. ICD-9-CM classifies hyperthyroidism to category 242, with fourth digits to identify the specific type and fifth digits to indicate thyrotoxic crisis.

Cystic Fibrosis

Cystic fibrosis is an inherited multisystem disorder found in both children and adults. Characterized by chronic obstruction and infection of airways and by maldigestion, cystic fibrosis also affects other body systems, including the pulmonary system, cardiac system, biliary system, and reproductive system. In addition, it affects the functioning of the pancreas. Moreover, intra-abdominal complications are common, including meconium ileus, rectal prolapse, ileocolic intussusception, inguinal hernia, gallstones, and gastroesophageal reflux. Treatment includes antibiotics to control lung infections, bronchodilators to relieve reversible airway symptoms, and anti-inflammatory agents to slow progression of moderate lung infections. Chest physical therapy helps to clear mucus from large airways.

ICD-9-CM classifies cystic fibrosis to subcategory 277.0, with fifth digits to indicate whether meconium ileus, pulmonary manifestations, or gastrointestinal manifestations are present. Additional codes may need to be assigned to identify accompanying conditions or complications, such as acute bronchitis (466.0) or pneumothorax (512.8).

Code V83.81 is used to indicate that a patient is a cystic fibrosis gene carrier.

Metabolic Disorders

Category 276, Disorders of fluid, electrolyte, and acid-base balance, includes the following conditions:

276.0	Hyperosmolality and/or hypernatremia
276.1	Hyposmolality and/or hyponatremia
276.2	Acidosis
276.3	Alkalosis
276.4	Mixed acid-base balance disorder
276.5x	Volume depletion
276.6	Fluid overload
276.7	Hyperpotassemia
276.8	Hypopotassemia
276.9	Electrolyte and fluid disorders not elsewhere classified

Generally, the preceding conditions are symptoms of a larger disease process and, as such, are usually coded as additional diagnoses when documented in the health record.

V Codes

Several V codes may relate to chapter 3. These include:

V12.1	Personal history of nutritional deficiency
V12.2	Personal history of endocrine, metabolic, and immunity disorders
V18.0	Family history of diabetes mellitus

V18.1	Family history of other endocrine and metabolic diseases
V45.85	Insulin pump status
V53.91	Fitting and adjustment of insulin pump
V65.46	Encounter for insulin pump training
V77.x	Special screening for endocrine, nutritional, metabolic, and immunity disorders
V83.81	Cystic fibrosis gene carrier

Chapter 7 Exercises

Review the following statements and cases and assign the appropriate codes:

1. Iatrogenic hypothyroidism

2. Protein-calorie malnutrition

3. Vitamin B$_{12}$ deficiency

4. Diabetic nephropathy

5. Familial hyperlipidemia

6. Polyuria, polydipsia; rule out diabetes mellitus (outpatient visit)

7. Cystic fibrosis

8. Addison's disease

9. Diabetes mellitus with hypoglycemic coma

10. Graves' disease with thyrotoxic crisis

11. Gangrene, left great toe, due to peripheral vascular disease second to diabetes mellitus, type I

12. Hypercholesterolemia

13. Gouty arthritis

(Continued on next page)

105

Chapter 7 Exercises (Continued)

14. Acute infantile rickets

15. Hypopituitarism secondary to radiation therapy for brain tumor 18 months ago; physician documents condition as a late effect.

16. Stein-Leventhal syndrome

17. Nutritional marasmus

18. Inpatient admission: Patient has a history of nausea with severe vomiting for the past two to three days. This 31-year-old male patient has a history of type I diabetes mellitus (since 1986) and is on 15 units of NPH and 10 of Regular in the morning and 10 units of NPH and 5 of Regular in the evening. He started having symptoms of nausea and had increased frequency of urination and polydipsia. An examination of the extremities showed no evidence of thrombophlebitis, varicosities, or edema. The patient was treated, and his blood sugar decreased from more than 600 to normal levels.

    Discharge diagnoses: Diabetes mellitus, type I; diabetic ketoacidosis

    Code(s):

19. Outpatient visit: Patient was evaluated for severe malnutrition and iron deficiency anemia secondary to her previously diagnosed amyotrophic lateral sclerosis. Social services were contacted for help with meals.

    Impression: Malnutrition; anemia; amyotrophic lateral sclerosis

    Code(s):

20. Outpatient visit #1: Patient was seen with complaints of nausea and vomiting, and anorexia. The physician orders a complete blood count and schedules the patient for a return visit.

    Impression: Suspected gastroenteritis

    Code(s):

    Outpatient visit #2: Patient continued to experience nausea and vomiting. The physician reviews the lab work with the patient, which shows increased levels of aldosterone. The physician prescribes potassium supplements and arranges for outpatient intravenous fluids for severe dehydration.

    Impression: Hypokalemia: severe dehydration

    Code(s):

Review Questions

Answer the following questions:

1. What are the two categories of diabetes mellitus?

2. What is diabetic ketoacidosis, and how is it coded?

3. How is end-stage renal disease due to diabetes coded?

4. How are diabetic foot ulcers coded?

5. What is the difference between codes 648.0x, Diabetes mellitus complicating pregnancy, and 648.8x, Abnormal glucose tolerance complicating pregnancy?

6. What do the fifth digits indicate in subcategory 277.0, Cystic fibrosis?

7. What do the fourth and fifth digits signify in category 242, Hypothyroidism?

Chapter 8

Mental Disorders

Objectives

After completing this lesson, the student should be able to do the following:

- Apply knowledge of current, approved ICD-9-CM coding guidelines to assign and sequence accurate codes for diagnoses related to mental disorders

- Identify the various types of mental disorders

- Differentiate between alcohol/drug abuse and alcoholism/drug dependence

Introduction

Chapter 5 of the ICD-9-CM codebook classifies mental disorders into the following categories:

Categories	Section Titles
290–299	Psychoses
300–316	Neurotic Disorders, Personality Disorders, and Other Nonpsychotic Mental Disorders
317–319	Mental Retardation

These conditions are generally treated by a psychologist or a psychiatrist.

The ICD-9-CM codes in this chapter are compatible with those included in the *Diagnostic and Statistical Manual of Mental Disorders, Fourth Edition (DSM-IV),* published by the American Psychiatric Association (APA). *DSM-IV* uses a multiaxial system involving an assessment on five different axes. Axes I, II, and III provide diagnostic information. Axis I, Clinical Disorders and Other Conditions That May Be a Focus of Attention, includes all psychiatric disorders except personality disorders and mental retardation, which make up Axis II. Axis III identifies the presence of general medical conditions. Axis IV is used to note clinically relevant psychosocial and environmental problems. Axis V is used to indicate the individual's overall psychological, social, and occupational functioning (APA 1994).

Descriptions of the various diagnostic categories in *DSM-IV* enable clinicians and investigators to diagnose, communicate about, study, and treat people with various mental disorders. All *DSM-IV* categories are listed in chapter 5 of the ICD-9-CM codebook; however, there are many differences between ICD-9-CM and DSM-IV in the organization and the narrative text of the codes.

Multiple Coding of Mental Disorders

Instructional notes indicating that additional codes must be assigned to fully describe the patient's condition are frequently encountered in mental health code listings. For example:

299.1 Childhood disintegrative disorder
Heller's syndrome

Use additional code to identify any associated neurological disorder

---

The instructional note in the preceding example indicates the need to assign an additional code to describe any associated neurological disorder. The instructional note in the next example indicates that an additional code must be assigned to describe any associated mental disorder, as well as any accompanying physical condition.

---

301 Personality disorders
Includes: character neurosis

Use additional code to identify any associated neurosis or psychosis, or physical condition

---

The instructional note in the next example states the specific code to assign for the presence of cerebral atherosclerosis.

> **290.4** **Vascular dementia**
>
> Multi-infarct dementia or psychosis
>
> Use additional code to identify cerebral atherosclerosis (437.0)

Fifth-Digit Subclassification for Coding Mental Disorders

Fifth digits are used quite frequently in the mental disorders chapter of ICD-9-CM to provide more specific information about the severity or course of a patient's illness. Although this specificity exists in the classification system, the documentation in the health record often does not provide the information required for assigning a specific fifth digit. The fifth digit for an unspecified course of illness is assigned when further information is unavailable. The course or extent of illness should never be assumed from general statements made in the health record.

Inclusion and Exclusion Notes for Coding Mental Disorders

Chapter 5 of the ICD-9-CM codebook contains numerous special inclusion notes. For example:

> **295** **Schizophrenic disorders**
>
> Includes: schizophrenia of the types described in 295.0–295.9
> occurring in children

The note in the preceding example instructs that codes 295.0–295.9 may be assigned in the pediatric population, when applicable. The inclusion note in the next example states that psychotic conditions due to or provoked by emotional stress (for example, divorce) or environmental factors (for example, forest fire) should be assigned to category 298.

> **298** **Other nonorganic psychoses**
>
> Includes: psychotic conditions due to or provoked by:
> emotional stress
> environmental factors as major part of etiology

Exclusion notes also are frequently used in chapter 5 to warn that specified forms of a condition are classified elsewhere. For example:

> **290.0** **Senile dementia, uncomplicated**
>
> Senile dementia:
> NOS
> simple type
>
> | *Excludes:* | *mild memory disturbances, not* |
> |---|---|
>
> *amounting to dementia, associated with senile*
> *brain disease (310.1)*
> *senile dementia with:*
> *delirium or confusion (290.3)*
> *delusional [paranoid] features (290.20)*
> *depressive features (290.21)*

This exclusion note advises that mild memory disturbances associated with senile brain disease and senile dementia with specific features—such as confusion, paranoia, and depression—are classified elsewhere.

Psychoses/Neuroses

A variety of mental conditions, both acute and chronic, which are related to psychiatric symptoms and impaired function, can be differentiated by the terms *psychoses* and *neuroses,* as demonstrated by the following ICD-9-CM classification:

Psychoses (290–299)
    Organic Psychotic Conditions (290–294)
    Other Psychoses (295–299)
Neurotic Disorders, Personality Disorders, and Other Nonpsychotic Mental Disorders (300–316)

The first step in coding is often to determine whether a condition is psychotic or nonpsychotic in nature.

> **EXAMPLE:**   291.81, Alcohol withdrawal
>   303.0, Acute alcholic intoxication
>
> **EXAMPLE:**   296.3, Major depressive disorder, recurrent episode
>   309.1, Prolonged depressive reaction
>
> **EXAMPLE:**   298.3, Acute paranoid reaction
>   301.0, Paranoid personality disorder

Generally, psychosis is characterized by personality problems and loss of contact with the real world. Moreover, it is often associated with illusions, hallucinations, or delusions. When the diagnostic statement notes "with dementia," "delirium," or "psychotic," the condition should be coded as a psychotic condition. Codes indicating psychosis should not be assigned unless the psychosis is clearly documented in the patient's medical record.

Categories 300–316 classify neurotic and personality disorders as well as other nonpsychotic mental illnesses such as:

300	Anxiety, dissociative, and somatoform disorders
301	Personality disorders
302	Sexual and gender identity disorders
303	Alcohol dependence syndrome
304	Drug dependence
305	Nondependent abuse of drugs
306	Physiological malfunction arising from mental factors
307	Special symptoms or syndromes, not elsewhere classified
308	Acute reaction to stress
309	Adjustment reaction
310	Specific nonpsychotic mental disorder due to brain damage
311	Depressive disorder, not elsewhere classified

312 Disturbance of conduct, not elsewhere classified
313 Disturbance of emotions specific to childhood and adolescence
314 Hyperkinetic syndrome of childhood
315 Specific delays in development
316 Psychic factors associated with diseases classified elsewhere

Dementia

Dementia is characterized by a permanent or progressive decline in several dimensions of intellectual function that interferes with the individual's normal social or economic activity. Dementias are considered to be of physical rather than psychiatric etiology, brought about by either a general medical condition, a substance, or a combination of these factors.

While the DSM-IV no longer uses the terminology *organic mental disorder* to refer to dementias, ICD-9-CM classifies dementias by type in the organic psychotic conditions subsection as follows:

- 290.0, Senile dementia, uncomplicated

- 290.10, Presenile dementia, uncomplicated

- 290.11, Presenile dementia with delirium

- 290.12, Presenile dementia with delusional features

- 290.13, Presenile dementia with depressive features

- 290.20, Senile dementia with delusional features

- 290.21, Senile dementia with depressive features

- 290.3, Senile dementia with delirium

- 290.40–290.43, Vascular dementia

- 290.8, Other specified senile psychotic conditions

- 290.9, Unspecified senile psychotic condition

When the dementia is present as a result of a specific disease, that condition is reported first, followed by a code from subcategory 294.1, Dementia in conditions classified elsewhere. Code 294.10 is used to report dementia without behavioral disturbance, whereas code 294.11 is used when behavioral disturbance or problems (aggressive, combative, or violent behavior, or wandering off) are present. A note under code 294.1 instructs the coder to "code first any underlying physical condition."

> **EXAMPLE:** Patient diagnosed as having Alzheimer's dementia
> with combative behavior: 331.0, 294.11

Alcohol/Drug Dependence and Abuse

Alcoholism (alcohol dependence) is a chronic condition in which a patient has become dependent on alcohol, demonstrates increased tolerance for the effects of alcohol, and is unable to stop using it even when facing strong incentives such as impaired health, deteriorating social interactions, and decreasing job performance. Such patients often experience physical signs of withdrawal during any sudden cessation of drinking. Drug dependence or drug addiction is a chronic mental and physical condition related to the patient's pattern of taking a drug or a combination of drugs. Drug dependence is characterized by behavioral and physiological responses such as a compulsion to take the drug, experience its psychic effects, or avoid the discomfort of its absence. There is increased tolerance and an inability to stop using the drug, even with strong incentives.

Alcoholism and Alcohol Abuse

Alcohol-related disorders can be both psychotic and nonpsychotic in nature. Category 291, Alcohol-induced mental disorders, includes the psychotic conditions characterized by organic symptoms such as delirium, dementia, amnesia, and hallucinations that are associated with severe chronic alcohol abuse and alcohol withdrawal.

Alcoholism per se is considered a nonpsychotic condition and classified to the category 303, Alcohol dependence syndrome, with a fourth digit to identify a state of acute intoxication (303.0) or other and unspecified forms (303.9). The fifth digits identify the stage of the alcoholism—unspecified, continuous, episodic, or in remission. An additional code should be assigned to identify any of the following associated conditions:

- 291.0–291.9, Alcohol-induced mental disorders
- 3040–304.9, Drug dependence
- 331.7, Cerebral degeneration in diseases classified elsewhere
- 345.0–345.9, Epilepsy
- 535.3, Alcoholic gastritis
- 571.1, Acute alcoholic hepatitis
- 571.2, Alcoholic cirrhosis of liver
- 571.3, Alcoholic liver damage, unspecified

Reported with code 305.0x, acute alcohol abuse is described as problem drinking. It includes those patients who drink to excess but have not reached a stage of physical dependency. Again, the fifth digit identifies the stage of the condition—unspecified, continuous, episodic, or in remission.

The exclusion note appearing below code 305.0 indicates that a diagnosis of acute alcohol intoxication in a patient with alcoholism is reported with code 303.0x.

Drug Dependence and Abuse

As with alcohol-related conditions, mental disorders related to substance misuse can be either psychotic or nonpsychotic in nature. Category 292 classifies drug-related conditions that are psychotic in nature and accompanied by organic symptoms such as delusions, hallucinations, delirium, and dementia. Drug withdrawal syndrome is included in this category.

Category 304 classifies drug addiction, with the fourth digit identifying the specific drug or class of drug involved. The fifth digit identifies the stage of dependence—unspecified, continuous, episodic, or in remission. When several drugs are involved in the addiction, ICD-9-CM provides the following codes for use:

- 304.7x, Combinations of opioid-type drug with any other

- 304.8x, Combinations of any drug dependence excluding opioid-type drug

Nondependent drug abuse represents problem drug taking. It includes those patients who take drugs to excess but have not yet reached a state of dependence. ICD-9-CM classifies nondependent drug abuse to codes 305.2x–305.9x. The fourth digit identifies the specific class of drug, and the fifth digit indicates the stage of the addiction.

Fifth Digits for Alcohol/Drug Dependence and Abuse

The following information can serve as a guide to selecting the appropriate fifth digit for categories 303–304 and code 305.0x. As always, the documentation in the health record should serve as the final determination for the code selected.

0	Unspecified	Inadequate documentation in the health record
1	Continuous	Alcohol: Refers to daily intake of large amounts of alcohol or regular heavy drinking on weekends or days off from work
		Drugs: Daily or almost daily use of drug(s)
2	Episodic	Alcohol: Refers to alcoholic binges lasting weeks or months, followed by long periods of sobriety
		Drugs: Indicates short periods between drug use or use on the weekends
3	In remission	Refers to either a complete cessation of alcohol or drug intake or to the period during which a decrease toward cessation is taking place (*Coding Clinic*, 2nd Quarter 1991)

Schizophrenic Disorders

Category 295 outlines schizophrenic disorders, referring to a group of psychoses where there is a personality disturbance or distortion of thinking, delusions, or autism.

The fourth digits under category 295 refer to the type of schizophrenia, namely:

.0 Simple type
.1 Disorganized type
.2 Catatonic type
.3 Paranoid type
.4 Schizophreniform disorder
.5 Latent schizophrenia
.6 Residual type
.7 Schizoaffective disorder
.8 Other specified types of schizophrenia
.9 Unspecified schizophrenia

The fifth-digit subclassification for use with category 295 includes:

0 Unspecified
1 Subchronic

2   Chronic
3   Subchronic with acute exacerbation
4   Chronic with acute exacerbation
5   In remission

Affective Disorders

Affective disorders are characterized as common mental diseases with mood disturbances. Category 296 deals with episodic mood disorders that are classified according to the symptoms that a patient exhibits.

The following fifth-digit subclassification is for use with categories 296.0–296.6 and provides information on the severity of the disorder:

0   Unspecified
1   Mild
2   Moderate
3   Severe, without mention of psychotic behavior
4   Severe, specified as with psychotic behavior
5   In partial or unspecific remission
6   In full remission

Documentation of severity should be included in the medical record before assigning fifth digits 1 through 6.

Usually, code 311, Depressive disorder, not elsewhere classified, is assigned for other nonpsychotic depressive disorders and covers conditions such as depression, depressive disorder, and depressive state, not otherwise specified.

Developmental Disorders

Category 315 covers disorders where there is a specific delay in development. For most patients, the developmental delay cannot be explained in terms of general intellectual retardation or a lack of or poor schooling but, rather, is in some way related to biological maturation as well as some nonbiological factors. The delays may be disorders relating to reading, speech or language coordination, learning difficulties, mixed development, or other specified developmental delays.

Chapter 8 Exercises

Review the following statements and cases and assign the appropriate codes:

1.   Acute exacerbation of residual-type schizophrenia

____

2.   Reactive depressive psychosis due to death of child

____

3.   Anxiety reaction manifested by fainting

____

Chapter 8 Exercises (Continued)

4. Alcoholic gastritis due to chronic alcoholism, episodic

5. Acute senile depression

6. Attention deficit disorder with hyperactivity (ADDH)

7. Alcohol dependence syndrome in remission resulting in cirrhosis of liver

8. Cerebral vascular dementia

9. Bipolar II disorder, NOS

10. Hypochondriac with continuous laxative habit

11. A 69-year-old female has been under the care of the Mental Hygiene Clinic in the past due to chronic anxiety problems. She is brought to emergency services today with severe depression. In addition, she is hypertensive.

    Discharge diagnoses: Severe depression; hypertension; chronic anxiety problems

    Code(s):

12. A 14-year-old male is seen by his physician because of problems he is having at his new school. The boy's teachers have called his parents to report disruptive conduct in all of his classes. Upon questioning the patient, the physician determines that the patient is having difficulty adjusting to his new environment in which he is being taught by all new teachers and having to make all new friends.

    Impression: Adolescent adjustment disorder; severe disturbance of conduct

    Code(s):

13. A 16-year-old female is seen by a physician in emergency services showing symptoms of severe vomiting and an unstable gait. An examination of the patient indicates that she is suffering from acute intoxication. A talk with the parents further reveals that this patient has chronic problems with alcoholism. Because this episode is so much worse than any previous episodes, the physician suggests detoxification and a rehabilitation facility. The parents readily agree, and the patient is released and will be admitted into a detox unit the next day.

    Discharge diagnoses: Acute alcohol intoxication; chronic alcoholism

    Code(s):

Review Questions

Answer the following questions:

1. How is dementia resulting from a specific disease coded and sequenced?

2. What is the difference between alcoholism and alcohol abuse?

3. In the coding of many mental disorders, what must be first determined?

4. What key words can indicate a psychotic condition in a health record?

5. When coding alcohol/drug dependence and abuse, what do the fifth digits indicate?

Chapter 9

Diseases of the Nervous System

Objectives

After completing this lesson, the student should be able to do the following:

- Apply knowledge of current, approved ICD-9-CM coding guidelines to assign and sequence accurate codes for diagnoses related to diseases of the nervous system and sense organs

- Delineate the various types of conditions related to this system

- Discuss the assignment of late effect codes in category 326

Introduction

Chapter 6 of the ICD-9-CM codebook includes conditions that affect the brain and spinal cord as well as the peripheral nervous system. In addition, it classifies a variety of eye and adnexal disorders and diseases of the ear and mastoid process.

The chapter is divided into the following major sections:

Categories	Section Titles
320–326	Inflammatory Diseases of the Central Nervous System
330–337	Hereditary and Degenerative Diseases of the Central Nervous System
340–349	Other Disorders of the Central Nervous System
350–359	Disorders of the Peripheral Nervous System
360–379	Disorders of the Eye and Adnexa
380–389	Diseases of the Ear and Mastoid Process

Generally, these conditions are treated by a neurologist, an ophthalmologist, or an ear, nose, and throat doctor.

Meningitis (320–322)

Meningitis is the inflammation of the meninges, the three connective tissue membranes that cover the brain and the spinal cord. Meningitis can be caused by a variety of microorganisms or viruses. It is classified in two chapters of the ICD-9-CM codebook: chapter 6, Diseases of the Nervous System and Sense Organs; and chapter 1, Infectious and Parasitic Diseases. Because of this particular classification, the instructions provided in the Alphabetic Index must be followed to ensure accurate code assignment.

Meningitis . . . 322.9
    abacterial NEC (*see also* Meningitis, aseptic) 047.9
    actinomycotic 039.8 *[320.7]*
    adenoviral 049.1
    Aerobacter aerogenes 320.82
    anaerobes (cocci) (Gram-negative) (Gram-positive)
        (mixed) (NEC) 320.81
    arbovirus NEC 066.9 *[321.2]*
        specified type NEC 066.8 *[321.2]*

It should be noted in the preceding example that two codes are required in some cases and one code is sufficient in other cases. However, accurate sequencing of the two codes is imperative. It also should be noted that the second code listed is in brackets and set in italicized type. This is done to indicate that this code must always follow the code that describes the underlying cause.

Late Effects of Conditions (326)

Category 326 is used to identify late effects of conditions classified in categories 320–325. The note under category 326 must be reviewed carefully because some codes in this series are excluded. Instructions to "use additional code to identify the residual condition," such as hydrocephalus or paralysis, also must be followed.

EXAMPLE: Residual hemiplegia due to late effect of encephalitis
342.90, Hemiplegia, unspecified, affecting unspecified side
326, Late effects of intracranial abscess or pyogenic infection

Sleep Disorders (327)

Category 327 includes various organic sleep disorders including organic insomnia (327.0), excessive somnolence (327.1), and organic sleep apnea (327.2). Fifth digits provide additional specificity.

Paralytic Conditions (342–344)

Categories 342–344 include the following paralytic conditions: hemiplegia and hemiparesis, infantile cerebral palsy, and other paralytic syndromes.

Hemiplegia and Hemiparesis (342.0x–342.9x)

Hemiplegia and hemiparesis are conditions characterized by paralysis of one side of the body. This category is further subdivided to differentiate between flaccid and spastic hemiplegia. *Flaccid* refers to the loss of muscle tone in the paralyzed parts, with the absence of tendon reflexes. *Spastic* refers to the spasticity of the paralyzed parts, with increased tendon reflexes. These codes are often assigned when the health record provides no further information, when the cause of the hemiplegia and hemiparesis is unknown, or as an additional code when the condition results from a specified cause. The fifth-digit subclassification identifies whether the dominant or nondominant side is affected. This type of specificity may not be available in the health record; if not, the coder should assign the fifth digit 0.

Infantile Cerebral Palsy (343.0–343.9)

Infantile cerebral palsy is a nonprogressive, brain-damaging disturbance of the prenatal and perinatal period characterized by persistent, qualitative motor dysfunction, paralysis, and, in severe cases, mental retardation. The subcategories identify the side of the body affected, as well as the affected extremity.

Other Paralytic Syndromes (344.0–344.9)

Other paralytic syndromes include conditions such as quadriplegia, paraplegia, diplegia, and monoplegia. Also classified in this section are codes describing cauda equina syndrome, with or without neurogenic bladder.

Epilepsy (345)

The term *epilepsy* denotes any disorder characterized by recurrent seizures. A seizure is defined as a transient disturbance of cerebral function due to an abnormal paroxysmal neuronal discharge in the brain. Physicians often document "recurrent seizure" or "seizure disorder" in the health record. These statements are not synonymous with epilepsy and do not warrant the assignment of code 345. In addition, the administration of certain anticonvulsive medication may or may not imply that a patient has epilepsy. Category 345 is to be assigned only when the documentation in the health record states "epilepsy."

ICD-9-CM identifies several types of epilepsy, including grand mal and petit mal status. Again, documentation in the health record provides direction as to which code to select. When the health record does not identify a particular form, subcategory 345.9x, Epilepsy, unspecified, should be assigned.

The following fifth-digit subclassification is for use with categories 345.0–.1, and 345.4–.9:

    0   without mention of intractable epilepsy
    1   with intractable epilepsy

The physician must state "intractable epilepsy" in the health record before the fifth digit 1 can be assigned. Epilepsy should never be assumed to be intractable based on generalities in the health record.

Disorders of the Eye and Adnexa (360–379)

Categories 360–379 of chapter 6 classify conditions of the eye and adnexa such as cataracts, retinal disorders, glaucoma, corneal ulcers, conjunctivitis, and disorders of the eyelids, orbits, and optic nerve.

Glaucoma (365)

Glaucoma is a group of eye diseases characterized by an increase in intraocular pressure causing pathological changes in the optic disk and typical visual field defects. Category 365 is further subdivided to identify the various types of glaucoma. For example, patients developing glaucoma as a result of corticosteroid therapy are classified to subcategory 365.3. Glaucoma associated with a congenital anomaly, dystrophy, and systemic syndromes is classified to subcategory 365.4. The codes and code titles in subcategory 365.4 are set in italicized type, with an instruction to first code the associated disease or disorder, such as neurofibromatosis, aniridia, and Rieger's anomaly. Both subcategories 365.3 and 365.4 require fifth digits. Code 365.83, Aqueous misdirection, is used to report a form of glaucoma formerly known as malignant glaucoma. When documentation in the health record states "glaucoma only," code 365.9, Unspecified glaucoma, may be assigned.

Cataract (366)

A cataract is the opacity of the crystalline lens of the eye or its capsule resulting in a loss of vision. As with glaucoma, ICD-9-CM identifies many types of cataracts. The exclusion note under category 366, however, serves as direction to use codes 743.30–743.34 for congenital cataracts. The first two subcategories, 366.0 and 366.1, classify cataracts according to their onset in life—early in life versus late in life. Subcategory 366.4 describes cataracts associated with other disorders. Codes 366.41–366.44 are set in italicized type and, as such, are not used for primary tabulation. The underlying disease, such as calcinosis or craniofacial dysostosis, is coded first. When documentation in the health record states "cataract only," code 366.9, Unspecified cataract, should be assigned.

Diseases of the Ear and Mastoid Process (380–389)

Categories 380–389 of chapter 6 include conditions such as otitis media and externa, Meniere's disease, cholesteatoma, hearing loss, and tinnitus.

Otitis Externa

Otitis externa (external otitis), or swimmer's ear, is an infection of the external auditory canal and may be acute or chronic. Acute otitis externa is characterized by moderate-to-severe pain, fever, regional cellulitis, and partial hearing loss. Instead of pain, chronic otitis externa is characterized by pruritus, which leads to scaling and thickening of the skin.

ICD-9-CM classifies otitis externa to subcategories 380.1, Infective otitis externa, and 380.2, Other otitis externa. Both 380.1 and 380.2 are further subdivided with fifth digits, which offer more specificity.

Otitis Media

Otitis media (OM) is an inflammation of the middle ear that may be further specified as suppurative or secretory and acute or chronic. Acute suppurative OM is characterized by severe, deep, throbbing pain, as well as sneezing and coughing; mild-to-high fever; hearing loss, dizziness, and nausea and vomiting. Acute secretory OM results in severe conductive hearing loss and, in some cases, a sensation of fullness in the ear with popping, crackling, or clicking sounds on swallowing or with jaw movement. Chronic OM has its origin in the childhood years but usually persists into adulthood. Cumulative effects of chronic OM include thickening and scarring of the tympanic membrane, decreased or absent tympanic mobility, cholesteatoma, and painless purulent discharge.

ICD-9-CM classifies OM to categories 381, Nonsuppurative otitis media and Eustachian tube disorders, and 382, Suppurative and unspecified otitis media. Both categories are further subdivided to identify acute and chronic forms and other specific types of OM. The following codes are used with common forms of otitis media:

- 381.00, Acute nonsuppurative otitis media, unspecified
- 381.01, Acute serous otitis media
- 381.10, Chronic serous otitis media, simple or unspecified
- 381.3, Other and unspecified chronic nonsuppurative otitis media
- 381.4, Nonsuppurative otitis media, not specified as acute or chronic
- 382.00, Acute suppurative otitis media without spontaneous rupture of eardrum
- 382.01, Acute suppurative otitis media with spontaneous rupture of eardrum
- 382.3, Unspecified chronic suppurative otitis media
- 382.4, Unspecified suppurative otitis media
- 382.9, Unspecified otitis media
- 382.9, Unspecified acute otitis media
- 382.9, Unspecified chronic otitis media

Chapter 9 Exercises

Review the following statements and cases and assign the appropriate codes:

1. Hemiplegia of dominant side due to an old CVA

2. Partial retinal detachment with single retinal defect

3. Tonic-clonic epilepsy

4. Acute follicular conjunctivitis

5. Mature cataract

6. Chronic serous otitis media

7. Classical migraine

8. Cholesteatoma of middle ear

9. Aerobacter aerogenes meningitis

10. Intracranial abscess

11. Tay-Sachs disease with profound mental retardation

12. Congenital diplegic cerebral palsy

13. An 88-year-old male was transferred from a local nursing home with complaints of fatigue, fever, sinus congestion, and headaches. He also suffered from Alzheimer's disease and was recently diagnosed with Tic douloureux. While in the hospital, he was treated with decongestants and an antibiotic for the sinusitis.

    Discharge diagnoses: Acute frontal sinusitis; Alzheimer's disease; Tic douloureux

    Code(s):

Chapter 9 Exercises (Continued)

14. A 78-year-old male was seen in the physician's office for his annual eye exam. During the exam, it was discovered that he had a mature, asymptomatic senile cataract in his right eye. Moreover, the intraocular pressure in that eye was not within normal limits. The physician's recommendation was to have the patient schedule surgery for removal of the cataract.

    Impression: Mature, senile cataract, right eye; primary open-angle glaucoma with borderline intraocular pressure

    Code(s):

    ____

15. An eighth-grade student was seen in the physician's office because she was no longer able to clearly see the blackboard from her seat near the back of the classroom. After her eyes were dilated and examined, the physician determined that she was nearsighted and prescribed glasses to correct the problem.

    Impression: Myopia

    Code(s):

    ____

Review Questions

Answer the following questions:

1. To accurately code meningitis, two codes must often be used as indicated in the Alphabetic Index. What is the proper sequencing when more than one code must be used?

2. Should conditions documented as "recurrent seizure" or "seizure disorder" be assigned a code from category 345, Epilepsy?

3. How are congenital cataracts coded?

4. What is a synonymous term for otitis externa?

5. What types of conditions are classified to category 326?

6. What is the difference between flaccid and spastic hemiplegia?

Chapter 10

Diseases of the Blood and Blood-Forming Organs

Objectives

After completing this lesson, the student should be able to do the following:

- Apply knowledge of current, approved ICD-9-CM coding guidelines to assign and sequence accurate codes for diagnoses related to diseases of the blood and blood-forming organs, including hemorrhagic disorders and diseases of white blood cells

- Identify the various anemias and the coding guidelines for each type

- Discuss the three types of coagulation defects

- List V codes appropriate to disorders of the blood and blood-forming organs

Cannot code lab tests

Introduction

Fluids constitute more than one-half of an adult's weight under normal circumstances, and blood is one of the body's most important fluids. Blood is composed of a liquid called plasma, red blood cells (erythrocytes), white blood cells (leukocytes), and platelets. The study of blood and blood-forming tissues is called hematology, and the physician who studies blood is a hematologist.

Chapter 4 of the ICD-9-CM codebook, Diseases of the Blood and Blood-Forming Organs, includes anemias, coagulation defects, purpura, and other hemorrhagic conditions and diseases of the white blood cells.

Anemias

Anemia is characterized by a decrease in the number of erythrocytes, the quantity of hemoglobin, or the volume of packed red cells in the blood. Laboratory data reflect a decrease in red blood cells (RBCs), hemoglobin (Hgb), or hematocrit (Hct).

Deficiency Anemias

Codes used to describe deficiency anemias are included in categories 280–281. The most common type—iron deficiency anemia (category 280)—is caused by an inadequate absorption or excessive loss of iron. Iron deficiency anemia due to chronic blood loss is reported with code 280.0. The underlying cause of the bleeding, such as an ulcer, menorrhagia, or cancer, also should be coded when documented in the health record. Without further specification, iron deficiency anemia is reported with code 280.9. Iron deficiency anemia due to acute blood loss (also known as acute posthemorrhagic anemia) is reported with code 285.1. It is defined as a normocytic, normochromic anemia developing as a result of rapid loss of large quantities of RBCs during bleeding. It may occur as a result of trauma with severe bleeding, rupture of an aneurysm, arterial erosion, cancerous or ulcerative lesions, and complications of surgery from excessive blood loss.

Category 281 describes other deficiency anemias, including:

- 281.0, Pernicious anemia
- 281.1, Other vitamin B_{12} deficiency anemia
- 281.2, Folate-deficiency anemia
- 281.3, Other specified megaloblastic anemias, NEC
- 281.4, Protein-deficiency anemia
- 281.8, Anemia associated with other specified nutritional deficiency
- 281.9, Unspecified deficiency anemia

Hemolytic Anemias

Hemolytic anemia refers to an abnormal reduction of red blood cells caused by an increased rate of RBC destruction and the inability of the bone marrow to compensate. Hemolytic anemias may be hereditary (category 282) or acquired (category 283).

Hereditary Hemolytic Anemias

Hereditary hemolytic anemias are caused by intrinsic abnormalities involving structural defects of RBCs or defects of globin synthesis or structure. Category 282 includes the following common hematologic disorders:

- 282.41–282.49, Thalassemias (including Cooley's anemia and sickle-cell thalassemia)

- 282.5, Sickle-cell trait

- 282.60–282.69, Sickle-cell disease

It is important to understand the difference between sickle-cell trait and sickle-cell disease. When a child receives the sickle-cell genetic trait from only one parent, he or she is considered a carrier of the trait (282.5). When the child receives the trait from both parents, he or she has sickle-cell disease (282.6x). When the physician documents both sickle-cell trait and sickle-cell disease, only the code for the disease is reported.

Acquired Hemolytic Anemias

Acquired hemolytic anemias are usually caused by extrinsic factors such as trauma (surgery or burns), infection, systemic diseases (Hodgkin's lymphoma, leukemia, or systemic lupus erythematosus), drugs or toxins, liver or renal disease, or abnormal immune responses. ICD-9-CM classifies acquired hemolytic anemia to category 283, with fourth and fifth digits (when applicable) to describe the specific type or cause. For example, code 283.0 identifies autoimmune hemolytic anemias, and codes 283.10–283.19 identify nonautoimmune hemolytic anemias.

Aplastic Anemia

Aplastic anemia is caused by an abnormal reduction of red blood cells due to a lack of bone marrow blood production. When aplastic anemia is accompanied by neutropenia and thrombocytopenia, it is called pancytopenia and coded to 284.8. Half the aplastic anemia cases are attributed to exposure to a toxin and half are determined to be of unknown causes. Toxins that can result in aplastic anemia include radiation and chemotherapy. ICD-9-CM classifies aplastic anemias to category 284, with fourth digits to indicate the specific type. For example, congenital, constitutional, or primary aplastic anemia is reported with code 284.0. Aplastic anemia without further specification is reported with code 284.9.

Other and Unspecified Anemias

Category 285 classifies other and unspecified anemias, including acute blood loss anemia (285.1) and sideroblastic anemia (285.0). Anemia of chronic illness (for example, end-stage renal disease or neoplastic disease) is reported with codes 285.21–285.29. Without further specification, anemia is reported with code 285.9.

Coagulation Defects

Coagulation defects are disorders of the platelets resulting in serious bleeding due to a deficiency of one or more clotting factors. ICD-9-CM classifies coagulation defects to category

286, with a fourth digit to identify the specific type. Three types of coagulation defects are recognized:

- Hemophilia A (classic hemophilia) is the most common type of coagulation defect and occurs as a result of factor VIII deficiency. It is inherited as an X-linked recessive disorder that is transmitted by females and affects males. ICD-9-CM classifies classic hemophilia to code 286.0.

- Hemophilia B (Christmas disease) results from a deficiency of factor IX. Like hemophilia A, this type is transmitted as an X-linked recessive trait. ICD-9-CM classifies hemophilia B to code 286.1.

- Hemophilia C is an autosomal recessive disease caused by a deficiency in factor XI. ICD-9-CM classifies this condition to code 286.2.

Other conditions are often confused with coagulation defects. For example, a patient being treated with Coumadin, heparin, or another anticoagulant may develop bleeding or hemorrhage. When this occurs, a code for the condition and associated hemorrhage is assigned, with an additional code of E934.2 to indicate the drug responsible for the bleeding documented by the physician. Code 286.5 is not assigned for bleeding in a patient taking an anticoagulant drug because this is not a hemorrhagic disorder due to an intrinsic circulating anticoagulant.

Another condition confused with coagulation defects is prolonged prothrombin time or other abnormal coagulation profiles. This condition is not coded as a coagulation defect. Code 790.92 is assigned to report an abnormal coagulation profile. However, when a patient is receiving Coumadin therapy, it is expected that he or she will have a prolonged bleeding time. In such a case, code 790.92 is not assigned.

Purpura and Other Hemorrhagic Conditions

Codes describing purpura, thrombocytopenia, and other hemorrhagic disorders are included in category 287. Thrombocytopenia is diagnosed when the platelet count falls below 100,000 per millimeter. Two types of thrombocytopenia are recognized: primary and secondary. Primary thrombocytopenia may be idiopathic, congenital, or hereditary, and is classified to code 287.3x. Fifth digits designate specific types of primary thrombocytopenia. Secondary thrombocytopenia may result from drug use, massive blood transfusions, extracorporeal circulation of blood, malignancies, portal hypertension, damaged blood vessels, and infectious processes. ICD-9-CM classifies secondary thrombocytopenia to code 287.4. An additional E code should be assigned to identify the drug or external cause.

Diseases of the White Blood Cells

Category 288 classifies diseases of the white blood cells (WBCs) with a fourth digit to identify the specific type of disorder. Two types of WBCs circulate in the body: granular and nongranular (agranular) leukocytes. Granular leukocytes include neutrophils, eosinophils, and basophils. Nongranular leukocytes include lymphocytes and monocytes. Agranulocytosis (also known as neutropenia) is an acute condition characterized by the absence of neutrophils or severe neutropenia and an extremely low granulocyte count. The most common cause is drug toxicity or hypersensitivity caused by large-dose and long-duration drugs. Neutropenia commonly occurs in patients receiving chemotherapy. ICD-9-CM classifies neutropenia to code 288.0.

Other Blood and Blood-Forming Organ Diseases

The last category (289) in chapter 4 of ICD-9-CM includes conditions not classified elsewhere, including familial and secondary polycythemia, chronic lymphadenitis, hypersplenism, chronic congestive splenomegaly, methemoglobinemia, and primary and secondary hypercoagulable state. Secondary polycythemia occurs as a result of tissue hypoxia and is associated with chronic obstructive pulmonary disease, congenital heart disease, and prolonged exposures to high altitudes (more than 10,000 feet). ICD-9-CM classifies secondary polycythemia to code 289.0.

V Codes

Some of the V codes that are applicable to chapter 4 include:

V10.6x	Personal history of leukemia
	Physician documentation is necessary to differentiate between a history of leukemia and leukemia in remission. Leukemia in remission is classified to the neoplasm chapter, with the fifth digit indicating the remission status.
V12.3	Personal history of diseases of blood and blood-forming organs
V16.6	Family history of leukemia
V18.2	Family history of anemia
V18.3	Family history of other blood disorders
V18.9	Genetic disease carrier
V26.3x	Genetic counseling and testing
V42.81	Organ or tissue replaced by transplant, bone marrow
V42.82	Organ or tissue replaced by transplant, peripheral stem cells
V58.6x	Long-term (current) drug use
V59.01	Blood donor, whole blood
V59.02	Blood donor, stem cells
V59.09	Blood donor, other
V59.3	Bone marrow donor
V78.x	Special screening for disorders of blood and blood-forming organs
V83.01	Asymptomatic hemophilia A carrier
V83.02	Symptomatic hemophilia A carrier

Chapter 10 Exercises

Review the following statements and case and assign the appropriate codes:

1. Sickle-cell disease with crisis

    ____

2. Iron deficiency anemia secondary to blood loss

    ____

3. Idiopathic thrombocytopenia

    ____

4. Cooley's anemia

    ____

5. Deficiency of factor I

    ____

6. Familial polycythemia

    ____

7. Folate deficiency anemia due to dietary causes

    ____

8. Fanconi's anemia

    ____

9. Idiopathic eosinophilia

    ____

10. Chronic mesenteric lymphadenitis

    ____

11. Screening for iron deficiency anemia

    ____

12. Anemia due to chronic blood loss from chronic gastric ulcer

    ____

13. Inpatient admission: An 89-year-old man with heart palpitations and abdominal pain was brought by his daughter to see the physician. The physician ordered an EKG, a CBC, and an upper GI workup. The GI workup revealed significant gastritis. The EKG was not significantly abnormal. The CBC revealed the following: Hct: 25%; Hgb: 6.4; and WBC: 5,000. The cardiologist indicated that he believed the palpitations were a symptom of the patient's anemia. Social services were notified because the physician attributed the anemia to nutritional deficiency. The patient received three units of packed cells and was discharged with a prescription for Tagamet.

    Discharge diagnoses: Anemia; gastritis

    Code(s):

    ____

Review Questions

Answer the following questions:

1. What causes hemolytic anemia (HA)?

2. What are some causes of acquired hemolytic anemia?

3. What is the difference between sickle-cell trait and sickle-cell disease?

4. What code or codes are assigned when the patient has aplastic anemia, neutropenia, and thrombocytopenia?

5. How should iron deficiency anemia be coded?

6. How is prolonged prothrombin time coded?

7. How is hemorrhage associated with Coumadin use coded?

Chapter 11

Diseases of the Circulatory System

Objectives

After completing this lesson, the student should be able to do the following:

- Apply knowledge of current, approved ICD-9-CM coding guidelines to assign and sequence accurate codes related to diseases of the circulatory system

- Delineate the major types of circulatory disorders

- Use the hypertension table in the Alphabetic Index

- Differentiate among the various types of hypertension and understand the coding guidelines for each type

- Understand the appropriate use of the fifth digits for category 410

- List V codes appropriate to disorders of the circulatory system

Introduction

Chapter 7 of the ICD-9-CM codebook provides a separate group of diagnostic codes for disorders of the circulatory system. These disorders are generally treated by cardiologists and cardiovascular surgeons.

Chapter 7 is divided into the following sections:

Categories	Section Titles
390–392	Acute Rheumatic Fever
393–398	Chronic Rheumatic Heart Disease
401–405	Hypertensive Disease
410–414	Ischemic Heart Disease
415–417	Diseases of Pulmonary Circulation
420–429	Other Forms of Heart Disease
430–438	Cerebrovascular Disease
440–448	Diseases of Arteries, Arterioles, and Capillaries
451–459	Diseases of Veins and Lymphatics and Other Diseases of Circulatory System

Circulatory system codes are often difficult to apply because a variety of nonspecific terminology is used to describe circulatory conditions. The coder should review carefully all the inclusion and exclusion notes in this chapter before assigning a code.

Valvular Heart Disease

Valvular heart disease occurs in different forms. Three types of mechanical disruption can occur: stenosis, or narrowing of the valve opening; incomplete closure of the valve; or prolapse of the valve. These conditions can result from disorders such as endocarditis, congenital defects, and inflammation, and may be coded as rheumatic or nonrheumatic. ICD-9-CM provides codes that specify single- or multiple-valve involvement, as follows:

- 94.0   Mitral stenosis

- 394.1   Rheumatic mitral insufficiency

- 395.0   Rheumatic aortic stenosis

- 396.1   Mitral valve stenosis and aortic valve insufficiency

- 397.0   Diseases of tricuspid valve

- 424.0   Mitral valve disorders

- 424.2   Tricuspid valve disorders, specified as nonrheumatic

Acute Rheumatic Fever and Rheumatic Heart Disease

Acute and chronic diseases of rheumatic origin are classified to categories 390–398. This section also covers diseases of mitral and aortic valves.

Acute Rheumatic Fever (390–392)

Rheumatic fever occurs after a streptococcal sore throat (Group A streptococcus hemolyticus). The acute phase of the illness is marked by fever, malaise, sweating, palpitation, and polyarthritis, which varies from vague discomfort to severe pain felt chiefly in the large joints. Most patients have elevated titers of antistreptolysin antibodies and increased sedimentation rates.

The importance of rheumatic fever derives entirely from its capacity to cause severe heart damage. Salicylates markedly reduce fever, relieve joint pain, and may reduce joint swelling, when present. Because rheumatic fever often recurs, prophylaxis with penicillin is recommended and has markedly reduced the incidence of rheumatic heart disease in the general population.

Chronic Rheumatic Heart Disease (393–398)

Rheumatic heart disease develops with an initial attack of rheumatic fever in about 30 percent of cases. The cardiac involvement may affect all three layers, causing pericarditis, scarring and weakening of the myocardium, and endocardial involvement of heart valves. The latter condition occurs in almost 66 percent of children who have had rheumatic fever and in about 20 percent of adults with rheumatic fever. A murmur heard over the heart is symptomatic of a valvular lesion. Rheumatic fever causes inflammation of the valves, thus damaging the valve cusps so that the opening may become permanently narrowed (stenosis). The mitral valve is involved in 75 to 80 percent of such cases; the aortic valve in 30 percent; and the tricuspid and pulmonary valves in less than 5 percent. In about 10 percent of patients, two of these valves are involved.

When stenosis affects the mitral valve, blood flow decreases from the left atrium into the left ventricle. As a result, blood is held back, first in the lungs, then in the right side of the heart, and, finally, in the veins of the body. Incompetence of a valve also may occur because the cusps will not retract. When the mitral valve cannot close, blood escapes back into the left atrium from the mitral valve. In the case of the aortic valve, blood escapes from the aorta into the left ventricle. In such cases, plastic and metal replacement valves that function as well as normal valves may be inserted surgically.

In coding diseases of the mitral valve and diseases affecting both the mitral and aortic valves, the Alphabetic Index to Diseases offers direction to codes from categories 393–398. Remember to always trust the Alphabetic Index and assign the code it indicates.

Hypertension

Hypertension is an elevation of systolic and/or diastolic blood pressure. A table is used to index the terms and codes associated with hypertension.

Hypertension, hypertensive (arterial) (arteriolar) (crisis) (degeneration) (disease) (essential) (fluctuating) (idiopathic) (intermittent) (labile) (low renin) (orthostatic) (paroxysmal) (primary) (systemic) (uncontrolled) (vascular)	Malignant	Benign	Unspecified
	401.0	401.1	401.9
with			
heart involvement (conditions classifiable to 429.0–429.3, 429.8, 429.9 due to hypertension) (*see also* Hypertension, heart)	402.00	402.10	402.90
with kidney involvement—*see* hypertension, cardiorenal			
renal involvement (only conditions classifiable to 585, 586, 587) (excludes conditions classifiable to 584) (*see also* Hypertension, kidney)	403.00	403.10	403.90
renal sclerosis or failure	403.00	403.10	403.90
with heart involvement—*see* Hypertension, cardiorenal			
failure (and sclerosis) (*see also* Hypertension, kidney)	403.01	403.11	403.91
sclerosis without failure (*see also* Hypertension, kidney)	403.00	403.10	403.90
accelerated—(*see also* Hypertension, by type, malignant)	401.0	—	—

The first column of the table identifies the hypertensive condition, such as accelerated, antepartum, cardiovascular disease, cardiorenal, and cerebrovascular disease. The remaining three columns are titled "malignant," "benign," and "unspecified," and they constitute the subcategories of hypertensive disease. Often the documentation in the patient's health record will not specify a hypertensive condition as malignant or benign; therefore, the unspecified code to describe that hypertensive condition must be assigned.

A threshold of blood pressure that an individual could overshoot and then be considered hypertensive has not been defined. Commonly, however, a sustained diastolic pressure above 90 mm Hg and a sustained systolic pressure above 140 mm Hg constitute hypertension. The prevalence of hypertension increases with age. About 90 percent of hypertension is primary (essential hypertension), and its cause is unknown. The remaining 10 percent is secondary to renal disease. Both essential and secondary hypertension can be either benign or malignant. Complications of hypertension include left ventricular failure, arteriosclerotic heart disease, retinal hemorrhages, cerebrovascular insufficiency, and renal failure.

Benign Hypertension

In most cases, benign hypertension remains fairly stable over many years and is compatible with a long life. When untreated, however, it becomes an important risk factor in coronary heart disease and cerebrovascular disease. Benign hypertension is also asymptomatic until complications develop. Effective antihypertensive drug therapy is the treatment of choice.

Malignant Hypertension

Malignant hypertension is far less common, occurring in only about 5 percent of patients with elevated blood pressure. The malignant form is frequently of abrupt onset and runs a course measured in months. It often ends with renal failure or cerebral hemorrhage. Usually a person with malignant hypertension will complain of headaches and difficulties with vision. Blood pressures of 200/140 are common, and an abnormal protrusion of the optic nerve (papilledema) occurs with microscopic hemorrhages and exudates seen in the retina. The initial event appears to be some form of vascular damage to the kidneys. This may result from long-standing benign hypertension with damage of the arteriolar walls, or it may derive from arteritis of some form. The chances for long-term survival depend on early treatment before significant renal insufficiency has developed.

Hypertensive Heart Disease

Hypertensive heart disease refers to the secondary effects on the heart of prolonged sustained systemic hypertension. The heart has to work against greatly increased resistance in the form of high blood pressure. The primary effect is thickening of the left ventricle, finally resulting in heart failure. The symptoms are similar to those of heart failure from other causes. Many persons with controlled hypertension do not develop heart failure.

Chapter-Specific Coding Guidelines

The following guidelines are applicable in coding hypertensive diseases:

- Hypertension, essential or NOS: Assign hypertension (arterial) (essential) (primary) (systemic) (NOS) to category 401, with the appropriate fourth digit to indicate malignant (.0), benign (.1), or unspecified (.9). Do not use either .0 (malignant) or .1 (benign) unless the documentation in the health record supports such a designation.

- Hypertension with heart disease: Certain heart conditions (429.0–429.3, 429.8, 429.9), when due to hypertension, are assigned a code from category 402. When a causal relationship is stated or implied, use only the code from category 402.

  In ICD-9-CM, a *stated* causal relationship is usually documented using the term *due to* (for example, congestive heart failure due to hypertension). An *implied* causal relationship is documented using the term *hypertensive.* In ICD-9-CM, hypertensive is interpreted to mean "due to." Therefore, hypertensive cardiomegaly also can be described as cardiomegaly due to hypertension.

  In category 402, Hypertensive heart disease, the fourth-digit subcategory describes whether the hypertensive condition is malignant, benign, or unspecified. The fifth-digit subclassification states the absence or presence of heart failure. The coder is advised to "Use additional code to specify type of heart failure."

  Although hypertension is frequently the cause of various forms of heart and vascular disease, ICD-9-CM does not presume a cause-and-effect relationship. The mention of "heart disease with hypertension only" should not be interpreted as a "due to" condition. Use of the terms *and* and *with* in the diagnostic statement does not imply cause and effect.

  > **EXAMPLE:**   Cardiomegaly and hypertension
  > 429.3, Cardiomegaly
  > 401.9, Essential hypertension, unspecified

- Hypertensive kidney disease: Assign codes from category 403, Hypertensive kidney disease, when conditions classified to categories 585–587 are present. Unlike hypertension with heart disease, ICD-9-CM presumes a cause-and-effect relationship and classifies chronic kidney disease with hypertensive disease. As with hypertensive heart disease, the fourth-digit subcategory describes whether the hypertensive condition is malignant, benign, or unspecified. The fifth-digit subclassification identifies the presence or absence of chronic kidney disease.

> **EXAMPLE:** Hypertension and chronic kidney disease
> 403.91, Hypertensive kidney disease, unspecified with chronic kidney disease

The coder is instructed to "Use additional code to identify the stage of chronic kidney disease (585.1–585.6), if known."

- Hypertensive heart and kidney disease: Assign codes from category 404, Hypertensive heart and kidney disease, when both hypertensive renal disease and hypertensive heart disease are stated in the diagnosis. Assume a causal relationship between the hypertension and the kidney disease, whether or not the condition is designated that way. Remember, the fourth-digit subcategory describes whether the hypertensive condition is malignant, benign, or unspecified. The fifth-digit subclassification identifies the presence, absence, or combination of heart failure and/or chronic kidney disease.

> **EXAMPLE:** Hypertensive cardiomegaly and hypertensive chronic kidney disease
> 404.92, Hypertensive heart and kidney disease, unspecified with chronic kidney disease

In this example, the fifth digit 2 reflects the presence of chronic kidney disease alone.

The coder is instructed to "Use additional code to identify the stage of chronic kidney disease (585.1–585.6), if known."

- Hypertensive cerebrovascular disease: Two codes are required to fully describe a hypertensive cerebrovascular condition. The first code assigned describes the cerebrovascular disease (430–438), followed by the appropriate code describing the hypertension (401–405).

> **EXAMPLE:** Cerebrovascular accident and benign hypertension
> 436, Acute, but ill-defined cerebrovascular disease
> 401.1, Benign essential hypertension

- Hypertensive retinopathy: Two codes are required to identify hypertensive retinopathy. First, assign code 362.11, Hypertensive retinopathy, followed by the appropriate code from categories 401–405 describing the hypertension.

- Hypertension, secondary: When a physician documents that the hypertension is due to another disease (secondary hypertension), two codes are required to describe the condition completely. One code describes the underlying condition, and the other is selected from category 405, Secondary hypertension.

Category 405 is subdivided at the fourth-digit level to describe whether the hypertensive condition is malignant, benign, or unspecified. The fifth-digit subclassification identifies the underlying condition of renovascular origin or of another origin.

Renovascular origin can include renal artery aneurysm, anomaly, embolism, fibromuscular hyperplasia, occlusion, stenosis, or thrombosis. Other types of diseases causing secondary hypertension can include a calculus of the ureter or kidney, a brain tumor, polycystic kidneys, or polycythemia.

EXAMPLE: Hypertension due to a malignant neoplasm of the brain
191.9, Malignant neoplasm of brain, unspecified
405.99, Other unspecified secondary hypertension

- Hypertension, transient and elevated blood pressure: Assign code 796.2, Elevated blood pressure reading without diagnosis of hypertension, when the diagnosis states either "elevated blood pressure reading" or "transient elevated blood pressure reading." When the patient has a diagnosis of hypertension, report the appropriate code from categories 401–404.

Ischemic Heart Disease

Ischemic heart disease (categories 410–414) is synonymous with arteriosclerotic heart disease, coronary ischemia, and coronary artery disease. It is the generic name for three forms of heart disease: myocardial infarction, angina pectoris, and chronic ischemic heart disease. All three diseases result from an imbalance between the need of the myocardium for oxygen and the oxygen supply. Usually the imbalance results from insufficient blood flow due to arteriosclerotic narrowing of the coronary arteries.

At the beginning of the ischemic heart disease section in chapter 7 of the ICD-9-CM codebook, the inclusion note states that the section includes ischemic heart conditions with mention of hypertension. The statement "Use additional code to identify presence of hypertension" also appears at the beginning of this section as an instruction to assign an additional code to describe hypertension, when present.

Myocardial Infarction

Myocardial infarction (MI) usually occurs as a result of sudden inadequacy of coronary blood flow. The first symptom of acute MI is the development of deep substernal pain described as an ache or pressure, often with radiation to the back or left arm. The patient is pale, diaphoretic (sweaty), and in severe pain. Major complications include tachycardia, frequent ventricular premature beats, Mobitz II heart block, and ventricular fibrillation. Heart failure occurs in about two-thirds of hospitalized MI patients. MI is reported with a code from category 410, Acute myocardial infarction. The fourth digit describes the specific location affected in the heart (that is, lateral wall or anterior wall).

Diagnostic Tools

The diagnosis of acute myocardial infarction (AMI) depends on the patient's clinical history, the physical examination, interpretation of electrocardiogram (ECG), chest radiograph, and measurement of serum levels of cardiac enzymes.

Diagnostic uncertainty frequently arises because of various factors. Many patients with AMI have atypical symptoms. Other people with typical physical symptoms do not have AMI. Electrocardiograms may also be nondiagnostic. Laboratory tests known as biochemical or serum markers of cardiac injury are commonly relied upon to diagnose or exclude an acute myocardial infarction.

Creatine kinase and lactate dehydrogenase have been the "gold standard" for the diagnosis of AMI for many years. However, single values of these tests have limited sensitivity and specificity. Newer serum markers in use today are Troponin T and I, myoglobin, and the MB isoenzyme of creatine kinase. These new markers are now being used instead of, or along with, the standard markers.

Electrocardiograms (EKGs) also prove useful in diagnosing myocardial infarctions. The initial EKG may be diagnostic in acute transmural myocardial infarction, but serial EKGs may be necessary to confirm the diagnosis for other myocardial infarction sites.

Fourth-Digit Subcategories and Fifth-Digit Subclassifications

ICD-9-CM classifies myocardial infarction to category 410, with the following fourth-digit subcategories describing the specific site involved:

410.0   Of anterolateral wall
410.1   Of other anterior wall
410.2   Of inferolateral wall
410.3   Of inferoposterior wall
410.4   Of other inferior wall
410.5   Of other lateral wall
410.6   True posterior wall infarction
410.7   Subendocardial infarction
410.8   Of other specified sites
410.9   Unspecified site

The fifth-digit subclassifications to category 410, Acute myocardial infarction, indicate the episode of care:

<table>
<tr><td>0</td><td>Episode of care unspecified
Use when the source of documentation does not contain sufficient information for the assignment of fifth digit 1 or 2.</td></tr>
<tr><td>1</td><td>Initial episode of care
Use fifth digit 1 to designate the first episode of care (regardless of facility site) for a newly diagnosed myocardial infarction. The fifth digit 1 is assigned regardless of the number of times a patient may be transferred during the initial episode of care.</td></tr>
<tr><td>2</td><td>Subsequent episode of care
Use the fifth digit 2 to designate an episode of care following the initial episode when the patient is admitted for further observation, evaluation, or treatment for an MI that has received initial treatment but is still less than eight weeks old.</td></tr>
</table>

In the physician's office and outpatient setting, the most appropriate fifth digit to identify subsequent episodes of an MI is 2. The assignment of fifth digit 0 should be avoided because the documentation in the health record should reflect the circumstances of the encounter.

When the patient has unstable angina leading to an MI, only the code describing the infarction is reported. The angina is considered symptomatic and thus is not coded. Code 412 may be assigned to indicate a previous ("old") myocardial infarction. This code is appropriate when the patient's MI is documented as old or healed with no current symptoms. No fourth or fifth digits are applicable for this code. When a patient is still symptomatic after eight weeks following a myocardial infarction, code 414.8, Other specified forms of chronic ischemic heart disease, is used.

Angina

Angina may be classified as either unstable angina or angina pectoris. Unstable angina, also known as crescendo and preinfarction angina, is the development of prolonged episodes of anginal discomfort, usually occurring at rest and requiring hospitalization to rule out myocardial infarction. Unstable angina is classified to code 411.1, Intermediate coronary syndrome.

Angina pectoris refers to chest pain as a result of heart ischemia. ICD-9-CM classifies this type of angina to category 413. This category further subdivides to identify the specific type of angina, such as angina decubitus and Prinzmetal angina. Without further specification, angina pectoris is assigned to code 413.9.

Chronic Ischemic Heart Disease

Arteriosclerosis or atherosclerosis is the narrowing of an arterial wall caused by the deposition of plaque-forming cholesterol and other lipids within the lumen. The large arteries—the aorta and its main branches—are primarily affected, but smaller arteries such as the coronary and cerebral arteries also can be affected. In such a case, the patient experiences chest pain, shortness of breath, and sweating. Blood pressure is high; pulse is rapid and weak. An x-ray reveals cardiomegaly and narrowing, or occlusion, of the affected vessel wall. Blood tests may show hypercholesterolemia.

Atherosclerosis is the major cause of ischemia of the heart, brain, and extremities. Its complications include stroke, congestive heart failure, angina pectoris, MI, and kidney failure. Treatment is directed toward the specific manifestation. Coronary atherosclerosis is reported with subcategory 414.0, which is further expanded to identify involvement of the native coronary arteries, bypassed grafts, or a combination of both, as follows:

- 414.00, Coronary atherosclerosis of unspecified type of vessel, native or graft

- 414.01, Coronary atherosclerosis of native coronary artery

- 414.02, Coronary atherosclerosis of autologous vein bypass graft

- 414.03, Coronary atherosclerosis of nonautologous biological bypass graft

- 414.04, Coronary atherosclerosis of artery bypass graft

- 414.05, Coronary atherosclerosis of unspecified type of bypass graft

- 414.06, Coronary atherosclerosis of native coronary artery of transplanted heart

- 414.07, Coronary atherosclerosis of bypass graft (artery) (vein) of transplanted heart

These fifth-digit codes are vessel specific and should be assigned when the physician's documentation states that atherosclerosis has been found in that specific vessel. A fifth-digit code should not be assigned based solely on the fact that a patient has atherosclerosis and a history of bypass surgery. An explanation of the fifth-digit codes follows:

- Code 414.00 is assigned when the documentation in the health record does not indicate whether the disease is present in a native vessel or a graft.

- Code 414.01 is assigned to show coronary artery disease in a native coronary artery. This code is used when a patient has coronary artery disease and no history of coronary artery bypass (CABG) surgery. It may be used when a patient, who previously had a percutaneous transluminal coronary angioplasty (PTCA), has vessels that have reoccluded as demonstrated by a recent cardiac catheterization.

- Code 414.02 is assigned to show coronary artery disease in an autologous vein bypass graft. Vein bypass grafts have been the most commonly performed coronary bypass grafts in the past. Patients who had a CABG procedure several years ago probably had saphenous veins used for graft material. Often these patients are readmitted for a "redo" CABG procedure.

- Code 414.03 is assigned to show coronary artery disease in a nonautologous biological bypass graft.

- Code 414.04 is assigned when the physician documents the diagnosis of coronary atherosclerosis in an internal mammary artery used for a bypass graft.

- Code 414.05 is assigned when the physician documents the diagnosis of coronary atherosclerosis in a bypass graft and the patient has a history of CABG surgery. This code is used when there is no further documentation of the type of bypass graft used.

- Code 414.06 is assigned when there is evidence of coronary atherosclerosis in the native coronary arteries of a patient who has had a heart transplant.

- Code 414.07 is assigned when there is evidence of coronary atherosclerosis in the bypass graft of a patient who has had a heart transplant.

Subcategory code 414.8, Other specified forms of chronic ischemic heart disease, includes an important note:

414.8   Other specified forms of chronic ischemic heart disease
Chronic coronary insufficiency
Ischemia, myocardial (chronic)
Any condition classifiable to 410 specified as chronic, or
    presenting with symptoms after 8 weeks from date of infarction

Excludes: *coronary insufficiency (acute) (411.89)*

This note advises that code 414.8 should be assigned when a diagnosis states chronic myocardial infarction with symptoms presenting eight weeks or more after the date of the infarction.

Other Forms of Heart Disease

The other forms of heart disease category includes codes 420–429. The following subsections describe three forms of heart disease: cardiomyopathy, cardiac dysrhythmias, and heart failure.

Cardiomyopathy

Cardiomyopathy is a disease, often of an unknown cause, that involves the muscle of the heart. ICD-9-CM classifies most cardiomyopathies to category 425, with the fourth digits identifying specific types, as follows:

- 425.0, Endomyocardial fibrosis

- 425.1, Hypertrophic obstructive cardiomyopathy

- 425.2, Obscure cardiomyopathy of Africa

- 425.3, Endocardial fibroelastosis

- 425.4, Other primary cardiomyopathies, such as congestive, constrictive, familial, hypertrophic, idiopathic, nonobstructive, obstructive, and restrictive

- 425.5, Alcoholic cardiomyopathy

- *425.7, Nutritional and metabolic cardiomyopathy*

- *425.8, Cardiomyopathy in other diseases classified elsewhere*

- 425.9, Secondary cardiomyopathy, unspecified

Codes 425.7 and 425.8 appear in italicized print and thus should be reported only in the secondary position. The underlying cause, such as a nutritional disorder, should be reported first.

Ischemic cardiomyopathy, resulting from prolonged, persistent deficiency of blood to the heart muscle, is reported with code 414.8, Other specified forms of chronic ischemic heart disease (*Coding Clinic,* 2nd Quarter 1990).

Cardiac Dysrhythmias

Cardiac dysrhythmias identify disturbances or impairments of the normal electrical activity of heart muscle excitation. ICD-9-CM classifies cardiac dysrhythmias to several categories depending on the specific type. Without further specification as to type of cardiac dysrhythmia, code 427.9 may be reported. Some common dysrhythmias are discussed below:

- Atrial fibrillation (427.31) is commonly associated with organic heart disease, such as coronary artery disease, hypertension and rheumatic mitral valve disease, thyrotoxicosis, pericarditis, and pulmonary embolism. Treatment includes pharmacologic therapy (verapamil, digoxin, and propranolol) and cardioversion.

- Atrial flutter (427.32) is associated with ischemic heart disease and pulmonary disease. Treatment is similar to the treatment for atrial fibrillation.

- Ventricular fibrillation (427.41) involves no cardiac output and is associated with cardiac arrest. Treatment is consistent with the treatment for cardiac arrest.

- Paroxysmal supraventricular tachycardia (427.0) is associated with congenital accessory atrial conduction pathway, physical or psychological stress, hypoxia, hypokalemia, caffeine and marijuana use, stimulant use, and digitalis toxicity. Treatment includes pharmacologic therapy (quinidine, propranolol, verapamil) and cardioversion.

- Sick sinus syndrome (427.81), often abbreviated as SSS, has various characteristics and an imprecise diagnosis. It may be diagnosed when the patient presents with sinus arrest, sinoatrial exit block, or persistent sinus bradycardia. Often SSS is the result of drug therapy including digitalis, calcium channel blockers, beta-blockers, sympatholytic agents, and antiarrhythmics. Another presentation includes recurrent supraventricular tachycardia associated with bradyarrhythmias. Prolonged ambulatory monitoring may be indicated to establish a diagnosis of sick sinus syndrome. Treatment includes insertion of a permanent cardiac pacemaker.

- Wolff-Parkinson-White syndrome (426.7), often abbreviated as WPW, is caused by conduction from the sinoatrial node to the ventricle through an accessory pathway that bypasses the atrioventricular node. Patients with WPW syndrome present with tachyarrhythmias, including supraventricular tachycardia and atrial fibrillation or flutter. Treatment includes catheter ablation following electrophysiologic evaluation.

- Atrioventricular (AV) heart blocks are classified as being of first, second, or third degree:

  —First-degree AV block is associated with atrial septal defects or valvular disease. ICD-9-CM classifies first-degree AV block to code 426.11.

  —Second-degree AV block is further classified as follows: Mobitz type I (Wenckebach) is associated with acute inferior wall MI or digitalis toxicity. Treatment includes discontinuation of digitalis and administration of atropine. ICD-9-CM classifies Mobitz type I AV block to code 426.13. Mobitz type II is associated with anterior wall or anteroseptal MI and digitalis toxicity. Treatment includes temporary pacing and, in some cases, permanent pacemaker insertion, as well as discontinuation of digitalis and administration of atropine. ICD-9-CM classifies Mobitz type II AV block to code 426.12.

  —Third-degree AV block, also referred to as complete heart block, is associated with ischemic heart disease or infarction, postsurgical complication of mitral valve replacement, digitalis toxicity, and Stokes-Adams syndrome. Treatment includes permanent cardiac pacemaker insertion. ICD-9-CM classifies third-degree AV block to code 426.0. When this type of heart block is congenital in nature, code 746.86 is reported rather than 426.0. Without further specification, atrioventricular block is reported with code 426.10.

- Sinus tachycardia is associated with normal physiologic response to fever, exercise, anxiety, pain, and dehydration. It also may accompany shock, left ventricular failure, cardiac tamponade, anemia, hyperthyroidism, hypovolemia, pulmonary embolism, and anterior myocardial infarction. Treatment is geared toward correcting the underlying cause. ICD-9-CM classifies sinus tachycardia, as well as supraventricular tachycardia, to code 427.89.

Heart Failure

Heart failure is characterized by the inability of the heart to contract with enough force to pump blood properly. It may be caused by hypertension, incompetent heart valves, or weakness of the heart resulting from MI. Heart failure may develop gradually or occur acutely. Its effects include the following:

- Increased pressure in the lung as fluid collects in the lung tissue, inhibiting oxygen and carbon dioxide exchange

- Impaired kidney function as blood filters poorly and body sodium and water retention increase, resulting in edema

- Impaired blood circulation as fluid collects in tissues, resulting in edema of the feet and legs

Early signs of heart failure are tachycardia, fatigue, and dyspnea with exertion, nocturnal dyspnea, cough, and intolerance to cold. Symptoms deteriorate into wheezing; productive, blood-tinged cough; feelings of suffocation; and cyanosis. Patients are pale and perspiring, with moist rales heard at the base of the lungs. Respiration becomes labored and weak, with a rapid pulse and congested lungs with oliguria. ICD-9-CM classifies heart failure to category 428 with fourth digits indicating whether the heart failure is congestive, unspecified (428.0), left heart failure (428.1), systolic (428.2x), diastolic (428.3x), or combined systolic and diastolic (428.4x). Fifth digits for 428.2, 428.3, and 428.4 specify whether the heart failure is unspecified, acute, chronic, or acute on chronic. However, when the heart failure is due to hypertension, a code from category 402 is used (*Coding Clinic,* 2nd Quarter 1990).

Diagnostic Tests

Several diagnostic tests are important in diagnosing heart failure in a patient. Typical remarks on a chest x-ray include hilar congestion, "butterfly" or "batwing" appearance of vascular markings, bronchial edema, Kerley B lines signifying chronic elevation of left atrial pressure, and heart enlargement.

Vital capacity (amount of air that can be expelled from the lungs) is reduced. Oxygen content of the blood is reduced, and circulation time is longer (normal circulation time from arm to lung is 4 to 8 seconds).

Urinalysis results show slight albuminuria, increased concentration with specific gravity of 1.020, and urine sodium decreased. Laboratory findings may include BUN 60 mg/100 ml; acidosis pH <7.35 due to increased CO_2 in blood from pulmonary insufficiency; and increased blood volume with a decrease in chloride, albumin, and total protein.

Cerebrovascular Disease

Cerebrovascular disease (categories 430–438) is any condition pertaining to the blood vessels or blood flow of the brain, usually secondary to atherosclerotic disease, hypertension, or a combination of both. The inclusion note at the beginning of this section advises that it includes cerebrovascular diseases with mention of hypertension. The instruction "Use additional code to identify presence of hypertension" (when hypertension is present) also appears at the beginning of this section. ICD-9-CM classifies cerebrovascular disease according to type of condition, as follows:

- 430, Subarachnoid hemorrhage
- 431, Intracerebral hemorrhage
- 432, Other and unspecified intracranial hemorrhage
- 433, Occlusion and stenosis of precerebral arteries
- 434, Occlusion of cerebral arteries
- 435, Transient cerebral ischemia
- 436, Acute, but ill-defined, cerebrovascular disease
- 437, Other and ill-defined cerebrovascular disease
- 438, Late effects of cerebrovascular disease

It should be noted that codes 433, Occlusion and stenosis of precerebral arteries, and 434, Occlusion of cerebral arteries, require the assignment of a fifth digit to identify the presence or absence of cerebral infarction.

Category 436, Acute, but ill-defined, cerebrovascular disease, is assigned when the diagnosis states cerebrovascular accident (CVA) without further specification. The health record should be reviewed carefully to ensure that nothing more specific is available. Postoperative cerebrovascular accident is reported using code 997.02, Iatrogenic cerebrovascular infarction or hemorrhage.

Category 438, Late effects of cerebrovascular disease, is further subdivided to identify the specific effect, such as hemiplegia or monoplegia, aphasia, dysphagia, disturbances of vision, alteration of sensations, apraxia, ataxia, vertigo, or facial weakness.

Fourth digits in category 438 identify specific late effects of cerebrovascular disease, including neurologic deficits that persist after initial onset of conditions classifiable to 430–437. The neurologic deficits may be present from the onset or may arise at any time after the onset of the condition classifiable to 430–437.

> **EXAMPLE:** 438.11   Late effect of cerebrovascular disease, aphasia
> 438.21   Late effect of cerebrovascular disease, hemiplegia, affecting dominant side
> 438.40   Late effect of cerebrovascular disease, monoplegia of lower limb affecting unspecified side

When the documentation in the health record indicates late effect of cerebrovascular disease without further specification about type, code 438.9, Unspecified late effects of cerebrovascular disease, may be reported. When residuals from an earlier CVA are still present when a new CVA is diagnosed, codes from category 438 can be assigned as additional codes.

Diseases of Arteries, Arterioles, and Capillaries

The diseases of the arteries, arterioles, and capillaries category includes codes 440–448. Some of the conditions belonging to this category are described in the following subsections.

Atherosclerosis of the Peripheral Extremities

Atherosclerosis of the peripheral extremities is classified to subcategory 440.2, which is further subdivided to describe the progression of the disease with intermittent claudication (440.21), rest pain (440.22), ulceration (440.23), or gangrene (440.24). Notations appearing below codes 440.22–440.24 remind the coder that as the disease progresses, only the code describing the most severe stage is reported. An additional code from 707.10–707.9 should be used when 440.23 is selected.

> **EXAMPLE:** Atherosclerosis of the extremities with intermittent claudication and rest pain: 440.22

Only code 440.22 should be assigned in the preceding example because the note below code 440.22 specifies that it includes conditions classifiable to code 440.21, which include intermittent claudication. Without further specification, atherosclerosis of the extremities is reported with code 440.20.

Peripheral Vascular Disease

Peripheral vascular disease (PVD) is a narrowing of the arterial wall by arteriosclerotic plaque. ICD-9-CM classifies PVD to category 443, which is further subdivided to identify specific types, such as Raynaud's syndrome, erythromelalgia, or thromboangiitis obliterans. Without further specification, PVD is reported with code 443.9.

Arterial Embolism and Thrombosis of Extremities

Arterial embolism and thrombosis of extremities are reported with subcategory 444.2, with the fifth digits identifying upper or lower extremity involvement. An embolism is defined as a blood clot or foreign substance blocking an artery. A thrombosis is an abnormal aggregation of blood factors causing an arterial obstruction. Atheroembolism, obstruction of a blood vessel by a cholesterol-containing embolism, is reported with category 445, Atheroembolism.

Diseases of Veins and Lymphatics and Other Diseases of the Circulatory System

Codes 451–459 are used to report diseases of veins and lymphatics and other diseases of the circulatory system. The following subsections discuss conditions that are classified to this category of codes.

Phlebitis and Thrombophlebitis

Phlebitis and thrombophlebitis are characterized by inflammation and thrombus formation in the deep (intermuscular or intramuscular) veins or superficial (subcutaneous) veins. Both conditions are characterized by edema, dusky cyanosis, dilation of superficial veins, local heat, redness, tenderness, and pain. More severe complications may result, such as pulmonary embolism, bacteremia, and septic emboli. ICD-9-CM classifies phlebitis and thrombophlebitis to category 451, which further subdivides to identify the specific sites involved.

Varicose Veins

Varicose veins are characterized by tortuous and dilated veins of the affected site. The most common site of varicose vein development is the lower extremities, usually of the saphenous system and its branches. The valves are absent or become incompetent (due to venous dilatation) to prevent venous pooling (venostasis) from reversed blood flow in the veins. Symptoms of varicose veins include: visible, prominent, elongated, tortuous superficial veins; dull, heavy, aching discomfort in the legs at the end of the day, relieved by elevation; superficial phlebitis; and hemorrhage from superficial variceal erosion or rupture.

ICD-9-CM classifies varicose veins of the lower extremities to category 454, with a fourth digit to identify the severity of the disease, such as that with inflammation, ulcer, or both. Varicose veins involving other sites, such as esophagus, pelvis, vulva, or scrota, are classified to category 456.

Hemorrhoids

Hemorrhoids are characterized by enlarged or thrombosed veins in the lower rectum or anus resulting in rectal bleeding and vague discomfort. They may be specified as internal or external. Internal hemorrhoids include varicosities of the superior and middle venous plexuses (those proximal to the anorectal line) that protrude, under the rectal mucosa, into the rectal lumen. External hemorrhoids are dilated inferior plexus veins (located distal to the anorectal line) that protrude from the rectum through the anus, are covered by squamous epithelium, and are more susceptible to thrombosis. Symptoms of both types of hemorrhoids include intermittent bleeding, usually after defecation; protrusion; pruritus ani due to incomplete cleansing of the anal region; painful acute prolapse, thrombosis, and ulceration; severely painful strangulation; mucus discharge; and a feeling of incomplete evacuation of the rectum.

ICD-9-CM classifies hemorrhoids to category 455, with the fourth digits identifying the specific type (internal versus external) and the presence of complications such as bleeding, strangulation, prolapse, and ulceration. Without further specification and with no complications present, hemorrhoids are reported with code 455.6.

Hypotension

Hypotension is an abnormally low blood pressure. Orthostatic hypotension, also known as postural hypotension, occurs upon arising from a recumbent position or when standing still. ICD-9-CM classifies hypotension to category 458, with the fourth digits indicating the specific type. When the underlying cause of the hypotension cannot be identified, a code from category 458 is assigned. When the underlying cause is known, a code for the hypotension is unnecessary.

Esophageal and Gastric Varices

Esophageal and gastric varices are the cause of death due to upper gastrointestinal bleeding in 30 percent of patients during initial hospitalization. There is a higher incidence of esophageal varices than gastric varices. There are numerous therapeutic procedures for esophageal and gastric varices, with a new one introduced each decade, indicating that none has a high success rate.

To develop varices, an individual's portal pressure must reach a hepatic vein pressure of 12 mm Hg (normal = 3 to 6 mm Hg). For bleeding to occur, a varix must be over 5 mm in diameter to have the tendency to burst. When a varix is under 5 mm, pressure from coughing or straining could cause rupture.

Most patients with varices have cirrhosis of the liver, which is usually alcoholic in origin. Patients also may have splenic vein thrombosis or hypersplenic states, predisposing them to develop more gastric varices.

> **EXAMPLE:** A patient admitted for bleeding esophageal varices and who also has Laennec's cirrhosis would have the following code assignments: Alcoholic cirrhosis of liver, 571.2; Bleeding esophageal varices, 456.20; Alcoholism, 303.9x (with fifth-digit designation as to type)

When bleeding varices are suspected, an endoscopy is performed within 12 hours of any signs of bleeding in order to document the source of hemorrhage. In addition to rupture of a varix, other causes of bleeding may include Mallory-Weiss tears, gastritis, peptic ulcers, and noninflammatory vascular lesions peculiar to portal hypertension (for example, congestive gastropathy).

Treatment for bleeding varices includes the following in the order that the physician considers them:

- Endoscopic injection sclerotherapy

- Intravenous infusion of vasopressin

- Balloon tamponade techniques

- Percutaneous obliteration (embolization)

- Surgery performed to insert a portal-systemic shunt (such as transjugular intrahepatic portosystemic shunt [TIPS])

Prevention of recurrent bleeding varices consists of surgical placement of a shunt, repeated injections of a sclerosing agent, or administration of propranolol (Inderal) that lowers the portal venous pressure.

Other Disorders of Circulatory System

Postphlebitic syndrome is classified to 459.1, with fifth digits indicating the presence or absence of complications including ulcers and inflammation. Idiopathic chronic venous hypertension is classified to 459.3, with fifth digits indicating the presence or absence of complications including ulcers or inflammation.

Circulatory V Codes

Some of the V codes that apply to the circulatory system include:

Personal history of diseases of circulatory system (V12.5x)
Family history of circulatory disease:
    Stroke (cerebrovascular) (V17.1)
    Ischemic heart disease (V17.3)
    Other cardiovascular diseases (V17.4)
Presence of heart valve transplant or prosthesis (V42.2 and V43.3)
Cardiac device in situ (V45.0x)
Aortocoronary bypass status (V45.81)
Awaiting organ transplant status (V49.83)
Fitting and adjustment of cardiac device (V53.3x)
Encounter for aftercare for long-term (current) use of anticoagulants (V58.61)
Encounter for aftercare for long-term (current) use of antiplatelet antithrombotic (V58.63)
Encounter for aftercare for long-term (current) use of aspirin (V58.66)
Observation for suspected cardiovascular disease (V71.7)
Special screening for cardiovascular diseases:
    Ischemic heart disease (V81.0)
    Hypertension (V81.1)
    Other and unspecified cardiovascular conditions (V81.2)

Chapter 11 Exercises

Review the following statements and cases and assign the appropriate codes:

1. Mitral valve stenosis with aortic valve insufficiency

   ____

2. Hypertensive cardiomegaly and hypertensive stage IV chronic kidney disease

   ____

3. Old myocardial infarction

   ____

4. Unstable angina with acute subendocardial infarction, initial episode

   ____

5. Acute systolic heart failure; benign hypertension

   ____

6. Hypertension due to Cushing's disease

   ____

7. Congestive heart failure and end-stage renal disease due to accelerated hypertension

   ____

8. Acute cerebrovascular accident due to stenosis and infarction of right carotid artery

   ____

9. Arteriosclerosis of right lower leg with claudication

   ____

10. Atrioventricular block, Mobitz type II

    ____

11. Benign hypertensive cardiomegaly

    ____

12. Bleeding esophageal varices in patient with portal hypertension

    ____

13. Internal hemorrhoids with bleeding and prolapse

    ____

14. Thrombophlebitis of deep femoral vein

    ____

Chapter 11 Exercises (Continued)

15. An 83-year-old male was readmitted to an acute care hospital from a local nursing home for treatment of a UTI due to E. coli. He is three weeks status post an inferior wall myocardial infarction. During his hospitalization, he experienced cardiac arrhythmia and was placed on a telemetry unit for monitoring. The arrhythmia resolved spontaneously.

    Discharge diagnoses: Urinary tract infection due to E. coli; myocardial infarction, inferior wall; cardiac arrhythmia

    Code(s):

16. A 78-year-old female, who had taken Lotensin as treatment for hypertension for three years, was admitted for evaluation of severe nausea and vomiting. A complete workup confirmed that these symptoms were due to stage V chronic kidney disease. The patient was started on renal dialysis and steadily improved.

    Discharge diagnoses: Stage V chronic kidney disease; hypertension; nausea and vomiting due to chronic kidney disease

    Code(s):

17. A 69-year-old female with previous MI, known hypertensive, began complaining of cough, chills, and fever about four days prior to admission. One day prior to admission, she started to complain of progressive dyspnea, associated with hemoptysis. She went to emergency services and was noted to be extremely dyspneic and wheezing. However, a chest x-ray showed evidence of bilateral lower lobe pneumonia with a PO_2 of 66 and white blood count of 12,400, for which admission was advised. The patient had an inferior wall MI 10 months ago. She also is known to have chronic anxiety problems and had been under the care of the Mental Hygiene Clinic. With medication and improvement in her respirations and x-ray findings, she was discharged. Her blood pressure was 154/110 on discharge, which was not considered unusual because her blood pressure was quite unstable as an outpatient, with variable high and low readings. This will be followed up in the office.

    Discharge diagnoses: Bilateral basilar pneumonia; old myocardial infarction with angina; hypertension; chronic anxiety; acute systolic heart failure

    Code(s):

Review Questions

Answer the following questions:

1. When the documentation in the patient's record does not specify the hypertensive condition as malignant or benign, how should the condition be coded?

2. When establishing a cause-and-effect relationship between hypertension and certain heart conditions, what terms should be documented in the diagnostic statement?

3. What do the fifth digits in category 403, Hypertensive kidney disease, indicate?

4. What two codes are necessary for correct coding of hypertensive cerebrovascular disease?

5. What is secondary hypertension, and how is it coded?

6. When is it appropriate to code 414.8, Other specified forms of chronic ischemic heart disease?

7. What do the fourth digits specify in category 438, Late effects of cerebrovascular disease?

8. What code is assigned when the physician indicates "an elevated blood pressure reading" or "transient elevated blood pressure reading"?

Chapter 12

Diseases of the Respiratory System

Objectives

After completing this lesson, the student should be able to do the following:

- Apply knowledge of current, approved ICD-9-CM coding guidelines to assign and sequence codes related to diseases of the respiratory system

- Identify the various types of respiratory disorders

- Differentiate among the various types of pneumonia

- Understand the appropriate use of the status asthmaticus fifth digits in category 493

- Explain the differences between alkalosis and acidosis

Introduction

Chapter 8 of the ICD-9-CM codebook includes the following sections:

Categories	Section Titles
460–466	Acute Respiratory Infections
470–478	Other Diseases of the Upper Respiratory Tract
480–487	Pneumonia and Influenza
490–496	Chronic Obstructive Pulmonary Diseases and Allied Conditions
500–508	Pneumoconioses and Other Lung Diseases due to External Agents
510–519	Other Diseases of Respiratory System

These diseases are most often treated by internists, allergists, and otorhinolaryngologists.

Bronchitis

Bronchitis is an inflammation of the bronchi and can be acute or chronic in nature. Acute bronchitis involves the tracheobronchial tree and is often due to exposure to cold, inhalation of irritating substances, or acute infections. Chronic bronchitis is associated with prolonged exposure to nonspecific bronchial irritants and is accompanied by mucous hypersecretion and certain structural changes in the bronchi. Usually associated with cigarette smoking, one form of bronchitis is characterized clinically by a chronic productive cough. ICD-9-CM classifies acute bronchitis to code 466.0, which includes the following diagnoses:

- Acute tracheobronchitis

- Croupous bronchitis

- Viral bronchitis

- Septic bronchitis

- Pneumococcal bronchitis

- Purulent bronchitis

- Fibrinous bronchitis

- Membranous bronchitis

- With tracheitis

ICD-9-CM classifies chronic bronchitis to category 491, which further subdivides to identify the specific type of chronic bronchitis, such as mucopurulent, simple, and obstructive. Without further specification as to type or severity (acute versus chronic), bronchitis is reported with code 490. When chronic bronchitis is described as obstructive or is associated with chronic obstructive pulmonary disease (COPD), code 491.20 (without exacerbation), 491.21 (with [acute] exacerbation), or 491.22 (with acute bronchitis) should be reported. Code 491.22 is used to report acute bronchitis with chronic obstructive pulmonary disease.

Chronic Obstructive Pulmonary Disease

Chronic obstructive pulmonary disease (COPD) is characterized by the decreased ability of the lungs to perform ventilation due to diffuse obstruction of the smaller bronchi and bronchioles, which results in coughing, wheezing, shortness of breath, and disturbances of gas exchange (O_2 and CO_2). Exacerbations of COPD, such as episodes of increased shortness of breath and cough, are often treated on an outpatient basis. More severe exacerbations, such as pneumonia, bronchitis, or other infections, usually result in admission to the hospital.

Treatment consists of oxygen support, arterial blood gas monitoring, intravenous or aerosol medication, and chest physical therapy as well as possible intubation with mechanical ventilation or tracheostomy. Medications frequently prescribed include inhaled bronchodilators (Alupent, Proventil, Ventolin, Atrovent) or oral bronchodilators (Theophylline, Albuterol).

The clinical course of COPD is extremely varied. However, two patterns of symptoms are often superimposed on each other: a progressive worsening of underlying lung function (progressive dyspnea, fatigue, and exacerbations) with recurring upper respiratory infections or lung infections. Stress caused by congestive heart failure (CHF) may lead to rapid deterioration of COPD.

Without further specification, COPD is classified to code 496. However, the exclusion note under code 496 reminds the coder that 496 is not to be used with any other code from categories 491–493. The excludes note directs the coder to more specific categories to be used as appropriate.

Excludes:	*chronic obstructive lung disease [COPD] specified (as) (with):* *allergic alveolitis (495.0–495.9)* *asthma (493.2)* *bronchiectasis (494.0–494.1)* *bronchitis (491.20–491.22)* *with emphysema (491.20–491.22)* *emphysema (492.0–492.8)*

Pneumonia

Pneumonia is inflammation of the lung with exudate. It is classified by the underlying cause (bacterial, viral, protozoal, fungal, mycobacterial, mycoplasmal, or rickettsial infection) or as a result of aspiration or surgery. ICD-9-CM classifies pneumonias to the following categories, most of which are subdivided to identify specific types or specific organisms:

- Category 480, Viral pneumonia

- Category 481, Pneumococcal pneumonia [Streptococcus pneumoniae pneumonia]

- Category 482, Other bacterial pneumonia

- Category 483, Pneumonia due to other specified organism

- Category 484, Pneumonia in infectious diseases classified elsewhere

- Category 485, Bronchopneumonia, organism unspecified

- Category 486, Pneumonia, organism unspecified

- Category 507, Pneumonitis due to solids and liquids (aspiration pneumonia)

The codes in category 484 are in italics, which signifies that they are always secondary codes and the underlying disease is coded first. More often, the underlying organism is not identified or not known at the time of coding. Without further specification, pneumonia is reported with code 486, Pneumonia, organism unspecified.

Viral Pneumonia

Viral pneumonia (category 480) is subdivided to fourth-digit subcategories that identify the specific virus. It is a highly contagious disease affecting both the trachea and the bronchi of the lungs. Inflammation destroys the action of the cilia and causes hemorrhage. Isolation of the virus is difficult, and x-rays do not reveal any pulmonary changes.

Pneumococcal Pneumonia

Pneumococcal pneumonia [Streptococcus pneumoniae pneumonia] (category 481) describes pneumonia caused by the pneumococcal bacteria. The bacteria lodge in the alveoli and cause an inflammation. When the pleura are involved, the irritated surfaces rub together and cause painful breathing. On examination, pleural friction can be heard. A chest x-ray demonstrates a consolidation of the lungs that results from pus forming in the alveoli and replacing the air. Approximately 90 percent of lobar pneumonia is due to pneumococcal bacteria.

Other Bacterial Pneumonia

Other bacterial pneumonia (category 482) is subdivided to fourth-digit subcategories that identify specific bacteria such as Klebsiella pneumoniae (482.0), Pseudomonas (482.1), Hemophilus influenzae (482.2), Streptococcus (482.3x), and Staphylococcus (482.4x). Bacteria are the most common cause of pneumonia in adults. Gram staining is a rapid and cost-effective method for diagnosing bacterial pneumonia, when a good sputum sample is available.

Pneumonia Due to Other Specified Organism

Codes for pneumonia due to other specified organism are included in category 483. Among the conditions in this category are Mycoplasma pneumoniae (483.0) and pneumonia due to Chlamydia (483.1). Code 483.8, Other specified organism, is used when the organism cannot be classified elsewhere.

Pneumonia in Infectious Diseases Classified Elsewhere

Pneumonia in infectious diseases classified elsewhere (category 484) is subdivided to fourth-digit subcategories that identify the specific infectious disease. These codes are set in italic type and thus are not meant for primary tabulation. In addition, instructional notations in this category direct coders to assign an additional code to describe the underlying disease.

Bronchopneumonia, Organism Unspecified

Category 485, Bronchopneumonia, organism unspecified, is a three-digit code that describes the site of the pneumonia. Bronchopneumonia usually begins in the terminal bronchioles of the lung and causes the air space to become filled with exudates.

Pneumonia, Organism Unspecified

Category 486, Pneumonia, organism unspecified, is a three-digit code that should be assigned only when the health record does not identify the causative organism.

Pneumonitis Due to Solids and Liquids

Category 507, Pneumonitis due to solids and liquids, is subdivided to fourth-digit subcategories that describe the causative agent. This category also is referred to as aspiration pneumonia. When the causative agent is unspecified, the Alphabetic Index to Diseases offers direction to code 507.0. In cases where the patient develops both aspiration pneumonia and bacterial pneumonia, codes for both types of pneumonia should be assigned.

Sinusitis

Sinusitis is inflammation of a sinus, particularly the paranasal sinuses (maxillary, frontal, ethmoidal, or sphenoidal). Acute sinusitis is an acute inflammation of the air-filled sinuses that contributes to blockage of the sinus openings and obstruction of their ventilation and drainage. ICD-9-CM classifies acute sinusitis to category 461, with the fourth digits identifying the specific sinus affected. When the diagnosis indicates acute pansinusitis (all sinuses), code 461.8 is reported. Chronic sinusitis is a chronic inflammation of the paranasal sinuses following persistent bacterial infection. ICD-9-CM classifies chronic sinusitis to category 473, with the fourth digits identifying the specific sinus affected. When the diagnosis indicates chronic pansinusitis (all sinuses), code 473.8 is reported.

Diseases of the Tonsils and Adenoids

Tonsillitis is inflammation of the tonsils and may be classified as acute or chronic. Acute tonsillitis is characterized by sore throat, fever, chills, swollen and tender submandibular lymph glands, inflamed tonsils, malaise, pain referred to ears, and purulent drainage from the tonsillar pillars. ICD-9-CM classifies acute tonsillitis to code 463. Chronic tonsillitis is characterized by recurrent attacks of acute tonsillitis, recurrent colds, unexplained fever, loss of appetite, tiredness, and a scarred, fissured appearance on the tonsillar surface. Treatment includes antibiotic therapy and tonsillectomy. ICD-9-CM classifies chronic tonsillitis to subcategory 474.0, which is further subdivided to identify involvement of adenoids (474.02). When the diagnosis is identified as hypertrophy of the tonsils and/or adenoids, the following codes are available:

- 474.10, Hypertrophy of tonsils with adenoids
- 474.11, Hypertrophy of tonsils only
- 474.12, Hypertrophy of adenoids only

Asthma

Asthma is characterized by difficult and labored breathing with coughing and wheezing due to spasmodic contraction of the bronchi and/or inflammation of the mucous membrane lining of the bronchi. In some cases, it is an allergic manifestation in sensitized persons. The term *reactive airway disease* is considered synonymous with asthma.

Fourth-Digit Subcategories

ICD-9-CM classifies asthma to category 493, with the following subcategories that describe the specific types:

493.0   Extrinsic asthma (an asthmatic condition caused by environmental allergen factors)

493.1   Intrinsic asthma (a form of asthma caused by the body's own immunological response)

493.2   Chronic obstructive asthma and chronic asthmatic bronchitis (a chronic form of asthma coexisting with chronic obstructive pulmonary disease [COPD])

493.9   Asthma, unspecified (the subcategory used when the documentation does not specify one of the types listed above)

Fifth-Digit Subclassification

The fifth-digit subclassification of category 493 describes whether the patient was in status asthmaticus or presents with acute exacerbation. Status asthmaticus is an acute asthmatic attack in which the degree of bronchial obstruction is not relieved by usual treatments such as epinephrine or aminophylline. Other terms that may be used to describe status asthmaticus include intractable asthmatic attack, refractory asthma, severe prolonged asthmatic attack, airway obstruction not relieved by bronchodilators, and severe intractable wheezing.

The fifth digits for use with codes 493.0–493.2, 493.9 are:

0   unspecified
1   with status asthmaticus
2   with (acute) exacerbation

Code 493.8, Other forms of asthma, has the following fifth digits:

493.81   Exercise induced bronchospasm
493.82   Cough variant asthma

Keep in mind that documentation in the health record must support the use of the fifth digits 1 and 2. In the outpatient setting, especially the physician's office, the more appropriate fifth digit is 0, without mention of status asthmaticus.

Upper and Lower Respiratory Infections

Upper respiratory infection (URI) is the sudden, severe onset of inflammation of an undetermined site in the airway tract above the bronchi. Without further specification, URI is reported with code 465.9. Lower respiratory infection (LRI) requires identification of the specific disease and site, such as bronchitis, in order to assign the appropriate ICD-9-CM code. Without further specification, LRI is reported with 519.8.

Pleural Effusion

Pleural effusion is inflammation of the visceral and parietal layers of the pleural cavity. Pain develops when the visceral layer lining the lungs expands with breathing and moves over and irritates the inflamed sensory nerve endings in the fixed parietal layer lining the thoracic cavity. Common causes of pleural effusion include: pneumonia, tuberculosis, pneumothorax, viral infection, pulmonary embolism, malignant process, lung abscess, systemic lupus erythematosus, bronchiectasis, rheumatoid arthritis, and pulmonary infarction. ICD-9-CM classifies pleural effusion, or pleurisy, to category 511, with the fourth digits identifying associated conditions. Without further specification, pleural effusion is reported with code 511.9.

Malignant pleural effusion is considered metastatic and is reported with code 197.2 from the neoplasm chapter of the ICD-9-CM codebook. Pleural effusion described as traumatic is reported with codes 860.2–860.5, 862.29, or 862.39, as indicated by the excludes note under code 511.8.

Pneumothorax

Pneumothorax is the abnormal accumulation of air or gas in the space separating the visceral and parietal pleural layers. There are several types of pneumothorax, including spontaneous, iatrogenic, or traumatic. Spontaneous tension pneumothorax is characterized by the ability of air to enter the pleural space, but the inability for it to escape. Iatrogenic pneumothorax, also known as postoperative pneumothorax, occurs as a result of surgical treatment. Traumatic pneumothorax occurs as a result of trauma and may involve either an open or closed chest wound. ICD-9-CM classifies pneumothorax to category 512, which is further subdivided to specify the type, such as iatrogenic (512.1) or tension (512.0). Without further specification, pneumothorax is reported with code 512.8, Other spontaneous pneumothorax. Traumatic pneumothorax is reported with a code from category 860, depending on the extent of the injury.

Respiratory Failure and Insufficiency

Respiratory failure is the inability of the respiratory system to supply adequate oxygen to maintain proper metabolism and/or to eliminate carbon dioxide. Respiratory failure is assigned to a patient with normal lung tissue, a PO_2 below 50 mm Hg, and a PCO_2 above 50 mm Hg. However, these parameters do not apply to patients with chronic obstructive pulmonary disease who often have values that are higher or lower. Respiratory failure is classified into three categories:

- 518.81, Acute respiratory failure

- 518.83, Chronic respiratory failure

- 518.84, Acute and chronic respiratory failure

Respiratory failure is assigned when documentation in the health record supports its use. It may be due to, or associated with, other respiratory conditions such as pneumonia, chronic bronchitis, or COPD. Respiratory failure also may be due to, or associated with, nonrespiratory conditions such as myasthenia gravis, CHF, MI, or CVA.

Arterial blood gases may be useful in diagnosing respiratory failure; however, normal values may vary from person to person depending on individual health status (*Coding Clinic,* 2nd Quarter 1990).

Code 518.82, Other pulmonary insufficiency, not elsewhere classified, includes conditions described as:

- Acute respiratory distress

- Acute respiratory insufficiency

- Adult respiratory distress syndrome, not elsewhere classified

Pulmonary Edema

Pulmonary edema is an abnormal, diffuse accumulation of fluid in the tissues and alveolar spaces of the lung that is characterized clinically by dyspnea and, when severe, by cyanosis. For classification purposes, pulmonary edema can be described as acute pulmonary edema of cardiac origin, acute pulmonary edema of noncardiac origin, or chronic pulmonary edema.

Acute Pulmonary Edema of Cardiac Origin

Because this condition is a manifestation of heart failure, use subcategory codes 428.0–428.4x. Documentation in the health record of a patient with acute pulmonary edema of cardiogenic origin usually references cardiac enlargement, presence of S-3 gallop, elevated pulmonary artery wedge pressure, or associated cardiac diseases. Frequently, the chest x-ray will show pleural effusions. Treatment often includes diuretics and other cardiac medications.

Acute Pulmonary Edema of Noncardiac Origin

Other forms of acute pulmonary edema that are noncardiogenic in origin are classified to diseases of the lung or to trauma. Some examples are:

- Postoperative pulmonary edema due to fluid overload (518.4 and 276.6)

- Radiation pneumonitis with acute pulmonary edema (508.0)

- Acute pulmonary edema due to pneumonia (486 and 518.4)

Chronic Pulmonary Edema

Chronic pulmonary edema or pulmonary edema NOS that is not of cardiogenic origin is coded to 514, Pulmonary congestion and hypostasis. But the health record and/or the physician should be consulted for further information to ensure that the pulmonary edema was not actually the *acute* type.

Candidiasis

Candida is a yeast that reproduces by budding. Candida species number in the hundreds, but Candida albicans is one of the most prevalent. The most common clinical manifestation of candidal overgrowth is oropharyngeal infection, or thrush. Because candida are part of the normal flora of the oropharynx, the isolation of candida from sputum occurs, especially in patients with pneumonia who are receiving antibiotics. To establish a diagnosis of candidal pneumonia (112.4), documentation of pulmonary tissue invasion is required. This confirmation of diagnosis requires a transbronchial or open-lung biopsy.

Tuberculosis

Pulmonary tuberculosis (TB) is an infectious disease caused by the microorganism Mycobacterium tuberculosis. Individuals particularly susceptible to TB are those with poor nutrition or substandard, close living conditions; patients with silicosis, cancer (especially bronchogenic carcinoma), diabetes mellitus, or HIV coinfection; and persons receiving immunosuppressive corticosteroids or cytotoxic drugs. Chest x-rays show dense infiltrates in a lower or midlung field with large massive hilar or mediastinal lymphadenopathy in primary TB. Chest x-rays in chronic pulmonary TB show atypical calcified lesions in the region of the clavicle, often referred to as Simon's foci. Symptoms of TB include fever, night sweats, weight loss, dyspnea, cough, and hemoptysis.

Extrapulmonary TB occurs in persons who have no tuberculosis immunity. It can infect the meninges, pericardium, kidney, and lymph nodes. Treatment of TB consists of bacterial drugs such as rifampin and isoniazid (isonicotinic acid hydrazide [INH]) combined with streptomycin, pyrazinamide, and ethambutol.

Alkalosis versus Acidosis

Assessments of arterial blood gas results (ABGs) are performed to determine whether respiratory acidosis or alkalosis or metabolic acidosis or alkalosis has developed. Key components of ABGs, which are interpreted by the clinician, are the oxygen level (pO_2), the acid-base balance (pH), the buffer level of bicarbonate ions (HCO_3), and the oxyhemoglobin saturation (O_2) in the blood. The following are normal values for these key components:

pO_2	=	80–100 mm Hg
pCO_2	=	35–45 mm Hg
pH	=	7.35–7.45
HCO_3	=	22–27 mEq/L
O_2	=	96%–100%

The traditional method of interpreting the acid-base status of ABGs uses the terminology "uncompensated," "partially compensated," and "compensated," along with the normal ranges for pCO_2 and pH. Table 12.1 displays the values for pH, pCO_2, and HCO_3 for both respiratory acidosis and alkalosis and metabolic acidosis and alkalosis.

Causes of respiratory acidosis or primary hypercapnia (increase in CO_2) include:

- Cardiopulmonary disease (specifically asthma with status asthmaticus)

- Severe bilateral pneumonia or bronchopneumonia

- Severe pulmonary edema

- COPD (bronchitis, bronchiectasis, bronchiolitis, emphysema)

Table 12.1.   Values for acidosis and alkalosis

Status	pH	pCO$_2$	HCO$_2$
Respiratory Acidosis			
Uncompensated	<7.35	>45	normal
Partially compensated	<7.35	>45	>27
Compensated	7.35–7.45	>45	>27
Respiratory Alkalosis			
Uncompensated	>7.45	<35	normal
Partially compensated	>7.45	<35	<22
Compensated	7.40–7.45	<35	<22
Metabolic Acidosis			
Uncompensated	<7.35	normal	<22
Partially compensated	<7.35	<35	<22
Compensated	7.35–7.40	<35	<22
Metabolic Alkalosis			
Uncompensated	>7.45	normal	>27
Partially compensated*	>7.45	>45	>27
Compensated*	7.40–7.45	>45	>27

*Partially compensated and compensated metabolic alkalosis occur infrequently because of the body's mechanism to prevent hypoventilation.

- Interstitial fibrosis

- Severe chronic pneumonitis

- Central nervous system depression by drugs, trauma, or lesion

- Neurologic or neuromuscular disease resulting in weakness of respiratory muscles

- Fatigue following any acute lung disease

Clinical manifestations of respiratory acidosis include irritability, headache, mental cloudiness, apathy, confusion, incoherence, combativeness, hallucinations, and cardiac arrhythmias.

Causes of respiratory alkalosis or primary hypocapnia (reduction in CO$_2$) include:

- Compensation for primary metabolic acidosis

- Pneumonia

- Pulmonary edema

- Asthma

- Pneumothorax

- Pulmonary fibrosis

- Drugs such as Doxapram, salicylates, and progesterone

- Nicotinic hepatic failure

- Septicemia

Symptoms of respiratory alkalosis include lightheadedness and confusion.

Primary causes of metabolic acidosis are ketoacidosis, renal failure, and ingestion of base-depleting drugs such as alcohol and aspirin. Causes of metabolic alkalosis are hypokalemia, gastric vomiting or suctioning, massive doses of steroids, and diuretics.

The following ICD-9-CM codes are for classifying these conditions:

276.2   Respiratory acidosis
276.3   Respiratory alkalosis
276.2   Metabolic acidosis
276.3   Metabolic alkalosis
276.4   Mixed acid-base balance disorder

V Codes

Code V12.61 is used to report personal history of recurrent pneumonia. Code V15.87 is used to show a history of extracorporeal membrane oxygenation (ECMO). Code V46.1 is used to demonstrate dependence on a respirator or ventilator. Fifth digits describe circumstances unique to patients who are dependent on a respirator:

V46.11   Dependence on respirator, status
V46.12   Encounter for respiratory dependence during power failure
V46.13   Encounter for weaning from respirator
V46.14   Mechanical complication of respirator

Code V46.2 can be used to show the patient's dependence on supplemental or long-term oxygen.

Chapter 12 Exercises

Review the following statements and cases and assign the appropriate codes:

1. Obstructive chronic bronchitis

   ____

2. Chronic maxillary sinusitis

   ____

3. Asthma with status asthmaticus

   ____

4. COPD

   ____

5. Pneumococcal pleural effusion

   ____

6. Acute upper respiratory infection with flu

   ____

7. Chronic respiratory failure

   ____

8. Adult respiratory distress syndrome

   ____

9. Streptococcal group B pneumonia

   ____

10. Staphylococcal bronchopneumonia

    ____

11. Allergic pneumonitis

    ____

12. Pneumonia in cytomegalic inclusion disease

    ____

13. Respiratory failure due to acute exacerbation of myasthenia gravis

    ____

14. Acute and chronic respiratory failure with COPD

    ____

15. Pneumococcal pneumonia due to HIV infection/AIDS

    ____

Chapter 12 Exercises (Continued)

16. Pansinusitis with hypertrophy of nasal turbinates

---

17. An 84-year-old female was transferred from the nursing home on the day of admission. She has had a persistent left upper lobe pneumonia and has received oral antibiotics for the past two weeks. The patient has become increasingly dehydrated with a persistent productive cough, which is the reason she has been admitted today. Her past medical history is also significant for chronic atrial fibrillation. A review of the chest x-rays demonstrates a fairly stable left upper lobe infiltrate with no pleural effusion. The patient seemed to improve on intravenous fluids and IV antibiotics. She is now afebrile with clearing of the pneumonia, so she is being discharged.

Discharge diagnoses: Left upper lobe pneumonia; dehydration; chronic atrial fibrillation

Code(s):

---

18. This patient, a 78-year-old male, was seen in emergency services because of acute respiratory failure. He also has a long history of chronic bronchitis. He was in his usual state of health until 7 to 10 days prior to admission, when he developed the acute onset of fever, wheezing, and shortness of breath. The patient had been started on broad-spectrum antibiotics prior to admission but did not respond. After being admitted, he was started on nebulizer breathing treatments and IV Solu-Medrol and Prednisone, and his condition improved. His lungs showed poor air entry. In addition, he was hypertensive.

Discharge diagnoses: Acute respiratory failure due to an acute exacerbation of chronic obstructive bronchitis; hypertension

Code(s):

---

19. A 67-year-old female presented to emergency services with a gradual increase in shortness of breath that was unresponsive to her home nebulizer treatments. In emergency services, she received more respiratory treatments but failed to clear and was therefore admitted to the hospital. A chest x-ray showed no evidence of active infiltrates. After being admitted, the patient received IV steroids and frequent respiratory therapy treatments. She gradually cleared and was discharged on Aminophylline by mouth and Ventolin treatments, and her Prednisone was reduced to 10 mg.

Discharge diagnoses: Status asthmaticus; chronic obstructive pulmonary disease

Code(s):

Review Questions

Answer the following questions:

1. For coding purposes, how is pneumonia classified?

2. What code(s) would be assigned to a patient who develops both aspiration pneumonia and bacterial pneumonia?

3. In the coding of both acute and chronic sinusitis, what do the fourth digits indicate?

4. What is a synonymous term for asthma?

5. What other terms in a health record can be used to describe status asthmaticus?

6. Respiratory failure may be due to, or associated with, what nonrespiratory conditions?

Chapter 13

Diseases of the Digestive System

Objectives

After completing this lesson, the student should be able to do the following:

- Apply knowledge of current, approved ICD-9-CM coding guidelines to assign and sequence accurate codes related to diseases of the digestive system

- Identify the major types of digestive disorders

- Discuss the categories that classify cholecystitis and cholelithiasis

Introduction

Chapter 14 of the ICD-9-CM codebook classifies diseases of the digestive system, including angiodysplasia, cholelithiasis, hernia, hepatitis, gastritis, and ulcer. The chapter is divided into the following sections:

Categories	Section Titles
520–529	Diseases of Oral Cavity, Salivary Glands, and Jaws
530–537	Diseases of Esophagus, Stomach, and Duodenum
540–543	Appendicitis
550–553	Hernia of Abdominal Cavity
555–558	Noninfectious Enteritis and Colitis
560–569	Other Diseases of Intestines and Peritoneum
570–579	Other Diseases of Digestive System

The diseases described in chapter 14 are treated primarily by gastroenterologists, internists, and proctologists. Many of the codes in this chapter include fourth and fifth digits to identify the severity (acute versus chronic) and the presence of hemorrhage and obstruction.

EXAMPLE:	531.01	Acute gastric ulcer with obstruction and hemorrhage
	533.50	Chronic or unspecified peptic ulcer with perforation without mention of obstruction
	535.31	Alcoholic gastritis with hemorrhage

Esophagitis

Esophagitis is an inflammation of the esophageal lining. Underlying causes include:

- Infection

- Irritation from a nasogastric (NG) tube

- Backflow of gastric juice from the stomach (most common cause)

ICD-9-CM classifies esophagitis to subcategory 530.1, with a fifth digit to describe the specific type. The codebook reminds coders to assign an additional code to identify the cause of the condition when induced by a chemical or drug (E code). Subcategory code 530.2, Ulcer of esophagus, has been expanded to include the following codes:

530.20	Ulcer of esophagus without bleeding
530.21	Ulcer of esophagus with bleeding

> *Excludes:* bleeding esophageal varices (456.0, 456.20)

Code 530.85 identifies Barrett's esophagus.

Mechanical Complications of Esophagostomy

Complications of esophagostomy are identified using codes 530.86, Infection of esophagostomy, and 530.87, Mechanical complication of esophagostomy.

Gastrointestinal Ulcers

Ulcers of the gastrointestinal tract are characterized by an inflammatory, necrotic, sloughing defect. ICD-9-CM classifies these ulcers to categories 531–534, which further subdivide to indicate severity (acute versus chronic) and associated complications, such as hemorrhage, perforation, and obstruction. The categories classifying gastrointestinal ulcers include:

- 531, Gastric ulcer

- 532, Duodenal ulcer

- 533, Peptic ulcer, site unspecified

- 534, Gastrojejunal ulcer

Diverticular Disease

A diverticulum of the intestine is a mucosal pouch, or sac, that herniates through a defect in the muscular layer of the intestinal wall. ICD-9-CM classifies diverticula to category 562, with a fourth digit to identify the specific site and a fifth digit to indicate the presence or absence of hemorrhage and the progression of the disease (diverticulosis versus diverticulitis). Diverticulosis is the presence of diverticula in the intestines, especially in the colon. It also results from herniation of the mucosa through defects in the muscular wall, usually at the site of blood vessel entry. Diverticulitis is the inflammation and infection of a diverticulum.

Appendicitis

Acute appendicitis (category 540) is inflammation of the appendix with the onset being sudden and severe. It is the most common disease requiring major surgery and may occur at any age, affecting both sexes equally. Appendicitis begins with generalized or localized abdominal pain in the upper right abdomen, followed by anorexia, nausea, and vomiting. The pain eventually localizes in the lower right abdomen with abdominal boardlike rigidity, retractive respirations, increasing tenderness, and increasingly severe abdominal spasm. Appendectomy is the only effective treatment.

ICD-9-CM classifies appendicitis with generalized peritonitis to code 540.0. This code is reported when the appendicitis is further described as fulminating, gangrenous, obstructive, ruptured, with perforation, or peritonitis. Appendicitis with peritoneal abscess is reported with code 540.1.

Appendicitis, unqualified, is coded to 541. Appendicitis described as chronic, recurrent, relapsing, or subacute is coded to 542, Other appendicitis.

Hernias

Hernias of the abdominal cavity are classified to categories 550–553. Category 550, Inguinal hernia, further subdivides to identify severity, with a fifth digit to identify the hernia as unilateral or bilateral and/or recurrent. Categories 551–553 identify abdominal hernias with varying degrees of severity. Hernias described as strangulated or incarcerated are classified as obstructed.

> **EXAMPLE:** 550.91 Inguinal hernia, without mention of obstruction or gangrene, unilateral, or unspecified, recurrent

Diaphragmatic hernia, also known as hiatal hernia (553.3), is a defect in the diaphragm that permits a portion of the stomach to pass through the diaphragmatic opening into the chest. Code 553.3 excludes congenital conditions. When a diaphragmatic hernia or a hiatal hernia is designated as congenital, codes 756.6 and 750.6, respectively, are assigned.

Enteritis and Gastroenteritis

Regional enteritis, also known as Crohn's disease or granulomatous enteritis, is a chronic inflammatory disease commonly affecting the distal ileum and colon. It is characterized by chronic diarrhea, abdominal pain, fever, anorexia, weight loss, right lower quadrant mass or fullness, and lymphadenitis of the mesenteric nodes. ICD-9-CM classifies regional enteritis to category 555, with the fourth digit identifying the specific site affected (for example, the large intestine). Without further specification as to site, code 555.9 should be assigned.

Gastroenteritis is an inflammation of the stomach, small intestine, and/or colon. It is characterized by diarrhea, nausea and vomiting, and abdominal cramps. Gastroenteritis can be caused by bacteria, amoebae, parasites, viruses, ingestion of toxins, drug reactions, enzyme deficiencies, or food allergens. ICD-9-CM classifies gastroenteritis according to the cause:

- 003.0, Salmonella gastroenteritis

- 005.9, Food poisoning, unspecified

- 008.8, Viral gastroenteritis, NEC

- 009.0, Infectious gastroenteritis

- 556.9, Ulcerative colitis, unspecified

- 558.3, Allergic gastroenteritis and colitis

- 558.9, Other and unspecified noninfectious gastroenteritis and colitis

Note that gastroenteritis due to an infectious process is classified to chapter 1 of the ICD-9-CM codebook, Infectious and Parasitic Diseases.

Gastritis and Duodenitis

Gastritis is inflammation of the gastric mucosa and may be described as acute or chronic. ICD-9-CM classifies gastritis to category 535, which further subdivides at the fourth-digit level to identify the underlying cause or specific type, with the fifth digit indicating the presence or absence of hemorrhage. The subcategories include:

- 535.0x, Acute gastritis
- 535.1x, Atrophic gastritis
- 535.2x, Gastric mucosal hypertrophy
- 535.3x, Alcoholic gastritis
- 535.4x, Other specified gastritis
- 535.5x, Unspecified gastritis and gastroduodenitis
- 535.6x, Duodenitis

Ostomy Complications

A colostomy is a surgically created opening (stoma) between the colon and the abdominal wall. An enterostomy is a surgically created opening (stoma) between other parts of the intestines and the abdominal wall. Complications of a colostomy or enterostomy are classified to subcategory 569.6, which is further subdivided as follows:

- 569.60, Colostomy and enterostomy complication, unspecified
- 569.61, Infection of colostomy or enterostomy
- 569.62, Mechanical complication of colostomy and enterostomy
- 569.69, Other complication

When reporting code 569.61, Infection of colostomy or enterostomy, the coder also should assign a code to identify the underlying organism, such as Staphylococcus aureus. An additional code should be used to specify the type of infection, such as septicemia.

Anal Fissure and Fistula

An anal fistula is an opening at or near the anus, usually (but not always) into the rectum above the internal sphincter. An anal fissure is a crack or slit in the mucous membrane of the anus. Fissures are very painful and difficult to heal. ICD-9-CM classifies these conditions to category 565:

- 565.0, Anal fissure
- 565.1, Anal fistula

Liver Cirrhosis

Cirrhosis of the liver, a long-term condition characterized by a fiberlike tissue covering the liver, results in a breakdown of the liver tissue and subsequent replacement by fat. ICD-9-CM classifies liver cirrhosis to category 571, which further subdivides to identify specific types of liver conditions, including types of liver cirrhosis. Careful review of the health record is necessary to identify the severity of the disease (acute versus chronic) and the underlying cause (for example, alcohol consumption). Several types of cirrhosis exist, including:

- 571.5, Cryptogenic
- 571.5, Macronodular or micronodular
- 571.5, Posthepatic
- 571.5, Postnecrotic
- 571.5, Portal
- 571.2, Alcoholic (most common)
- 571.6, Biliary

Hemorrhage of Digestive Tract

Gastrointestinal (GI) hemorrhage is the abnormal escape of blood from the GI tract. Some common causes of upper GI bleeding include duodenal ulcer, gastric or duodenal erosions, varices, and gastric ulcer. Common causes of lower GI bleeding include diverticular disease, carcinoma of the colon, colon polyps, inflammatory bowel disease (ulcerative colitis, Crohn's disease), and angiodysplasia. The presentation of GI bleeding can vary from that of occult bleeding to acute hemorrhage. Upper GI bleeding may be identified when the patient vomits bright red blood or by analysis of gastric fluid obtained through a nasogastric tube. Lower GI bleeding may be identified by asymptomatic passage of maroon-colored stool or bright red blood. The bleeding may be brisk and intermittent over several days. ICD-9-CM classifies gastrointestinal hemorrhage to category 578, which further subdivides to identify the specific site of the bleeding, as follows:

- 578.0, Hematemesis (vomiting of blood)
- 578.1, Melena (bloody stool)
- 578.9, Unspecified gastrointestinal hemorrhage

A positive occult blood test without further specification as to cause is reported with code 792.1.

Rectal and anal hemorrhage is the abnormal escape of blood from the rectal and/or anal canal. ICD-9-CM classifies this type of hemorrhage to code 569.3. The exclusion note under code 569.3 reminds the coder that when the hemorrhage is specified as gastrointestinal, a code from category 578 should be assigned.

Peritonitis and Retroperitoneal Infections

Code 567, Peritonitis and retroperitoneal infections, is often used with other digestive system codes. Fourth digits differentiate among peritonitis in infectious diseases classified elsewhere

(567.0), Pneumococcal peritonitis (567.1), other suppurative peritonitis (567.2), retroperitoneal infections (567.3), other specified peritonitis (567.8), and unspecified peritonitis (567.9).

Subcategory codes 567.2, 567.3, and 567.8 are further divided into fifth-digit subcategory codes to provide increased specificity.

Cholecystitis and Cholelithiasis

Cholecystitis is an acute or chronic inflammation of the gallbladder. Cholelithiasis refers to gallstones in the gallbladder.

Two categories are available to classify cholecystitis and cholelithiasis:

- 574, Cholelithiasis

- 575, Other disorders of gallbladder

Category 574 is divided into the following four-digit subcategories to describe the existence of calculus or stones with acute or chronic cholecystitis:

574.0   Calculus of gallbladder with acute cholecystitis
574.1   Calculus of gallbladder with other cholecystitis
574.2   Calculus of gallbladder without mention of cholecystitis
574.3   Calculus of bile duct with acute cholecystitis
574.4   Calculus of bile duct with other cholecystitis
574.5   Calculus of bile duct without mention of cholecystitis
574.6   Calculus of gallbladder and bile duct with acute cholecystitis
574.7   Calculus of gallbladder and bile duct with other cholecystitis
574.8   Calculus of gallbladder and bile duct with acute and chronic cholecystitis
574.9   Calculus of gallbladder and bile duct without cholecystitis

In category 574, the fifth-digit subclassification describes the presence or absence of obstruction.

Category 575 contains the following two codes relating to cholecystitis:

575.0   Acute cholecystitis
575.1   Other cholecystitis

In subcategory 575.1, the fifth-digit subclassification indicates severity:

575.10   Cholecystitis, unspecified
575.11   Chronic cholecystitis
575.12   Acute and chronic cholecystitis

Chapter 13 Exercises

Review the following statements and cases and assign the appropriate codes:

1. Reflux esophagitis

2. Hemorrhagic alcoholic gastritis

   535.31

3. Diverticulosis of colon with bleeding

   550.03

4. Bilateral recurrent inguinal hernia with gangrene

5. Hiatal hernia

   555.2

6. Crohn's disease of the small and large intestines

   555.0   555.1

7. Acute gastroenteritis

8. Colostomy infection

   569.61

9. Alcoholic cirrhosis of liver

10. Chronic pancreatitis

    577.1

11. Blood in stool

12. Acute perforated peptic ulcer

    533.10

13. Acute appendicitis with perforation and peritoneal abscess

14. Acute cholecystitis with cholelithiasis

    574.00

15. Diverticulosis and diverticulitis of colon

Chapter 13 Exercises (Continued)

16. An elderly man came into Dr. Smith's office complaining of severe epigastric <u>pain</u>. He had experienced <u>some nausea, but no vomiting</u>. Dr. Smith decided to perform studies to rule out cholecystitis and ulcer perforation.

    Impression: Possible cholecystitis and/or perforated stomach ulcer

    Code(s): _789.06_ , _575.10_ , _531.50_

17. A 78-year-old woman was admitted to the hospital because of severe rectal bleeding. Because her hemoglobin count was so low, she also received three transfusions of whole blood. A colonoscopy was done and several ulcers of the rectum were found that later proved to be ulcerative proctitis.

    Discharge diagnoses: Rectal bleeding; acute blood loss anemia; ulcerative proctitis

    Code(s): _______________

18. A 25-year-old female patient came to emergency services with complaints of "yellow" eyes, very dark urine, and arm and shoulder pain. The following tests were done with indicated results: (a) liver function tests showed <u>profound jaundice</u>; (b) ultrasound of gallbladder revealed <u>no gallstones</u>; (c) blood work done was felt to be indicative of <u>sickle-cell anemia</u>. In consideration of these findings, along with the fact that her liver function continued to improve, it was felt that she should be monitored for <u>possible acute hepatitis B</u>.

    Discharge diagnosis: Jaundice due to sickle-cell anemia vs. possible acute hepatitis B

    Code(s): _782.4_ _282.60_ , _070.30_

Review Questions

Answer the following questions:

1. What code is assigned for appendicitis that is further described as "fulminating, gangrenous, obstructive, or with perforation"?

2. What is a synonymous term for diaphragmatic hernia?

3. What are some common causes of upper gastrointestinal bleeding?

4. How would a positive occult blood test be coded?

5. What do the fourth digits under category 574, Cholelithiasis, specify?

6. How are complications of a colostomy or enterostomy coded?

1. 540.0

2. Hiatal Hernia

3. Duodenal ulcer, gastric erosions, varices gastric ulcer

4. 578.1

5. Existance of calculus

6. 569.62

Chapter 14

Diseases of the Genitourinary System

Objectives

After completing this lesson, the student should be able to do the following:

- Apply knowledge of current, approved ICD-9-CM coding guidelines to assign and sequence accurate codes related to diseases of the genitourinary system
- Discuss the major disorders of the genitourinary system
- Identify documentation in the health record that may signify renal failure
- Understand the major gynecologic disorders

Introduction

Chapter 10 of the ICD-9-CM codebook includes the following sections:

Categories	Section Titles
580–589	Nephritis, Nephrotic Syndrome, and Nephrosis
590–599	Other Diseases of Urinary System
600–608	Diseases of Male Genital Organs
610–611	Disorders of Breast
614–616	Inflammatory Disease of Female Pelvic Organs
617–629	Other Disorders of Female Genital Tract

These conditions are most often treated by urologists, gynecologists, and general surgeons.

Nephritis, Nephrosis, and Nephrotic Syndrome

Categories 580–589 include codes for nephritis, nephrosis, and nephrotic syndrome. The codes further subdivide to identify the specific disease and the severity (acute versus chronic).

> **EXAMPLE:** 584.6   Acute renal failure with lesion of renal cortical necrosis
> 585   Chronic kidney disease (CKD)
> 586   Renal failure, unspecified

Chronic Kidney Disease

Chronic kidney disease (CKD) is usually the result of a gradually progressive loss of renal function. Its causes include chronic glomerular diseases, chronic infections, congenital anomalies, vascular diseases, obstructive processes, collagen diseases, nephrotic agents, and endocrine diseases. CKD produces major changes in all body systems, resulting in a multitude of complications, including anemia, cardiomyopathy, brittle fingernails, pulmonary edema, increased susceptibility to respiratory infections, metabolic acidosis, and fluid overload. Hemodialysis or peritoneal dialysis can help to control some of the manifestations of end-stage renal disease (ESRD).

ICD-9-CM classifies chronic kidney disease to category 585. Fourth-digit subcategory codes identify the stage of the disease:

585.1   Chronic kidney disease, Stage I
585.2   Chronic kidney disease, Stage II (mild)
585.3   Chronic kidney disease, Stage III (moderate)
585.4   Chronic kidney disease, Stage IV (severe)
585.5   Stage V chronic kidney disease
585.6   End stage renal disease
585.9   Chronic kidney disease, unspecified

Additional codes should be reported to identify any associated manifestations and kidney transplant status. Acute renal disease and acute renal insufficiency are both assigned code 593.9.

> **EXAMPLE:** End-stage renal disease with anemia and congestive heart failure:
> 585.6, ESRD; 285.21, Anemia in end-stage renal disease; 428.0, Congestive heart failure, unspecified

Documentation that may signify renal failure in the health record includes:

- Significantly elevated values of serum creatinine or BUN, or diminished creatinine clearance
- Specific clinical and laboratory findings such as anemia, hyperphosphatemia, hypo-calcemia, hyperkalemia, acidemia, renal osteodystrophy, and uremic symptoms, including nausea, vomiting, itching, hemorrhagic conditions, hypertension, edema, dyspnea, lethargy, and coma

However, the coder needs more than an abnormal lab finding to add an additional diagnosis. Remember to always query the physician regarding the specific diagnosis being treated when it is not clearly documented.

Nephrotic Syndrome

Nephrotic syndrome is characterized by proteinuria, hypoalbuminemia, hyperlipidemia, and edema. It is not a disease itself but, rather, results from a specific glomerular disease that indicates renal damage. ICD-9-CM classifies nephrotic syndrome to category 581, which further subdivides to identify the specific type of lesion involved, such as membranous glomeru-lonephritis. In addition, code 581.81, Nephrotic syndrome in diseases classified elsewhere, is reported when nephrotic syndrome occurs secondary to another disease, such as diabetes mellitus. The underlying disease should be coded and sequenced first.

Renal insufficiency (593.9) refers to the early stages of renal impairment. It is usually diagnosed by mildly elevated values of serum creatinine or BUN or diminished creatinine clearance. Clinical symptoms or other abnormal laboratory parameters may or may not be present but are usually minimal. To a large extent, treatment depends on the underlying cause with the goal of preventing progression to renal failure.

Other Diseases of Urinary System

Categories 590–599 include codes for urinary tract infections. Other urinary symptoms are generally coded to category 788, Symptoms involving urinary system.

Urinary Tract Disorders

Urinary tract disorders include pyelonephritis, cystitis, calculus of urinary tract, vesicoureteral reflux, and urethral stricture.

Pyelonephritis

Pyelonephritis, also known as pyelitis, is a pus-forming infection of the kidney. Acute pyelonephritis (590.1x) is usually caused by an infection that moves upward from the lower urinary tract into the kidneys. Its symptoms include fever, chills, pain, nausea, and the frequent need to urinate. Urinalysis will reveal many bacteria and white blood cells, and antibiotic therapy is prescribed. Chronic pyelonephritis (590.0x) develops after a bacterial kidney infection. Most cases are linked to some form of blockage, such as a stone in the ureter. Treatment includes removal of the blockage and long-term use of antibiotics. Without further specification, pyelonephritis is reported with code 590.80. Code 590.81, Pyelitis or pyelonephritis in diseases classified elsewhere, is reported when the pyelonephritis occurs secondary to another disease, such as tuberculosis. The underlying disease should be coded and sequenced first.

Cystitis

Cystitis is inflammation of the urinary bladder and ureters. Symptoms include dysuria, suprapubic pain, lower back pain, hematuria, and the need and desire to urinate often. It may be caused by bacterial infection, a stone, or a tumor. Most common in women, this condition is often recurrent. Most cases are due to a vaginal infection that extends through the urethra to the bladder. Cystitis in men is due to urethral or prostatic infections or catheterizations. Depending on the diagnosis, treatment may include antibiotics, drinking more liquids, bed rest, drugs to control bladder spasms, and, when needed, surgery.

ICD-9-CM classifies cystitis to category 595, with the fourth-digit subcategories describing type, severity, and location. An instruction at the beginning of this category advises that an additional code from chapter 1 of the ICD-9-CM codebook, Infectious and Parasitic Diseases, should be assigned to identify the organism involved.

595.0	Acute cystitis
595.1	Chronic interstitial cystitis
595.2	Other chronic cystitis
595.3	Trigonitis
595.4	*Cystitis in diseases classified elsewhere*
595.8x	Other specified types of cystitis
595.9	Cystitis, unspecified

Without further specification, cystitis is reported with code 595.9.

Urinary tract infection without further specification as to site is reported with code 599.0. An additional code should be assigned when the underlying organism is identified. The coder should not arbitrarily add an additional diagnosis on the basis of an abnormal lab finding alone. The physician should always be queried when the specific diagnosis is not clearly stated in the health record.

> **EXAMPLE:** Urinary tract infection due to E. coli: 599.0, Urinary tract infection; 041.4, Escherichia coli

Calculus of Urinary Tract

Calculi of the urinary tract can occur in the kidney, ureter, urethra, or bladder. The renal pelvis or calyces of the kidneys are a common place of formation. Calculi can vary in size and may be solitary or multiple. They may remain in the renal pelvis or enter into the ureter. In some instances, calculi can cause obstruction, which may result in hydronephrosis. Calculi are classified to several different codes in ICD-9-CM, depending on the location of the calculus, as follows:

- 592.0, Calculus of kidney
- 592.1, Calculus of ureter
- 592.9, Urinary calculus, unspecified
- 594.0, Calculus in diverticulum of bladder
- 594.1, Other calculus in bladder
- 594.2, Calculus in urethra
- 594.8, Other lower urinary tract calculus
- 594.9, Calculus of lower urinary tract, unspecified

Vesicoureteral Reflux

Vesicoureteral reflux is a backflow of urine from the bladder into the ureter. It is characterized by abdominal or flank pain, persistent or recurrent urinary infection, dysuria (pain with voiding), and frequency or urgency of urination. Moreover, pyuria, hematuria, proteinuria, or bacteriuria may accompany vesicoureteral reflux. ICD-9-CM classifies vesicoureteral reflux to subcategory 593.7, with the fifth digit specifying the extent of involvement. Additional codes should be used to report chronic pyelonephritis, renal agenesis, or renal dysplasia.

Urethral Stricture

Urethral stricture is an abnormal narrowing of the urethra due to inflammation, scarring, or pressure from outside the body. ICD-9-CM classifies urethral stricture to category 598, which further subdivides to identify the underlying cause, such as infection or postoperative development. Additional codes may be assigned to indicate any urinary incontinence that may be due to, or a result of, urethral stricture. When the urethral stricture is specified as congenital, code 753.6, Atresia and stenosis of urethra and bladder neck, should be assigned.

Urinary Obstruction

Urinary obstruction is reported with code 599.6x. Urinary obstruction due to prostatic hyperplasia is reported using codes 600.0–600.9 with a fifth digit of 1.

Other Urinary Symptoms

Other urinary symptoms include hematuria, urinary retention, urinary dysuria, and urinary incontinence.

Hematuria

Hematuria, blood in the urine, can produce a red-to-brown discoloration depending on the amount of blood in the urine and the acidity of the urine. Slight hematuria may cause no discoloration and would only be detected by chemical testing or a microscopic examination. This condition may present with pain or may be painless. ICD-9-CM classifies hematuria to code 599.7.

Urinary Retention

Urinary retention is a buildup of urine in the bladder. Its causes may be related to loss of muscle tone in the bladder, nerve damage, a blocked urethra, or use of a narcotic painkiller, such as morphine. ICD-9-CM classifies urinary retention to category 788, which is located in chapter 16 of the ICD-9-CM codebook, Symptoms, Signs, and Ill-Defined Conditions. The category further subdivides to identify specific types of urine retention, including:

- 788.20, Retention of urine, unspecified
- 788.21, Incomplete bladder emptying
- 788.29, Other specified retention of urine

Urinary retention associated with prostatic hyperplasia is reported using codes 600.0–600.9 with a fifth digit of 1.

Urinary Dysuria

Urinary dysuria is painful urination. This condition may suggest an inflammation or irritation of the urethra or bladder neck. ICD-9-CM classifies this condition to code 788.1, which is also located in chapter 16.

Urinary Incontinence

Urinary incontinence is a loss of urine without warning and may be associated with many conditions. ICD-9-CM classifies urinary incontinence to subcategory 788.3, which further subdivides to type, such as urge or stress incontinence, continuous leakage, and nocturnal enuresis. Not to be confused with urge incontinence, code 788.63, Urgency of urination, identifies the intense feeling of having to urinate.

Other symptoms related to the genitourinary system include urinary frequency (788.41), polyuria (788.42), nocturia (788.43), and oliguria and anuria (788.5).

Disorders of the Prostate

Category 600, Hyperplasia of prostate, includes many forms of hyperplasia, some of which may be indicative of the need for further testing. Fourth digits for category 600 distinguish between simple enlargement of the prostate and more complex forms of prostatic enlargement. Category 600 includes the following subcategories:

600.0x Hypertrophy (benign) of prostate
600.1x Nodular prostate
600.2x Benign localized hyperplasia of prostate
600.3   Cyst of prostate
600.9x Hyperplasia of prostate, unspecified

Benign Prostatic Hypertrophy

Code 600.0x, Benign prostatic hypertrophy (BPH), commonly occurs in men over 60 years old. The prostate gland, which encircles the urethra at the base of the bladder, becomes enlarged and presses on the urethra, obstructing the flow of urine from the bladder. Symptoms of BPH include urinary frequency, urgency, nocturia, incontinence, and hesitancy; decreased size and force of stream; and/or complete urinary retention. Straining to void may rupture veins of the prostate, causing hematuria.

A diagnosis of BPH is made by a rectal examination that finds the prostate enlarged and with a rubbery texture. Urinalysis shows WBC, RBC, albumin, bacteria, and blood. Cystoscopy reveals the extent of enlargement. A postvoiding cystogram shows the amount of residual urine in the bladder.

Benign and malignant neoplasms of the prostate are excluded from this category. The note under code 600 reminds the coder that additional codes should be reported for any associated urinary incontinence (788.30–788.39).

Fifth digits for subcategory code 600.0, Hypertrophy (benign) of prostate, include:

600.00 Hypertrophy (benign) of prostate without urinary obstruction
        Hypertrophy (benign) of prostate NOS
600.01 Hypertrophy (benign) of prostate with urinary obstruction
        Hypertrophy (benign) of prostate with urinary retention

Additional fifth digits have been added to subcategory codes 600.1, Nodular prostate, 600.2, Benign localized hyperplasia of prostate, and 600.9, Hyperplasia of prostate, unspecified, to indicate whether urinary obstruction/retention is present.

Prostatitis

Prostatitis is inflammation of the prostate that may present in an acute form (601.0) or a chronic form (601.1). Additional codes may be assigned to identify the underlying organism, such as Staphylococcus aureus (041.1x) or Streptococcus (041.0x).

Mild and moderate prostatic intraepithelial neoplasia (PIN I and PIN II) should be coded to 602.3. An excludes note directs the coder to use code 233.4 when severe prostatic dysplasia (PIN III) is diagnosed.

Hydrocele

A hydrocele is an accumulation of fluid in any saclike cavity or duct, specifically in the membrane surrounding the testicles or along the spermatic cord. ICD-9-CM classifies hydroceles to category 603, which includes hydrocele involving the spermatic cord, testis, or tunica vaginalis. This category further subdivides to identify specific types, such as encysted or infected. When the hydrocele is described as congenital, the correct code assignment is 778.6, Congenital hydrocele.

Breast Disorders

Disorders of the breast that are not neoplastic in nature are classified to categories 610 and 611. Category 610, Benign mammary dysplasias, includes the following conditions:

- 610.0, Solitary cyst of the breast
- 610.1, Diffuse cystic mastopathy (including fibrocystic breast disease)
- 610.2, Fibroadenosis of breast
- 610.3, Fibrosclerosis of breast
- 610.4, Mammary duct ectasia (including periductal mastitis)
- 610.8, Other specified benign mammary dysplasias (including sebaceous breast cyst)
- 610.9, Benign mammary dysplasia, unspecified

Category 611, Other disorders of breast, includes the following conditions:

- 611.0, Inflammatory disease of breast (including mastitis and abscess)
- 611.1, Hypertrophy of breast (including gynecomastia)
- 611.2, Fissure of nipple
- 611.3, Fat necrosis of breast
- 611.4, Atrophy of breast
- 611.5, Galactocele

- 611.6, Galactorrhea not associated with childbirth

- 611.71, Mastodynia

- 611.72, Lump or mass in breast

- 611.79, Other signs and symptoms in breast (including nipple discharge, inversion, or retraction)

- 611.8, Other specified disorders of breast (including hematoma, infarction, or subinvolution of breast and occlusion of breast duct)

- 611.9, Unspecified breast disorder

Inflammatory Disease of Female Pelvic Organs

Categories 614–616 include codes for reporting infections of the female pelvic organs. The note at the beginning of the section reminds the coder to "Use additional code to identify organism, such as Staphylococcus or Streptococcus."

> **EXAMPLE:** Acute salpingitis; organism involved—streptococcus: 614.0, Acute salpingitis and oophoritis; 041.00, Unspecified streptococcus infection in conditions classified elsewhere and of unspecified site

Gynecologic Disorders

Gynecologic disorders include endometriosis, cervicitis, genital prolapse, cervical dysplasia, ovarian cysts, and ovarian dysfunction.

Endometriosis

Endometriosis is the presence of endometrial tissue outside the lining of the uterine cavity. It is generally confined to the pelvic area but can appear anywhere in the body. The classic symptom of endometriosis is dysmenorrhea, which can cause constant pain in the lower abdomen, vagina, posterior pelvis, and back. ICD-9-CM classifies endometriosis to category 617, which further subdivides to identify the specific sites affected.

Cervicitis

Cervicitis (616.0) is a sudden or long-term inflammation of the cervix, which is the lower, narrow end of the uterus. In the acute phase, swelling, redness, and bleeding occur. This condition also can produce a foul-smelling discharge, pelvic pain, itching, and/or a burning of the outer genital area. Chronic cervicitis, a persistent inflammation of the cervix, produces symptoms similar to the acute type. ICD-9-CM classifies cervicitis to code 616.0, which includes both the acute and chronic types.

Genital Prolapse

Genital prolapse is the falling, sliding, or sinking of the uterus and/or vagina from its normal position or place. ICD-9-CM classifies genital prolapse to category 618, which further subdivides to identify the extent of the disease and associated conditions, such as cystocele, cystourethrocele, rectocele, urethrocele, and proctocele. Subcategory code 618.0, Prolapse of vaginal walls without mention of uterine prolapse, has fifth digits that provide additional detail on the types of prolapses. Subcategory code 618.8, Other specified genital prolapse, is also subdivided to provide additional detail. Additional codes to indicate associated urinary incontinence should be reported when supported by documentation in the health record.

Cervical Dysplasia

Cervical dysplasia is the condition of abnormal cell structure in the cervical epithelium. This condition is classified to code 622.1x in ICD-9-CM. Often cervical dysplasia is the precursor of more serious conditions, such as carcinoma in situ of the cervix or cervical intraepithelial neoplasia (CIN) III. The types of conditions classified to 622.1x include:

- Anaplasia of cervix

- Cervical atypism

- Cervical intraepithelial neoplasia I [CIN I]

- Cervical intraepithelial neoplasia II [CIN II]

- Cervical dysplasia, NOS

- Mild dysplasia of cervix [CIN I]

- Moderate dysplasia of cervix [CIN II]

Cervical intraepithelial neoplasia III (CIN III) and severe dysplasia are classified to 233.1, Carcinoma in situ of breast and genitourinary system, cervix uteri.

Ovarian Cysts

Ovarian cysts may be nonneoplastic or neoplastic in origin. Nonneoplastic cysts include follicular, lutein, corpus luteum, and endometrial or chocolate cysts. Endometrial and chocolate cysts are classified to code 617.1, Endometriosis of the ovary. Follicular, lutein, and corpus luteum ovarian cysts are classified to the following codes:

- 620.0, Follicular cyst of the ovary (including graafian follicular cyst)

- 620.1, Corpus luteum cyst or hematoma (including lutein cyst)

- 620.2, Other and unspecified ovarian cyst (including corpus albicans, serous, retention, and theca-lutein)

Benign ovarian neoplasms are classified to code 220, Benign neoplasm of ovary.

Other Gynecologic Disorders

Category 626, Disorders of menstruation and other abnormal bleeding from female genital tract, includes the following conditions:

- 626.0, Absence of menstruation (including primary or secondary amenorrhea)

- 626.1, Scanty or infrequent menstruation (including oligomenorrhea)

- 626.2, Excessive or frequent menstruation (including menometrorrhagia, menorrhagia, and polymenorrhea)

- 626.3, Puberty bleeding

- 626.4, Irregular menstrual cycle

- 626.5, Ovulation bleeding (regular intermenstrual bleeding)

- 626.6, Metrorrhagia (bleeding unrelated to menstrual cycle)

- 626.7, Postcoital bleeding

- 626.8, Other disorders of menstruation and other abnormal bleeding, including dysfunctional uterine bleeding (DUB) and retained menstruation

- 626.9, Unspecified disorders of menstruation and other abnormal bleeding

Category 627, Menopausal and postmenopausal disorders, includes codes to identify symptomatic menopausal states due to either natural or artificial menopause. Asymptomatic postmenopausal status is assigned code V49.81.

- 627.2, Symptomatic menopausal or female climacteric states

- 627.4, Symptomatic states associated with artificial menopause

Chapter 14 Exercises

Review the following statements and cases and assign the appropriate codes:

1. Chronic kidney disease, stage III

2. Acute pyelonephritis due to E. coli

3. Staghorn calculus of kidney

4. Hematuria, frequency of urination, and nocturia

5. Fibroadenosis of breast

6. Cervical dysplasia

7. Vesicoureteral reflux with bilateral reflux nephropathy

8. Acute glomerulonephritis with necrotizing glomerulitis

9. Actinomycotic cystitis

Chapter 14 Exercises (Continued)

10. Absence of menstruation

    626.0

11. Postmenopausal bleeding

    627.1

12. Infected hydrocele

    603.1

13. Diabetic nephrotic syndrome, Type I

    250.41 , 581.81

14. Female infertility secondary to Stein-Leventhal syndrome

    256.4 , 628.0

15. Acquired multiple cysts of the kidney

    593.2.

16. A 77-year-old female was admitted to the hospital with intense pain described as renal or ureteral colic. An IVP revealed a relatively large stone in the left kidney with some renal dysfunction and another stone in the distal ureter on the left side. During the IVP, the patient began to complain of some chest pain and a cardiology consultation was requested.

    Discharge diagnoses: Left ureteral calculus; left renal calculus; chest pain

    Code(s):

    592.1   592.0 , 786.50

17. A 27-year-old female complaining of elevated temperature was seen in emergency services by her family physician; the high was 102. She also complained of lower back pain and frequent urination. A urinalysis was done and a bacterial organism (Pseudomonas) identified. She was given a prescription for antibiotics and released.

    Discharge diagnosis: Severe, acute cystitis

    Code(s):

    595.0 , 041.7

18. A 36-year-old female was admitted to the hospital with complaints of severe and constant pain in the lower abdomen and back. Upon questioning by the physician, the patient stated that her menstrual periods were very painful, often causing her to have to miss work. A diagnostic workup revealed endometriosis that involved the fallopian tubes, both ovaries, and the uterus. A hysterectomy and bilateral salpingo-oophorectomy was done, and the patient was later discharged from the hospital in good condition.

    Discharge diagnosis: Endometriosis of the fallopian tubes, both ovaries, and uterus

    Code(s):

    617.2 , 617.1 , 617.0

Review Questions

Answer the following questions:

1. What do the fourth digits identify in code 585, Chronic kidney disease?

2. What additional code is needed when a code for urinary tract infections is assigned?

3. In the coding of vesicoureteral reflux (593.7), what additional codes should be used?

4. How is benign prostatic hypertrophy diagnosed?

5. When codes from category 600, Hyperplasia of prostate, are used, what additional codes should be assigned?

6. How are breast disorders coded that are not neoplastic in nature?

Chapter 15

Complications of Pregnancy, Childbirth, and the Puerperium

Objectives

After completing this lesson, the student should be able to do the following:

- Apply knowledge of current, approved ICD-9-CM coding guidelines to assign and sequence accurate codes for diagnoses related to complications of pregnancy, childbirth, and the puerperium

- Apply knowledge of ICD-9-CM coding guidelines to assign and sequence accurate codes for the different types of abortions and the possible complications of each

- Define the terms *preterm, postterm,* and *prolonged* as they relate to the gestational period

- Understand the appropriate use of the fifth digits for categories 640–648, 651–659, 660–669, and 670–676

- List the criteria for assignment of category 650, Normal delivery

- Discuss the V codes that are appropriate to abortion, pregnancy, childbirth, and the post-partum period

Introduction

Chapter 11 of the ICD-9-CM codebook classifies conditions that affect the management of pregnancy, childbirth, and the puerperium (or postpartum period). Many conditions that are classified to other chapters in the codebook are reclassified to chapter 11 when they occur during pregnancy, childbirth, or in the postpartum period. Any condition occurring during these periods is considered a complication unless the physician specifically states that it is unrelated to the pregnancy. When a physician states that the pregnancy is unrelated to the condition being treated, the condition is coded and V22.2, Pregnant state, incidental, is assigned as an additional code.

Chapter 11 includes the following sections:

Categories	Section Titles
630–633	Ectopic and Molar Pregnancy
634–639	Other Pregnancy with Abortive Outcome
640–648	Complications Mainly Related to Pregnancy
650–659	Normal Delivery, and Other Indications for Care in Pregnancy, Labor, and Delivery
660–669	Complications Occurring Mainly in the Course of Labor and Delivery
670–677	Complications of the Puerperium

The conditions described in these categories are most often treated by obstetricians and gynecologists.

Ectopic Pregnancy

An ectopic pregnancy is a pregnancy that arises from implantation of the ovum outside the uterine cavity. Ninety-eight percent of ectopic pregnancies are tubal (occurring in the fallopian tube). Other sites include the peritoneum, the ovary, or the cervix. Category 633, Ectopic pregnancy, further subdivides into subcategories identifying the site of the ectopic pregnancy, for example, tubal (633.1) or ovarian (633.2).

Fifth digits for use with code 633 indicate whether there is a coexisting intrauterine pregnancy.

> **EXAMPLE:** 633.0 Abdominal pregnancy
> 633.00 Abdominal pregnancy without intrauterine pregnancy
> 633.01 Abdominal pregnancy with intrauterine pregnancy

Abortion

An abortion is the expulsion or extraction from the uterus of all or part of the products of conception: the embryo or a nonviable fetus weighing less than 500 grams. When fetus weight cannot be determined, an estimated gestation of less than 22 completed weeks is considered an abortion. Abortions and the complications that follow abortions, ectopic pregnancies, and molar pregnancies are classified to categories 634–639, as follows:

- 634, Spontaneous abortion

- 635, Legally induced abortion

- 636, Illegally induced abortion

- 637, Unspecified abortion

- 638, Failed attempted abortion

- 639, Complications following abortion and ectopic and molar pregnancies

The fourth digits of categories 634–638 indicate the presence or absence of a complication arising during the same admission or encounter as that of the abortion. A complete listing of the fourth-digit subdivision can be found at the beginning of the section, Other Pregnancy with Abortive Outcome (634–639).

.0   **Complicated by genital tract and pelvic infection**
Endometritis
Salpingo-oophoritis
Sepsis NOS
Septicemia NOS
Any condition classifiable to 639.0, with condition classifiable to 634–638

> | *Excludes:* | urinary tract infection (634–638 with .7) |

.1   **Complicated by delayed or excessive hemorrhage**
Afibrinogenemia
Defibrination syndrome
Intravascular hemolysis
Any condition classifiable to 639.1, with condition classifiable to 634–638

.2   **Complicated by damage to pelvic organs and issues**
Laceration, perforation, or tear of:
     bladder
     uterus
Any condition classifiable to 639.2, with condition classifiable to 634–638

.3   **Complicated by renal failure**
Oliguria
Uremia
Any condition classifiable to 639.3, with condition classifiable to 634–638

.4   **Complicated by metabolic disorder**
Electrolyte imbalance with conditions classifiable to 634–638

.5   **Complicated by shock**
Circulatory collapse
Shock (postoperative) (septic)
Any condition classifiable to 639.5, with condition classifiable to 634–638

.6   **Complicated by embolism**
Embolism:
     NOS
     amniotic fluid
     pulmonary
Any condition classifiable to 639.6, with condition classifiable to 634–638

.7   **With other specified complications**
Cardiac arrest or failure
Urinary tract infection
Any condition classifiable to 639.8, with condition classifiable to 634–638

.8   **With unspecified complication**

.9   **Without mention of complication**

Complications of Abortion

As indicated earlier, complications are classified according to the body system involved or specific type, such as "complicated by genital tract and pelvic infection." The fourth digit 7 is assigned when a specific complication is stated in the health record but cannot be classified to the previous six subcategories. In such cases, the abortion code is listed first, followed by a code specifying the complication.

> **EXAMPLE:** Incomplete spontaneous abortion due to severe preeclampsia: 634.71, Spontaneous abortion with other specified complications; 642.53, Severe preeclampsia complicating pregnancy, childbirth, and the puerperium

The fourth digit 8 is assigned when the documentation indicates the presence of a complication of an abortion without further specification as to type. The physician should be queried to determine a specific complication before this code is assigned. The fourth digit 9 is assigned when a complication is not mentioned.

Codes from categories 640–648 and 651–657 may be used with an abortion code to indicate the pregnancy complication that resulted in the abortion. In this circumstance, the fifth digit 3, antepartum condition or complication, should be assigned with the pregnancy code. Codes from series 660–669 must not be used for complications of abortion.

Category 639, Complications following abortion and ectopic and molar pregnancies, is used when a complication occurs after the abortion itself was completed during a previous encounter. When such complications require care and/or evaluation in either the inpatient or outpatient setting, a code from category 639 is reported, as noted:

Note: This category is provided for use when it is required to classify separately the complications classifiable to the fourth-digit level in categories 634–638; for example:

(a) when the complication itself was responsible for an episode of medical care, the abortion, ectopic, or molar pregnancy itself having been dealt with at a previous episode

(b) when these conditions are immediate complications of ectopic or molar pregnancies classifiable to 630–633 where they cannot be identified at the fourth-digit level

---

The fourth-digit subcategories in category 639 parallel those in categories 634–638; however, a code from categories 634–638 cannot be assigned with a code from category 639.

Fifth-Digit Subclassification for Abortion

Three fifth digits are available for use with categories 634–637:

0 Unspecified (as to complete or incomplete)
1 Incomplete
2 Complete

ICD-9-CM defines complete and incomplete abortions as follows: A complete abortion is the expulsion of all of the products of conception from the uterus prior to the episode of care. An incomplete abortion is the expulsion of some, but not all, of the products of conception from the uterus. When placenta or secundines remain, the abortion is considered incomplete.

The fact that a dilation and curettage was performed following an abortion does not necessarily mean that the abortion is incomplete. A review of the pathology report will confirm a complete or incomplete abortion.

Category 638 does not require the use of a fifth digit because the code describes a failed attempted abortion and, as such, the abortion did not occur.

Abortion Resulting in Live Fetus

The National Center for Health Statistics, in consultation with the American College of Obstetricians and Gynecologists, has confirmed that code 644.21, Early onset of delivery, should be assigned for an abortion resulting in a liveborn infant. By definition, an abortion (termination of pregnancy) cannot result in a liveborn infant. In addition to code 644.21, a code to describe the outcome of delivery (V27) may be assigned. If the abortion was induced, a code for the procedure performed for the termination of pregnancy also should be assigned.

> **EXAMPLE:** Spontaneous abortion resulting in liveborn fetus: 644.21, Early onset of delivery; V27.0, Outcome of delivery, single liveborn

Missed Abortion

A missed abortion (632) occurs when the fetus has died before completion of 22 weeks' gestation, with retention in the uterus for four or more weeks. After six weeks in the uterus, dead fetus syndrome (641.3x) may develop, with disseminated intravascular coagulation (DIC) and progressive hypofibrinogenemia. Massive bleeding may occur when delivery is finally completed. During this time, symptoms of pregnancy disappear. A brownish vaginal discharge may occur, but no bleeding. Missed abortions should be completed by physician intervention as soon as the diagnosis is certain with Doppler ultrasound or other methods.

Threatened Abortion

A threatened abortion (640.0x) is characterized by intrauterine bleeding occurring before the twenty-second completed week of gestation without expulsion of the products of conception and without dilation of the cervix.

Habitual or Recurrent Abortion

A habitual or recurrent abortion is the spontaneous expulsion of a dead or nonviable fetus in three or more consecutive pregnancies at about the same period of development. If the recurrent abortion is current, that is, when the patient's admission or encounter is for a recurrent abortion, use abortion codes (634–638). When the current hospital admission or encounter involves a problem with the pregnancy, but with no current abortion, assign code 646.3x, Habitual aborter. When the current hospital admission or encounter does not involve a pregnancy, assign code 629.9, Unspecified disorder of female genital organs. Code V23.2, Pregnancy with history of abortion, is used to describe supervision of a high-risk pregnancy with no problems.

Pregnancy

Normal pregnancies are intrauterine. Following is a guide for determining preterm, term, and prolonged postterm pregnancies:

- Preterm describes delivery before 37 completed weeks of gestation.

- Term describes delivery between 38 and 40 weeks of gestation.

- Postterm describes delivery between 40 and 42 completed weeks of gestation.

- Prolonged describes delivery after 42 completed weeks of gestation.

The postpartum period, or puerperium, begins immediately after delivery and continues for six weeks. In the Alphabetic Index to Diseases, long listings of conditions appear under **"Pregnancy," "Labor," "Delivery,"** and **"Puerperium."** Indentations often are used under these main terms, so extreme care should be taken in locating and selecting the appropriate code.

Obstetric encounters in the outpatient setting often are described more appropriately with the use of V codes. For example, category V22, Normal pregnancy, which includes codes to describe encounters for supervision of normal pregnancy, is often reported for routine prenatal visits. However, in some cases, the circumstances of the encounter or admission require assignment of a code from chapter 11 of ICD-9-CM. Such circumstances may include:

- Complications of the pregnancy, childbirth, or puerperium that affect the management and care of the mother

> **EXAMPLE:** Pregnancy with urinary tract infection that requires antibiotic therapy: 646.6x, 599.0
>
> **EXAMPLE:** Pregnancy with bleeding at 20 weeks' gestation: 640.9x
>
> **EXAMPLE:** Pregnancy with mild preeclampsia at 22 weeks' gestation: 642.4x

- Medical conditions (which may or may not be preexisting) that affect the management and care of the mother

> **EXAMPLE:** Type I diabetic at 25 weeks' gestation: 648.0x, 250.01
>
> **EXAMPLE:** Pregnancy at 20 weeks' gestation with a diagnosis of gonorrhea: 647.1x, 098.0
>
> **EXAMPLE:** Pregnancy at 23 weeks' gestation; patient dependent on cocaine: 648.3x, 304.20

It should be noted that all of the preceding examples required the assignment of two codes to fully describe the condition(s). When a condition develops that does not affect the pregnancy or its management, the condition is reported along with code V22.2, Incidental pregnancy. To assign code V22.2, the physician must state that the condition is unrelated to the pregnancy.

> **EXAMPLE:** Patient, at 20 weeks' gestation, with a sprained ankle: 845.00, Sprained ankle; V22.2, Incidental pregnancy

Fifth-Digit Subclassifications for Pregnancy

Assignment of the fifth digit centers on the episode of care, the encounter in which the patient is receiving care. Generally, an inpatient episode of care extends from time of admission until time of discharge. An outpatient episode of care involves a visit to a clinic or a private practitioner's office, or a home healthcare visit.

The following fifth-digit subclassification is required for use in categories 640–648, 651–659, 660–669, and 670–676:

0　**unspecified as to episode of care or not applicable**

1　**delivered, with or without mention of antepartum condition**
Antepartum condition with delivery

Delivery NOS

Intrapartum obstetric condition　(With mention of antepartum complication during current episode of care)

Pregnancy delivered

2　**delivered, with mention of postpartum complication**
Delivery with mention of puerperal complication during current episode of care

3　**antepartum condition or complication**
Antepartum obstetric condition, not delivered during current episode of care

4　**postpartum condition or complication**
Postpartum or puerperal obstetric condition or complication following delivery
　　that occurred:
　　　　during previous episode of care
　　　　outside hospital, with subsequent admission for observation or care

The fifth digit 0 is used for the rare occurrence where the episode of care is unspecified and/or not applicable. Note that the fifth digit 0 is applicable with all the categories (excluding those so stated). Fifth digits 1 and 2 indicate that the delivery occurred during the same admission. The fifth digit 1 is assigned whenever there is no mention of an antepartum condition or whenever an antepartum complication is present. The fifth digit 2 is assigned when a postpartum complication exists. Because both of these codes indicate that delivery occurred during this episode of care, they may be used together on the same record when both antepartum and postpartum conditions are present.

Fifth digits 3 and 4 both indicate that the delivery did not occur during this episode of care. The fifth digit 3 is assigned when an antepartum condition is present, and the fifth digit 4 is assigned when a postpartum condition exists. Because these digits indicate that delivery did not occur during this admission, they can never be combined with fifth digits 1 and 2. Moreover, they cannot be assigned together because the patient cannot be in both the antepartum and the postpartum state during the same episode of care.

Normal Delivery

Category 650, Normal delivery, is assigned when all the following criteria are met:

- Delivery of a full-term, single, healthy liveborn infant

- Delivery without prenatal or postpartum complications classifiable to categories 630–676 (which includes ante- and postpartum conditions such as multiple gestation and breast abscess. Code 650 may be used when the patient had a complication at some point during her pregnancy, but at the time of admission for delivery, the complication had been resolved.)

- Cephalic or occipital presentation with spontaneous, vaginal delivery requiring minimal or no assistance, with or without episiotomy, without fetal manipulation (for example, rotation, version) or instrumentation (forceps)

Outcome of Delivery (V Codes)

The outcome of delivery, as indicated by a code from category V27, should be included on all maternal delivery records. This is always an additional, not a principal, diagnosis code used to reflect the number and status of babies delivered. Category code V27 is referenced in the Alphabetic Index under **"Outcome of delivery."**

> **EXAMPLE:** Normal delivery and pregnancy, single liveborn: 650, Normal delivery; V27.0, Outcome of delivery, single liveborn

Obstetrical and Nonobstetrical Complications

Many preexisting conditions, such as diabetes, hypertension, or anemia, may affect or complicate the pregnancy or its management. Moreover, the pregnant state may aggravate the preexisting condition. For this reason, when the pregnancy aggravates the condition or when the condition aggravates the pregnancy, the preexisting or other nonobstetrical condition is reclassified to chapter 11 of the ICD-9-CM codebook. The categories representing such conditions are 642–643, 646–648, 671, and 673–676. In some cases, the code in the obstetrical chapter completely describes the condition. In other situations, a secondary code is needed to further specify the condition.

Category 642, Hypertension complicating pregnancy, childbirth, and the puerperium, provides specific subcategories as to the type of hypertension; therefore, a secondary code from category 401 is not required.

> **EXAMPLE:** Term pregnancy complicated by benign essential hypertension; undelivered: 642.03, Benign essential hypertension complicating pregnancy, childbirth, and the puerperium

Many women develop transient or gestational hypertension during pregnancy. This condition usually clears when the pregnancy is over. Gestational hypertension is coded to 642.3x. When the patient develops eclampsia or preeclampsia without preexisting hypertension, codes 642.4x–642.6x are used. When the preeclampsia or eclampsia is superimposed on existing hypertension, code 642.7x is assigned.

Category 643, Excessive vomiting in pregnancy, further subdivides to indicate at what point during the pregnancy the vomiting began and the presence or absence of metabolic disturbances. Code 643.0x, Mild hyperemesis gravidarum, is reported when vomiting starts before the end of week 22 of gestation. Code 643.1x, Hyperemesis gravidarum with metabolic disturbance, is reported when the vomiting starts before the twenty-second week with the presence of dehydration, electrolyte imbalance, or carbohydrate depletion. Code 643.2x, Late vomiting of pregnancy, is reported when the vomiting begins after the twenty-second week of gestation. Code 643.9x, Unspecified vomiting of pregnancy, is reported when the documentation in the health record does not indicate at what point in the pregnancy the vomiting began.

Category 645, Late pregnancy, is used to demonstrate that a woman is over forty weeks' gestation. Code 645.1x is used for a pregnancy over forty completed weeks to forty-two completed weeks' gestation, and code 645.2x is used for a pregnancy that has advanced beyond forty-two completed weeks of gestation.

Categories 646–648 include codes describing conditions and/or complications mainly related to pregnancy. For the most part, these categories require the assignment of an additional code to further specify the condition.

For example, subcategory 646.2, Unspecified renal disease in pregnancy, without mention of hypertension, requires the assignment of an additional code to specify the type of renal disease.

> **EXAMPLE:** Term pregnancy with chronic nephropathy, delivered:
> 646.21, Unspecified renal disease in pregnancy, without mention of hypertension; 582.9, Chronic glomerulonephritis with unspecified pathological lesion in kidney

Subcategory 646.6, Infections of genitourinary tract in pregnancy, requires the assignment of an additional code to specify the infection. A third code should be assigned to identify the specific organism involved, such as E. coli or pseudomonas.

> **EXAMPLE:** Pregnancy at 25 weeks' gestation with acute cystitis:
> 646.63, Infections of genitourinary tract in pregnancy;
> 595.0, Acute cystitis

Subcategory 646.8, Other specified complications of pregnancy, is used when the specified complication is not classified elsewhere in chapter 11, such as insufficient weight gain in pregnancy or uterine size–date discrepancy. Subcategory 646.9 is used when the diagnosis is identified as a "pregnancy complication" but is not specified as to type of complication.

Category 647, Infectious and parasitic conditions in the mother classifiable elsewhere, but complicating pregnancy, childbirth, or the puerperium, further subdivides to identify the general type of infectious or parasitic condition, such as gonorrhea, viral, or venereal disease. A second code should be assigned to describe the specific infectious or parasitic condition.

> **EXAMPLE:** Intrauterine pregnancy, 18 weeks' gestation with chronic gonorrhea:
> 647.13, Gonorrhea in the mother classifiable elsewhere, but complicating pregnancy, childbirth, or the puerperium;
> 098.2, Chronic gonococcal infection of lower genitourinary tract

Category 648, Other current conditions in the mother classifiable elsewhere, but complicating pregnancy, childbirth, or the puerperium, further subdivides to include a variety of conditions, such as diabetes mellitus, thyroid dysfunction, anemia, drug dependence, and mental disorders. These categories are quite broad and require the assignment of an additional code to further specify the condition.

> **EXAMPLE:** Intrauterine pregnancy, 20 weeks, active cocaine abuse:
> 648.43, Mental disorders in the mother complicating pregnancy, childbirth, or the puerperium; 305.60, Nondependent cocaine abuse

> **EXAMPLE:** Intrauterine pregnancy, 20 weeks, dependence on cocaine:
> 648.33, Drug dependence in the mother complicating pregnancy, childbirth, or the puerperium; 304.20, Cocaine dependence

It should be noted that ICD-9-CM reclassifies abuse of a drug to mental disorders in the obstetrical chapter (648.4x) and dependence on a drug to drug dependence in the obstetrical chapter (648.3x). This is another example of how careful review of the health record is needed to ensure accurate code assignment.

When reporting code 648.8x, Abnormal glucose tolerance, the coder is reminded to "Use additional code, if applicable, to identify long-term [current] use of insulin (V58.67)."

Other Indications for Care in Pregnancy, Labor, and Delivery

Categories 651–659 classify conditions that occur mainly during pregnancy and labor and delivery. Category 651, Multiple gestation, has fourth-digit subcategories that indicate the number of fetuses. Code 651.7x identifies women who have undergone fetal reduction for large number multiple pregnancies. Category 652 identifies malposition and malpresentation of the fetus, such as breech, shoulder, or brow presentation.

Category 653, Disproportion, addresses the difference in size between the fetal head and the mother's pelvis. The fourth-digit subcategories identify the type of disproportion. Category 654, Abnormality of organs and soft tissues of pelvis, classifies any abnormalities, congenital or acquired, affecting the delivery process.

Category 655, Known or suspected fetal abnormality affecting management of mother, is subdivided to fourth-digit subcategories that describe the type of abnormality.

> **EXAMPLE:** Patient admitted at 38 weeks' gestation for a scheduled cesarean delivery (classical) for known fetal hydrocephalus confirmed on ultrasound: 655.01, Central nervous system malformation in fetus

Category 656, Other fetal and placental problems affecting management of mother, is subdivided to fourth-digit subcategories that describe the specific problem.

> **EXAMPLE:** Patient admitted at 38 weeks' gestation in fetal distress; emergency cesarean delivery performed: 656.31, Fetal distress affecting management of mother

Codes from categories 655 and 656 are assigned only when the fetal condition is actually responsible for modifying the management of the mother, that is, by requiring diagnostic studies, additional observation, special care, or termination of the pregnancy. The fact that a fetal condition exists does not justify assigning a code from this series to the mother's health record.

Category 658, Other problems associated with amniotic cavity and membranes, is subdivided to fourth-digit subcategories that identify the types of conditions, such as polyhydramnios and infection of the amniotic cavity.

Complications Occurring Mainly in the Course of Labor and Delivery

Complications that can occur in the course of labor and delivery include obstructed labor and trauma to the perineum and vulva, among others. Category 660, Obstructed labor, is subdivided to describe various types of obstructed labor such as obstruction caused by malposition of fetus, obstruction caused by bony pelvis, obstruction caused by abnormal pelvic soft tissues, and locked twins. Subcategory codes 660.0, 660.1, 660.2, and 660.8 include a note to assign an additional code to further describe the position, disproportion, or abnormality.

Category 664, Trauma to perineum and vulva during delivery, includes perineal lacerations. The following five subcategories identify laceration degrees:

- Subcategory 664.0, First-degree perineal laceration, includes lacerations, ruptures, or tears involving the fourchette, hymen, labia, skin, vagina, and/or vulva.

- Subcategory 664.1, Second-degree perineal laceration, includes lacerations, ruptures, or tears (following episiotomy) that involve the pelvic floor, perineal muscles, and/or vaginal muscles.

- Subcategory 664.2, Third-degree perineal laceration, includes lacerations, ruptures, or tears (following episiotomy) that involve the anal sphincter, rectovaginal septum, and/or sphincter, not otherwise specified.

- Subcategory 664.3, Fourth-degree perineal laceration, includes lacerations, ruptures, or tears of sites classifiable to subcategory 664.2 and also involving the anal mucosa and/or the rectal mucosa.

- Subcategory 664.4, Unspecified perineal laceration, is available for use when the extent of the laceration is not specified in the health record.

Category 666, Postpartum hemorrhage, includes fourth-digit subcategories that identify third-stage hemorrhage (retained placenta), immediate postpartum hemorrhage, and delayed and secondary postpartum hemorrhage.

Category 669, Other complications of labor and delivery, not elsewhere classified, includes the following fourth-digit subcategories:

- Subcategory 669.5, Forceps or vacuum extractor delivery without mention of indication, is assigned when the reason for the forceps or vacuum extraction is not indicated.

- Subcategory 669.6, Breech extraction without mention of indication, is assigned when the reason for the breech extraction is not indicated.

- Subcategory 669.7, Cesarean delivery without mention of indication, is assigned when the reason for the cesarean delivery is not indicated.

When the specific reason for the breech extraction, or cesarean, forceps, or vacuum extractor delivery is documented, that code is assigned rather than the nonspecific 669.5, 669.6, and 669.7 codes.

Complications of the Puerperium Category

Category 671, Venous complications in pregnancy and the puerperium, is subdivided to identify the types of venous conditions/complications; therefore, no additional code assignment is required.

> **EXAMPLE:** Twenty-six-week intrauterine pregnancy, varicose veins of legs:
> 671.03, Varicose veins of legs complicating pregnancy and the
> puerperium

Category 672, Pyrexia of unknown origin during the puerperium, is not subdivided into fourth-digit subcategories but does require a fifth digit. A note instructs the coder to use "0" as the fourth digit.

Category 677, Late effect of complication of pregnancy, childbirth, or the puerperium, is used when a complication of an obstetrical experience results in a sequela requiring subsequent care or treatment. This code can be used at any time after the postpartum period. As with all late effects, the code for the residual condition is sequenced first and code 677 is assigned as an additional code.

V Codes

Several categories of V codes are pertinent to pregnancy, childbirth, and the puerperium. A detailed description of categories V20–V29 is given in chapter 2 of this book. Other V codes of interest include:

V13.21	Personal history of preterm labor
V13.29	Other genital system and obstetric disorders
V18.9	Genetic disease carrier
V23.41	Pregnancy with history of preterm labor
V23.49	Pregnancy with other poor obstetric history
V25.03	Encounter for emergency contraceptive counseling and prescription
V26.31	Screening for genetic disease carrier status
V26.32	Other genetic testing
V26.33	Genetic counseling
V59.7x	Egg donor
V61.5	Multiparity
V61.7	Other unwanted pregnancy
V65.11	Pediatric pre-birth visit for expectant mother
V72.40	Pregnancy examination or test, pregnancy unconfirmed
V72.41	Pregnancy exam, negative
V82.4	Maternal postnatal screening for chromosomal anomalies

Chapter 15 Exercises

Review the following statements and cases and assign the appropriate codes:

1. Hyperemesis gravidarum with dehydration, 12 weeks' gestation

2. Uterine pregnancy at 19 weeks' gestation with bleeding

3. Uterine pregnancy at 20 weeks' gestation with transient hypertension

4. Failure of lactation, delivered one week ago (patient discharged from hospital 5 days ago)

5. Uterine pregnancy, 22 weeks' gestation with acute cystitis due to E. coli

6. Twenty-five-week pregnancy with internal hemorrhoids

7. Thirty-week pregnancy with uncontrolled type I diabetes mellitus

8. Routine prenatal care, primigravida with no complications

9. Routine postpartum care, no complications

10. Elderly multigravida, prenatal care, no complications

11. Triplet pregnancy, delivered spontaneously; all liveborn

12. Late vomiting of pregnancy, undelivered

13. Preeclampsia complicating pregnancy, delivered this admission

14. Threatened abortion with hemorrhage at 15 weeks' gestation

15. Postpartum deep thrombophlebitis; developed two weeks following delivery

(Continued on next page)

Chapter 15 Exercises (Continued)

16. Twin delivery with malposition of one fetus; both liveborn

17. Prenatal visit at 12 weeks' gestation; pernicious anemia

18. Acute salpingo-oophoritis following spontaneous abortion two weeks ago

19. Missed abortion, 19 weeks' gestation

20. Patient seen by physician with bleeding due to retained placenta three days after spontaneous abortion

21. Intrauterine death at 21 weeks' gestation, undelivered

22. Normal delivery of single liveborn; first-degree perineal laceration

23. Inpatient admission: A 33-year-old patient delivered a baby boy weighing 11 lb., 1 oz. Patient had a third-degree perineal laceration that was subsequently repaired. The physician indicates that the baby was "large for dates," causing the laceration.

    Mother's chart:

    Baby's chart:

24. Outpatient visit: The patient was seen in the prenatal clinic at 30 weeks' gestation with preexisting benign hypertension. The patient reports that she has not felt any fetal movement in several days. The physician could not hear a heartbeat, so he performed an ultrasound that revealed a nonviable fetus.

    Impression: Intrauterine fetal death; hypertension

    Code(s):

25. Inpatient admission: A grand multipara patient delivers her eighth child and undergoes a bilateral partial salpingectomy for sterilization. Patient was moderately depressed during her last trimester.

    Discharge diagnoses: Delivery (vaginal) of single liveborn; grand multiparity; depression; tubal ligation

    Code(s):

Chapter 15 Exercises (Continued)

26. Outpatient visit: A patient is seen four weeks postpartum and treated for a severe urinary tract infection due to E. coli.

    Impression: UTI due to E. coli

    Code(s):

27. Inpatient admission: The patient is a 33-year-old, gravida 2, para 1 admitted for induction due to severe preeclampsia and decreased fetal movements. She was admitted at 32 weeks for induction. Because of the decreased fetal movements, a cesarean section was performed. She delivered a viable female. Postoperatively, the patient was treated with Aldomet and Apresoline for accelerated hypertension.

    Discharge diagnoses: Delivery; severe preeclampsia; decreased fetal movements; premature delivery

    Code(s):

28. Outpatient visit: The patient was seen for routine prenatal visit with complaint of hyperemesis. She is a primigravida at 18 weeks' gestation and has been unable to eat for several days. Moreover, she has been anemic during the past month. The physician prescribed medication and scheduled a return visit.

    Impression: Anemia; hyperemesis gravidarum

    Code(s):

29. Outpatient visit: The patient underwent a cesarean section 10 days prior to this outpatient visit. She presents with an elevated temperature and drainage at the incision site. Hemoglobin and hematocrit are both very low. The physician prescribes iron supplements and antibiotics. A repeat RBC is ordered.

    Impression: Postoperative wound infection

    Code(s):

30. Inpatient admission: The patient was at 31 weeks' gestation and was admitted in active labor. Ultrasound revealed that the fetus was in a breech presentation. Although the contractions stopped after 3 hours, the patient was observed overnight because of her history of being a habitual aborter. Contractions began again on the second day. Because of the obstructed labor, she was delivered prematurely of a viable infant via cesarean section.

    Discharge diagnoses: Breech delivery; obstructed labor; habitual aborter

    Code(s):

31. Outpatient visit: Patient sees her ENT physician for complaint of acute sore throat. The physician notes that she is pregnant, but the sore throat is treatable and does not affect the pregnancy.

    Impression: Acute sore throat; pregnancy

    Code(s):

Review Questions

Answer the following questions:

1. What is an ectopic pregnancy?

2. What do the fourth digits in categories 634–638 indicate? What do the fifth digits indicate?

3. What is a missed abortion?

4. Define preterm, term, prolonged, and postterm pregnancy.

5. What code is used for a routine prenatal visit?

6. What criteria must be met to assign code 650 for a delivery?

7. What code is used on the mother's chart to specify the outcome of delivery?

8. When is it appropriate to use a code from category 655, Known or suspected fetal abnormality affecting the management of mother, or category 656, Other fetal and placental problems affecting management of mother?

9. When is it appropriate to use a code from category 677, Late effect of complication of pregnancy, childbirth, or the puerperium?

10. What should the coder do when a code requires a fifth digit but is not subdivided into fourth-digit subcategories?

11. When is it appropriate to use category 639, Complications following abortion and ectopic and molar pregnancies?

Chapter 16

Congenital Anomalies and Certain Conditions Originating in the Perinatal Period

Objectives

After completing this lesson, the student should be able to do the following:

- Apply knowledge of current, approved ICD-9-CM coding guidelines to assign and sequence accurate codes for diagnoses related to congenital anomalies

- Apply knowledge of current, approved ICD-9-CM coding guidelines to assign and sequence accurate codes for diagnoses related to certain conditions originating in the perinatal period

- List the criteria used in determining whether a congenital anomaly or a perinatal condition is significant and reportable

- Differentiate between congenital anomalies and perinatal conditions

- Define the perinatal or newborn period

- List V codes appropriate to use in relation to congenital anomalies and conditions in the perinatal period

Introduction

The newborn period begins at birth and lasts through the twenty-eighth day following birth. All clinically significant conditions noted on routine newborn examination should be coded. A condition is significant when it requires any of the following:

- Clinical evaluation

- Therapeutic treatment

- Diagnostic procedures

- Extended length of hospital stay

- Increased nursing care and/or monitoring

- Implications for the future healthcare needs of the child

The preceding guidelines are identical to the general coding guidelines for selection of "other diagnoses," with the exception of the final item regarding implications for future healthcare needs. Only the physician can determine whether a condition is clinically significant. Pediatricians or neonatologists generally treat newborns and infants.

Congenital Anomalies

A congenital anomaly is present at, and exists from, the time of birth. Chapter 14 of the ICD-9-CM codebook classifies congenital anomalies (740–759). The chapter is organized by body system, beginning with the central nervous system. Because many conditions can be congenital or acquired in origin, careful review of the subterms in the Alphabetic Index is needed to ensure selection of the appropriate code to describe a congenital condition.

An appropriate code from the congenital anomalies category (codes 740–759) should be assigned when a specific abnormality is diagnosed for an infant. Such abnormalities may occur as a set of symptoms or as multiple malformations. A code should be assigned for each presenting manifestation of the syndrome when the syndrome is not specifically indexed in ICD-9-CM.

> **EXAMPLE:** A child was diagnosed with Sticker's syndrome. *Coding Clinic* (3rd Quarter 1999, 16–17) advised coders to assign code 756.89 for other specified anomalies of muscle, tendon, fascia, and connective tissue. Each manifestation of the syndrome is coded separately because this syndrome is not specifically indexed in ICD-9-CM. The patient may have myopia (367.1), retinal detachment (361.9), sensorneural hearing loss (389.10), and cleft palate (749.00), among other hereditary eye and joint disorders. Each documented condition would be coded separately in addition to 756.89.

If a congenital anomaly is noted during the hospital admission when the infant is born, the code describing the anomaly is assigned as an additional diagnosis. The principal diagnosis is a code from the category series V30–V39, Liveborn Infants According to Type of Birth.

> **EXAMPLE:** Liveborn male infant born in the hospital with tetralogy of Fallot: V30.00, Single liveborn, delivered in hospital without mention of cesarean delivery; 745.2, Tetralogy of Fallot

However, if the infant was transferred on the day of birth to another hospital for care of the congenital anomaly, the principal diagnosis at the second hospital would be the congenital anomaly.

> **EXAMPLE:** Liveborn male infant transferred for care of thoracic spina bifida with hydrocephalus: 741.02, Spina bifida of dorsal [thoracic] region with hydrocephalus

The following subsections describe several common congenital anomalies.

Spina Bifida

Spina bifida is a defective closure of the vertebral column. It ranges in severity from the occult type revealing few signs to a completely open spine (rachischisis). In spina bifida cystica, the protruding sac contains meninges (meningocele), the spinal cord (myelocele), or both (myelomeningocele). Commonly seen in the lumbar, low thoracic, or sacral region, spina bifida extends for three to six vertebral segments. When the spinal cord or lumbosacral nerve roots are involved in the spina bifida, as is usually the case, varying degrees of paralysis occur below the involved level. The result may be orthopedic conditions such as clubfoot or dislocated hip. The paralysis usually affects the sphincters of the bladder and rectum. Hydrocephalus, an excessive accumulation of cerebrospinal fluid within the ventricles, is associated with at least 80 percent of the lumbosacral type.

In ICD-9-CM, most types of spina bifida, excluding spina bifida occulta, are assigned to category 741. The category further subdivides to describe the presence or absence of hydrocephalus. The fifth-digit subclassification describes the site of the spina bifida. However, spina bifida occulta is coded 756.17.

When surgical repair is deemed necessary, closure of the defect takes place. When hydrocephalus exists, a shunt (most often a ventriculo-peritoneal shunt) also may be necessary.

Cardiac Conditions

Congenital heart defects can be divided into two types—cyanotic and acyanotic. Acyanotic defects continue to eject oxygenated blood from the heart. The following conditions are classified as acyanotic:

- Aortic stenosis (AS)
- Atrial septal defect (ASD)
- Coarctation of the aorta
- Endocardial cushion defect
- Patent ductus arteriosus (PDA)
- Pulmonary stenosis (PS)
- Ventricular septal defect (VSD)

Cyanotic heart defects allow right-to-left shunting of unoxygenated blood that mixes with oxygenated blood, resulting in arterial blood oxygen desaturation. The following defects are considered cyanotic:

- Hypoplastic left ventricle syndrome
- Hypoplastic right ventricle syndrome

- Persistent truncus arteriosus (PTA)

- Pulmonary atresia

- Tetralogy of Fallot (TOF)

- Total anomalous pulmonary venous return (TAPVR)

- Complete transposition of great vessels (TGV)

- Tricuspid atresia

Two of the most common congenital cardiac defects are ventricular septal defect and patent ductus arteriosus. Ventricular septal defect, the more common of the two, is an abnormal communication or opening in the ventricular septum that allows the blood to shunt from the left ventricle to the right ventricle. The defect may be small or large and can occur in several locations in the heart, most commonly in the area of the membranous septum. Although some of the smaller asymptomatic defects close spontaneously in some people by the age of seven or eight years, other people will require corrective surgery. In repair, a prosthetic material of Dacron or Teflon is used to patch the defect. ICD-9-CM classifies ventricular septal defects to code 745.4.

In patent ductus arteriosus, the fetal blood vessel that connects the aorta and the pulmonary artery, the ductus arteriosus, allows blood to bypass nonfunctioning fetal lungs. Within the first 72 hours of life, the ductus arteriosus begins to constrict, and within twelve weeks, it completely closes. In some patients, especially premature infants with respiratory distress syndrome, the ductus does not close. When the ductus remains open, heart failure and pulmonary congestion result. When surgical repair is required, ligation of the ductus is performed. ICD-9-CM assigns code 747.0 for patent ductus arteriosus.

Cleft Lip and Cleft Palate

Cleft lip, cleft palate, and combinations of the two are the most common congenital anomalies of the head and neck. A cleft is characterized by a fissure or elongated opening of a specified site, usually forming during the embryonic stage. Cleft lips and palates are classified as partial or complete, and can occur either bilaterally or unilaterally. The most common clefts are left unilateral complete clefts of the primary and secondary palate, and partial midline clefts of the secondary palate involving the soft palate and part of the hard palate. The incisive foramen serves as the dividing point between the primary and secondary palates.

In ICD-9-CM, cleft palate and cleft lip are classified to category 749. This category further subdivides to describe cleft palate (749.0x), cleft lip (749.1x), and a combination (749.2x). These subcategories further subdivide to identify unilateral, bilateral, and complete and incomplete. The documentation in the health record should be reviewed to determine whether the cleft is complete or incomplete (partial). The physician should be queried when the documentation is unclear. Surgical repair of cleft lips and/or palates is not conducted until after the twelfth week of life. Sometimes secondary revisions are required to correct any tissue deformities or scars.

Pyloric Stenosis

Pyloric stenosis results from hypertrophy of the circular and longitudinal muscularis of the pylorus and distal antrum of the stomach. In this case, the infant typically feeds well until about two weeks after birth, at which time regurgitation of food occasionally occurs. Several days later, projectile vomiting begins. Dehydration due to the vomiting is common. Surgery is the preferred treatment.

Fredet-Ramstedt pyloromyotomy is performed after the dehydration has been managed. Pyloric stenosis is assigned code 750.5.

Polycystic Kidney Disease

Polycystic kidney disease is an inherited disorder characterized by multiple, bilateral, grape-like clusters of fluid-filled cysts that grossly enlarge the kidneys, compressing and eventually replacing functioning renal tissue. The infantile form of this condition reveals an infant with pronounced epicanthal folds, a pointed nose, a small chin, and floppy, low-set ears. Signs of respiratory distress and congestive heart failure also may be present. This condition eventually deteriorates into uremia and renal failure. ICD-9-CM classifies cystic kidney disease to sub-category 753.1, with the following fifth-digit subclassifications:

- 753.10, Cystic kidney disease, unspecified
- 753.11, Congenital single renal cyst
- 753.12, Polycystic kidney, unspecified type
- 753.13, Polycystic kidney, autosomal dominant
- 753.14, Polycystic kidney, autosomal recessive
- 753.15, Renal dysplasia
- 753.16, Medullary cystic kidney
- 753.17, Medullary sponge kidney
- 753.19, Other specified cystic kidney disease

When there is no further specification as to the type of polycystic kidney disease, code 753.12 should be assigned. In addition, the coder should assign other complications that may be present, such as chronic kidney disease (585.x). Acquired cysts of the kidney are classified to code 593.2.

Certain Conditions Originating in the Perinatal Period

Chapter 15 of the ICD-9-CM codebook includes the following sections:

Categories	Section Titles
760–763	Maternal Causes of Perinatal Morbidity and Mortality
764–779	Other Conditions Originating in the Perinatal Period

As stated earlier, the perinatal, or newborn, period is defined as beginning before birth and lasting through 28 days after birth. The following inclusion note appears at the beginning of chapter 15:

> Includes: conditions which have their origin in the perinatal period
> before birth until the first 28 days after birth even though
> death or morbidity occurs later

Although the perinatal period lasts through 28 days after birth, the codes in chapter 15 may be assigned beyond the 28 days and may, in fact, be used for adults. The condition must have its origin in the perinatal period, although it could continue to affect the patient beyond that period.

> **EXAMPLE:** A two-month-old seen by a pediatrician is diagnosed with transitory tachypnea; the baby was first diagnosed with this condition at age three weeks: 770.6, Transitory tachypnea of newborn

In this example, the patient has transitory tachypnea that initially developed at the age of three weeks. Subsequent visits for evaluation or care of this condition, regardless of age, should be reported with code 770.6 because it meets the criteria set forth in the note.

Codes from Maternal Causes of Perinatal Morbidity and Mortality (760–763) are assigned only when the maternal condition has actually affected the fetus or newborn. The fact that the mother has an associated medical condition or experiences some complication of pregnancy, labor, or delivery does not justify the routine assignment of codes from these categories to the newborn record.

> **EXAMPLE:** Liveborn infant born (in hospital) with fetal alcohol syndrome to an alcohol-dependent mother: V30.00, Single liveborn, delivered in hospital without mention of cesarean delivery; 760.71, Alcohol affecting fetus via placenta or breast milk

> **EXAMPLE:** Delivery of a normal healthy infant (in hospital) to a mother who occasionally uses cocaine: V30.00, Single liveborn, delivered in hospital without mention of cesarean delivery

In the first example, the use of alcohol by the mother was manifested in the infant; therefore, a code for fetal alcohol syndrome is assigned. But in the second example, the infant was healthy and normal despite the mother's occasional use of cocaine; therefore, no code is assigned to describe noxious influences of cocaine affecting the fetus (760.75).

A number of substances are known to have effects on the development of the fetus when the mother is exposed to the substance during pregnancy. Subcategory code 760.7 identifies these substances:

760.70	Unspecified noxious substance
760.71	Alcohol
760.72	Narcotics
760.73	Hallucinogenic agents
760.74	Anti-infectives
760.75	Cocaine
760.76	Diethylstilbestrol [DES]
760.77	Anticonvulsants
760.78	Antimetabolic agents
760.79	Other

Categories 764 and 765 classify slow fetal growth and fetal malnutrition, and disorders related to short gestation and low birth weight. At the beginning of this section, the following fifth-digit subclassifications applicable to category 764 and codes 765.0 and 765.1 are introduced:

0   unspecified [weight]
1   less than 500 grams
2   500–749 grams
3   750–999 grams
4   1,000–1,249 grams
5   1,250–1,499 grams
6   1,500–1,749 grams
7   1,750–1,999 grams
8   2,000–2,499 grams
9   2,500 grams and over

More than one code from category 765, Disorders relating to short gestation and low birth weight, can be used on the same chart because codes 765.0x and 765.1x describe birth weight while code 765.2x indicates weeks of gestation. The following instruction is given under codes 765.0 and 765.1: Use additional code for weeks of gestation (765.20–765.29).

Other Respiratory Conditions of Fetus and Newborn

Category 770, Other respiratory conditions of fetus and newborn, contains many different newborn respiratory conditions such as subcategory 770.1, Fetal and newborn aspiration. Fifth digits for this subcategory include:

770.10   Fetal and newborn aspiration, unspecified
770.11   Meconium aspiration without respiratory symptoms
770.12   Meconium aspiration with respiratory symptoms
770.17   Other fetal and newborn aspiration without respiratory symptoms
770.18   Other fetal and newborn aspiration with respiratory symptoms

Meconium staining is reported with code 779.84 and meconium passage during delivery is reported with code 763.84.

Subcategory code 770.8, Other respiratory problems after birth, also contains many different newborn respiratory conditions. Fifth digits indicate the specific type of respiratory problem.

<table>
<tr><td>770.8</td><td colspan="2">Other respiratory problems after birth</td></tr>
<tr><td></td><td>770.81</td><td>Primary apnea of newborn</td></tr>
<tr><td></td><td></td><td>Apneic spells of newborn NOS</td></tr>
<tr><td></td><td></td><td>Essential apnea of newborn</td></tr>
<tr><td></td><td></td><td>Sleep apnea of newborn</td></tr>
<tr><td></td><td>770.82</td><td>Other apnea of newborn</td></tr>
<tr><td></td><td></td><td>Obstructive apnea of newborn</td></tr>
<tr><td></td><td>770.83</td><td>Cyanotic attacks of newborn</td></tr>
<tr><td></td><td>770.84</td><td>Respiratory failure of newborn</td></tr>
<tr><td></td><td></td><td>*Excludes:*   *respiratory distress syndrome (769)*</td></tr>
<tr><td></td><td>770.89</td><td>Other respiratory problems after birth</td></tr>
</table>

Infections

ICD-9-CM classifies perinatal infections to category 771, Infections specific to the perinatal period. Although the perinatal period extends through the twenty-eighth day of life, the following inclusion note appears at the beginning of the category:

Includes:　infections acquired before or during birth or via the umbilicus
or during the first 28 days after birth

Therefore, an infant who develops a urinary tract infection at the age of 20 days, for example, would be assigned code 599.0, Urinary tract infection, site unspecified. The infant would not have a diagnosis code from 771.8, Other infection specific to the perinatal period, because the infant acquired the infection after birth.

If a newborn has a condition that may be either due to the birth process or community acquired and the documentation does not indicate which it is, the default is due to the birth process and the code from chapter 15 should be used. If the condition is community acquired, a code from chapter 15 should not be assigned.

Subcategory code 771.8, Other infections specific to the perinatal period, is expanded to provide unique codes for the infections included in it.

771.81	Septicemia [sepsis] of newborn
771.82	Urinary tract infection of newborn
771.83	Bacteremia of newborn
771.89	Other infections specific to the perinatal period
	Intra-amniotic infection of fetus NOS
	Infection of newborn NOS

Newborns of HIV-positive mothers often test positive for HIV on ELISA or western blot tests. This finding may actually reflect the mother's HIV status and not the infant's. Infants may test positive as long as 18 months.

Fetal and neonatal hemorrhage, code 772, is used to report various types of hemorrhage in a fetus or neonate, with fourth digits identifying the specific location of the hemorrhage.

Neonatal cardiac dysrhythmias, such as neonatal bradycardia or neonatal tachycardia, are reported using codes 779.81 and 779.82, respectively. Code 779.83 is used for delayed separation of umbilical cord.

V Codes

A code from categories V30–V39 is assigned for any newborn. The appropriate code is selected based on whether the birth is single or multiple, and whether it occurred in the hospital, immediately before admission to the hospital, or outside the hospital with no subsequent admission. For live births in the hospital, a fifth digit indicates whether they were cesarean deliveries.

These codes are used only for newborns and only at birth. When a newborn is seen by the physician on an outpatient basis after birth in the hospital, these codes are not used. The code for the condition necessitating the encounter is used. Code V20.2 is assigned for routine health checks or care of a healthy infant or child. This is frequently called well-baby care.

Category V29 also is used to describe situations in which a newborn is suspected of having a particular condition, but without signs or symptoms. A full description of categories V29 and V30 can be found in chapter 2 of this book.

Chapter 16 Exercises

Review the following statements and cases and assign the appropriate codes:

1. Single liveborn male (born in the hospital via cesarean delivery) with congenital diaphragmatic hernia

2. Single liveborn male (normal delivery); polydactyly of fingers

3. Physician's office visit: Incomplete unilateral cleft lip and palate

4. Physician's office visit: Congenital talipes equinovalgus; Down's syndrome

5. Twin male (mate liveborn) born in hospital via cesarean section; cryptorchism

6. Physician's office visit: Hyperbilirubinemia of prematurity; baby weighed 2,000 grams at birth

7. Physician's office visit: Hypoglycemia in infant born of diabetic mother

8. Physician's office visit: Patent ductus arteriosus

9. Physician's office visit: Childhood-type polycystic kidney

10. Single liveborn (born in hospital via vaginal delivery); erythroblastosis fetalis due to ABO incompatibility

11. Routine well-baby visit

12. Single liveborn male (born in hospital via vaginal delivery); premature at 29 weeks (1,300 grams); hyaline membrane disease

13. Physician's office visit: Accessory digit, left hand

(Continued on next page)

Chapter 16 Exercises (Continued)

14. Single liveborn male (born in hospital via vaginal delivery); necrotizing enterocolitis discovered in a newborn at birth

15. Premature "crack" baby born in the hospital to a mother dependent on cocaine, birth weight of 1,247 grams; 34 weeks' gestation

16. Two-year-old diagnosed with fragile X syndrome

17. Physician's office visit: During a well-baby exam, the physician noted a heart murmur. An echocardiogram revealed peripheral branch pulmonary artery stenosis and a patent ductus foramen ovale.

18. Physician's office visit: The patient is a 19-month-old female who was seen for an evaluation of a right clubfoot. She is currently asymptomatic but tests positive for HIV.

    Impression: Talipes equinovarus; positive for HIV

    Code(s):

19. Inpatient admission: The two-day-old female was born prematurely by cesarean section at 31 weeks and 1,900 grams. She was found to have a congenital diaphragmatic hernia. Prior to corrective surgery, the infant developed respiratory distress and was subsequently intubated. Her condition improved, and she was discharged on the sixth hospital day.

    Discharge diagnoses: Prematurity; diaphragmatic hernia; respiratory distress

    Code(s):

20. Inpatient admission: The 6-week-old infant with Down's syndrome was admitted through emergency services with a 48-hour history of upper respiratory infection. The baby had been crying for several hours. Examination revealed acute suppurative otitis media and upper respiratory infection. The baby had been seeing the pediatrician weekly for failure to thrive. The baby was started on antibiotics and admitted.

    Discharge diagnoses: Earache; failure to thrive; upper respiratory infection; Down's syndrome

    Code(s):

21. Inpatient admission: The infant patient was born in the hospital to a 23-year-old primigravida. When induction of labor failed, the baby was delivered by cesarean section. The mother was a known chronic alcoholic; therefore, the newborn was placed in the NICU for observation for possible alcohol-related problems. The baby appeared to be fine.

    Discharge diagnosis: Single newborn

    Code(s):

Review Questions

Answer the following questions:

1. When a baby is born in the hospital with a congenital anomaly, what code is listed first?

2. What is the difference between cyanotic and acyanotic heart defects?

3. What series of codes is assigned for newborns when birth occurs in a hospital?

4. What code is assigned for well-baby care?

5. How is the perinatal period defined in ICD-9-CM?

Chapter 17

Diseases of the Skin and Subcutaneous Tissue

Objectives

After completing this lesson, the student should be able to do the following:

- Apply knowledge of current, approved ICD-9-CM coding guidelines to assign and sequence accurate codes for diagnoses related to disorders of the skin and subcutaneous tissue

- Discuss the organism responsible for causing cellulitis and the predisposing conditions for cellulitis

- Identify the major types of skin disorders

Introduction

Chapter 12 of the ICD-9-CM codebook includes conditions such as dermatitis, cellulitis, ulcers of the skin and subcutaneous tissue, urticaria, and diseases of the nails and hair. The following sections are included in chapter 12:

Categories	Section Titles
680–686	Infections of Skin and Subcutaneous Tissue
690–698	Other Inflammatory Conditions of Skin and Subcutaneous Tissue
700–709	Other Diseases of Skin and Subcutaneous Tissue

These conditions generally are treated by dermatologists, internists, and general practitioners.

Cellulitis

Cellulitis is an acute inflammation of a localized area of superficial tissue. Predisposing conditions are open wounds, ulcerations, tinea pedis, and dermatitis, but these conditions need not be present for cellulitis to occur. Physical findings reveal red, hot skin with edema at the site of infection. The area is tender, and the skin surface has a peau d'orange (skin of an orange) appearance with ill-defined borders. Nearby lymph nodes often become inflamed. Cellulitis clears within a few days when treated with antibiotics. In severe cases, abscesses may form that require drainage. However, coders should not assume that mention of redness at the edges of a wound or ulcer represents cellulitis. The normal hyperemia associated with a wound usually extends slightly beyond the wound's edges rather than in the diffuse pattern that characterizes cellulitis. Unless a diagnosis of cellulitis is documented by the physician, a code from categories 681–682 should not be assigned.

The organism responsible for cellulitis is usually streptococcus. There is ordinarily little or no necrosis, suppuration, or abscess, although these occasionally occur when other organisms, such as staphylococcus, are involved. Both abscess and lymphangitis are included in the code for cellulitis of the skin.

ICD-9-CM classifies cellulitis to categories 681 and 682. Category 681, Cellulitis and abscess of finger and toe, is further subdivided to identify the site. Category 682, Other cellulitis and abscess, also is further subdivided to identify the site. An additional code should be assigned to identify the organism involved.

> **EXAMPLE:** Cellulitis of the upper arm due to streptococcus:
> 682.3, Other cellulitis and abscess of upper arm and forearm;
> 041.00, Streptococcus infection in conditions classified elsewhere and of unspecified site

Coding of cellulitis secondary to superficial injury, burn, or frostbite requires two codes: one for the injury and one for the cellulitis. Note that code 958.3, Posttraumatic wound infection, NEC, is not assigned when the infection is identified as cellulitis (*Coding Clinic,* 2nd Quarter 1991).

Cellulitis frequently develops as a complication of chronic skin ulcers (707.0–707.9). These codes do not include any associated cellulitis, and two codes are required when both conditions are present.

Cellulitis described as gangrenous is classified to code 785.4, Gangrene, rather than to the 681–682 cellulitis categories, when it develops as the result of either injury or ulcer.

Cellulitis also may be present as a postoperative wound infection or as a result of the penetration of the skin involved in IV therapy. It may develop as early as five days postoperatively but often does not appear until a little later (*Coding Clinic,* 2nd Quarter 1991).

Dermatitis

Dermatitis is inflammation of the skin. ICD-9-CM classifies dermatitis to categories 690–694, depending on the underlying cause and type. Contact dermatitis resulting from substances such as detergents, solvents, oils and greases, drugs and medicines, plants, animal fur, and other chemical products, as well as solar radiation, is reported with a code from category 692. Contact dermatitis due to sunburn is coded as 692.7x, with fifth digits indicating the severity of the burn. Dermatitis resulting from substances taken internally, such as rashes due to drug reactions or food, is reported with a code from category 693. An E code should be used to identify the drug.

> **EXAMPLE:**　　Contact dermatitis due to detergents: 692.0, Contact dermatitis and other eczema due to detergents

> **EXAMPLE:**　　Dermatitis due to penicillin: 693.0, Dermatitis due to drugs and medicines; E930.0, Adverse effect of penicillin, therapeutic use

Chronic Ulcers of the Skin

Chronic ulcers of the skin are classified to category 707. Decubitus ulcer, or bedsore, is an ulceration due to prolonged pressure. Decubitus ulcers usually are located in the lower back or sacral area. ICD-9-CM classifies decubitus ulcers to code 707.0, with fifth digits identifying the specific site of the ulcer. Pressure ulcer is another synonym for decubitus ulcer.

Ulcers associated with arteriosclerosis of the limbs are classified to code 440.23, Atherosclerosis of the extremities with ulceration. An additional code from 707.10–707.9 is required. A note under subcategory code 707.1 reminds the coder to "code, if applicable, any causal condition first."

Chapter 17 Exercises

Review the following statements and cases and assign the appropriate codes:

1. Diaper rash

2. Cellulitis of the foot; culture reveals Staphylococcus aureus

   682 , 041.11

   682.7

3. Infected ingrowing toenail

4. Pilonidal cyst with abscess

   685.0

5. Postinfectional skin cicatrix

6. Allergic urticaria

   708.0

7. Circumscribed scleroderma

8. Erythema multiforme

   695.1

9. Acute lymphadenitis

10. A 24-year-old female patient is seen by her dermatologist for acne that has persisted since the birth of her baby some eight months ago. While reviewing the patient's medical record, the dermatologist notes that the patient had a history of high blood pressure during her pregnancy along with a history of hyperemesis gravidarum. The physician diagnoses her acne and prescribes medicine. In addition, he takes her blood pressure, which was within the normal range (120/80).

    Impression: Acne

    Code(s):

    706.1

11. An elderly female patient was seen in the nursing home due to the acute onset of erythema, tenderness, and swelling in the right posterior neck area. The provisional diagnosis was cellulitis, and she was begun on IV antibiotic treatment. A CT scan was ordered and revealed a medium-sized soft tissue mass in the right posterior neck with the possibility of some abscess formation.

    Diagnoses: Cellulitis; possible abscess formation

    Code(s):

Review Questions

Answer the following questions:

1. What are some of the predisposing conditions for cellulitis?

2. What organism is usually responsible for causing cellulitis?

3. How is dermatitis coded that results from substances taken internally?

4. What are synonymous terms for decubitus ulcer?

5. How is cellulitis coded when it is secondary to superficial injury, burn, or frostbite?

1. Open wounds ulcerations, tinea pedis, dermatitis

2. Streptococcus

3. with an E-code

4. Bedsores

5. One for the injury and one for the cellulitis

Chapter 18

Diseases of the Musculoskeletal System and Connective Tissue

Objectives

After completing this lesson, the student should be able to do the following:

- Apply knowledge of current, approved ICD-9-CM coding guidelines to assign and sequence accurate codes for diagnoses related to diseases of the musculoskeletal system and connective tissue such as arthritis, systemic lupus erythematosus, and intervertebral disk disorders

- Define pathologic fracture and explain the coding rules relating to a pathologic fracture

- List the V codes appropriate for use with disorders of the musculoskeletal system and connective tissue

Introduction

Chapter 13 of the ICD-9-CM codebook is divided into the following sections:

Categories	Section Titles
710–719	Arthropathies and Related Disorders
720–724	Dorsopathies
725–729	Rheumatism, Excluding the Back
730–739	Osteopathies, Chondropathies, and Acquired Musculoskeletal Deformities

The musculoskeletal system provides support and movement of body parts. The skeleton is the framework of the body and is composed of bone and cartilage. The bones provide a place for muscles and supporting structures to attach. The muscles allow the movement of the various body parts by means of contraction and relaxation of muscle fibers.

Orthopedics is the branch of medicine that deals with the preservation and restoration of bones and associated structures. An orthopedist or orthopedic surgeon is one who practices orthopedics. Rheumatology is the branch of medicine that deals with rheumatic disorders, which affect the connective tissues of the body, especially the joints and related structures. A rheumatologist is a specialist in rheumatology. Rheumatologists most often treat the various forms of arthritis.

To report musculoskeletal diseases accurately, the following information must be known:

- Anatomic site, such as cervical spine, hip, or ankle

- Severity (acute versus chronic)

- Underlying cause, such as neurogenic, drug induced, or postsurgical

The beginning of chapter 13 indicates that the fifth-digit subclassification must be used with the following categories: 711–712, 715–716, 718–719, and 730. The fifth-digit subclassification is repeated at the beginning of each of these series of codes.

Systemic Lupus Erythematosus

Systemic lupus erythematosus (SLE) is a chronic generalized connective tissue disorder ranging from mild to fulminating. It is marked by skin eruptions, arthralgia, fever, leukopenia, visceral lesions, and other constitutional symptoms. ICD-9-CM classifies SLE to code 710.0. Instructions indicate that an additional code should be assigned to identify any manifestations, such as nephritis, endocarditis, or nephrotic syndrome.

Arthritis

ICD-9-CM classifies the various types of arthritis to the following categories:

- 711, Arthropathy associated with infections

- 712, Crystal arthropathies

- 713, Arthropathy associated with other disorders classified elsewhere

- 714, Rheumatoid arthritis and other inflammatory polyarthropathies

- 715, Osteoarthrosis and allied disorders

- 716, Other and unspecified arthropathies

The first three categories describe arthropathies that, for the most part, are due to another disease process. Coders should be guided by the instructional notations and code first the underlying condition, followed by a code from categories 711, 712, or 713. Instructional notations also may indicate that the infectious organism should be coded.

> **EXAMPLE:** Arthropathy involving the knees in Behçet's syndrome:
> 136.1, Behçet's syndrome; 711.26, Arthropathy of the knees in
> Behçet's syndrome

Septic Arthritis

Septic (infectious) (bacterial) arthritis (711.0) is caused when pyogenic bacteria or other infectious agents invade the synovial tissue. The type of organism infecting the joint determines the course of the illness. Adults are most commonly infected with gonococci, staphylococci, streptococci, or pneumococci. Children are frequently infected with staphylococci, H. influenzae, and Gram-negative bacilli. Septic arthritis at any age may be caused by viral pathogens (for example, rubella, mumps, or hepatitis B).

Lyme Disease

Lyme disease, originally called Lyme arthritis, was recognized in 1975 because of the close geographic clustering of children in Lyme, Connecticut, who were thought to have juvenile rheumatoid arthritis. Lyme disease is caused by a spirochete, Borrelia burgdorferi, which is transmitted by ticks. Within a few weeks to two years after the tick bite, approximately 80 percent of the victims develop joint symptoms, such as joint pain, and intermittent attacks of arthritis. This nonrheumatoid arthritis is the third, or persistent, stage of Lyme disease.

When still in the active phase, Lyme disease is coded as 088.81, along with a code for the arthritis. Arthritis also can be considered as a late effect of Lyme disease. When this is the case, a late effect code should be used.

> **EXAMPLE:** Arthritis secondary to Lyme disease: 088.81 and 711.8x
>
> **EXAMPLE:** Arthritis after acute phase of Lyme disease: 139.8 and 711.8x

Code 139.8 is found in the Alphabetic Index under "**Late,** effect (s) (of), infectious diseases."

Lyme disease is now associated with other musculoskeletal syndromes and may cause osteomyelitis or myositis. Myocarditis, pericarditis, cardiac arrhythmias, and meningoencephalitis can be complications of Lyme disease.

Rheumatoid Arthritis

Category 714, Rheumatoid arthritis (RA) and other inflammatory polyarthropathies, classifies a chronic, crippling condition that affects the joints of the hands, feet, wrists, elbows, and ankles. Periods of remission and exacerbation occur in afflicted patients. Although the exact etiology of the disease is unknown, immunologic changes and tissue hypersensitivity, complicated by a cold and damp climate, may have a contributory effect. The synovial membranes are primarily affected. The joints become inflamed, swollen, and painful, as well as stiff and tender. A characteristic sign is the formation of nodules over body surfaces. During an active period, the patient suffers from malaise, fever, and sweating. Rheumatoid arthritis occurs in women two to three times more frequently than in men.

Category 714 is further subdivided to identify specific types of inflammatory conditions of the joints. The note under code 714.0, Rheumatoid arthritis, reminds the coder to also code any manifestations documented, such as myopathy and polyneuropathy. Juvenile rheumatoid arthritis, chronic or unspecified, is assigned to 714.30. Juvenile arthritis begins before the age of 16 and has similar characteristics to adult RA. Juvenile RA is clinically divided into various subtypes, such as systemic, pauciarticular, and polyarticular. Systemic onset is sometimes called Still's disease. High fever, rash, splenomegaly, adenopathy, and neutrophilic leukocytosis are characteristics of this subtype. Approximately 40 percent of children with the condition are affected by the pauciarticular subtype, which is characterized by iritis, joint deformity, and unequal leg length. The polyarticular type, which also affects approximately 40 percent of children with the disease, is characterized by symptoms and onset similar to adult RA.

Osteoarthrosis and Allied Disorders

Category 715, Osteoarthrosis and allied disorders, includes conditions described as osteoarthrosis, osteoarthritis, degenerative arthritis, and degenerative joint disease. Osteoarthritis is characterized by erosion of cartilage (either primary or secondary to trauma or other conditions), which becomes soft, frayed, and thinned. This condition also is known as degenerative joint disease and osteoarthrosis. The fourth digit identifies the type of osteoarthrosis, such as generalized or localized, and whether the arthritis is secondary or primary. When one body part, such as the knees (unilateral or bilateral), is documented in the health record, the coder should select localized osteoarthrosis, remembering also to assign the appropriate fifth digit to identify the specific site involved.

Category 716, Other and unspecified arthropathies, includes conditions such as traumatic arthropathy/arthritis (716.1x), transient arthropathy (716.4x), and arthropathy/arthritis without further specification (716.9x).

The appropriate fifth digit should be assigned to identify the specific site involved for all categories related to arthritis.

Other Joint Disorders

Category 719, Other and unspecified disorders of joint, includes a variety of codes to describe nonspecific conditions of the joints. The note under category 719 reminds the coder that valid fifth digits are listed under each subcategory code to which they apply. This fifth digit subclassification is for use with codes 719.0–719.6, 719.8–719.9. This category further divides into the following subcategories:

- 719.0, Effusion of joint

- 719.1, Hemarthrosis

- 719.2, Villonodular synovitis

- 719.3, Palindromic rheumatism

- 719.4, Pain in joint

- 719.5, Stiffness of joint, not elsewhere classified

- 719.6, Other symptoms referable to joint

- 719.7, Difficulty in walking

- 719.8, Other specified disorders of joint

- 719.9, Unspecified disorder of joint

The preceding subcategories require the assignment of a fifth digit to identify the specific site affected.

Dorsopathies

Codes describing intervertebral disk disorders and spondylosis, as well as other back disorders, are included in the section on dorsopathies (720–724). Intervertebral disk disorders are classified to category 722, which is further subdivided to identify the specific disorder, such as displacement or degeneration of an intervertebral disk or postlaminectomy syndrome. The subcategories are further divided to identify the specific site affected, such as cervical, thoracic, or lumbar, and the presence of myelopathy (functional disorder of the spinal cord).

Category 724 includes codes to describe other and unspecified disorders of the back, including back pain, sciatica, spinal stenosis, neuritis, radiculitis, and lumbago. The coder should not assign a nonspecific code from category 724 when the underlying cause is known.

Osteopathies, Chondropathies, and Acquired Musculoskeletal Deformities

The osteopathies, chondropathies, and acquired musculoskeletal deformities section (730–739) of chapter 13 includes codes describing osteomyelitis, bone cysts, malunion and nonunion of fractures, pathological fractures, acquired deformities of the limbs, and curvature of the spine.

Category 730, Osteomyelitis, periostitis, and other infections involving bone, is further subdivided to fourth-digit subcategories that describe acute or chronic osteomyelitis, as well as osteopathy or bone infections resulting from other diseases such as poliomyelitis. The fifth-digit subclassification identifies the site involved. An additional code should be assigned that describes the organism involved.

Pathologic fractures occur as a result of an existing disease process, such as osteoporosis or bone metastasis. This type of fracture often occurs spontaneously; however, minor injuries also may result in a fracture because the bone is already weakened. ICD-9-CM classifies pathologic fractures to subcategory 733.1, with the fifth digit identifying the specific bone affected. Two codes should be assigned to fully describe a pathologic fracture: one for the fracture and one for the underlying cause.

> **EXAMPLE:**   Fracture of T12 due to osteoporosis, with no history of injury:
> 733.13, Pathologic fracture of vertebra; 733.00, Osteoporosis, unspecified

Malunion of a fracture occurs when the bone ends of a reduced fracture do not align properly. It is classified to code 733.81. Nonunion of a fracture is the failure of the bone ends to align and is classified to code 733.82. Re-reduction of the fracture may be required for either condition. Stress fractures or stress reactions are coded to subcategory 733.93, 733.94, or 733.95, depending on the specific bone involved.

V Codes

Some of the V codes related to the musculoskeletal system and connective tissues include:

V13.4	Personal history of arthritis
V13.5	Personal history of other musculoskeletal disorders
V17.7	Family history of arthritis
V17.81	Family history of osteoporosis
V17.89	Family history of other musculoskeletal diseases
V43.6x	Organ or tissue replaced by other means, joint
V49.6x	Other conditions influencing health status, upper limb amputation status
V49.7x	Other conditions influencing health status, lower limb amputation status
V49.84	Bed confinement status
V52.0	Fitting and adjustment of prosthetic device and implant, artificial arm
V52.1	Fitting and adjustment of prosthetic device and implant, artificial leg
V53.7	Fitting and adjustment of orthopedic devices
V54.0x	Aftercare involving internal fixation device
V54.1x	Aftercare for healing traumatic fracture
V54.2x	Aftercare for healing pathologic fracture
V54.81	Aftercare following joint replacement (The coder is advised to identify the joint replacement site using codes V43.60–V43.69.)
V54.89	Other orthopedic aftercare
V58.4x	Other aftercare following surgery
V67.00	Follow-up examination following surgery, unspecified
V67.09	Follow-up examination following other surgery
V67.4	Follow-up examination following treatment of healed fracture
V82.1	Special screening for rheumatoid arthritis
V82.2	Special screening for other rheumatic disorders
V82.3	Special screening for congenital dislocation of hip
V82.81	Special screening for osteoporosis

Chapter 18 Exercises

Review the following statements and cases and assign the appropriate codes:

1. Displacement of thoracic intervertebral disk

2. Difficulty walking due to primary localized osteoarthrosis of the hip

3. Pathologic fracture of the vertebra due to osteoporosis

4. Acquired talipes equinovarus

5. Baker's cyst of knee

6. Systemic lupus erythematosus

7. Acute osteomyelitis of ankle due to staphylococcus

8. Pathologic fracture of the vertebra due to metastatic carcinoma of the bone from the lung

9. Nonpyogenic arthritis of the hip due to staphylococcal infection

10. Ankylosing spondylitis

11. Charcot's arthritis due to diabetes

12. Acute polymyositis; thoracogenic scoliosis

13. Nonunion fracture, left hip

14. Dupuytren's contracture

15. Outpatient visit: The patient sustained a cervical fracture in an automobile accident six years ago. He has been experiencing paresthesia at C3–C4 for two years. The symptoms are worsening with pain in his neck and radiating through his arms.

    Impression: Cervical stenosis

    Code(s):

(Continued on next page)

Chapter 18 Exercises (Continued)

16. Emergency services visit: This elderly farmer was brought to emergency services with severe nausea and vomiting. Two days ago, he developed diarrhea and now is slightly dehydrated. His past history reveals a history of arthritis for which he is on medication. The patient had a coronary artery bypass graft three months ago. Lab work revealed: Stool sample with Giardia lamblia. The patient was rehydrated and released on antidiarrheal medication. He was given pain medication for his arthritis.

    Impression: Gastroenteritis, Giardia; dehydration; arthritis

    Code(s):

    ____

17. Outpatient visit: A 76-year-old female was seen with complaints of severe joint pain in the hips and knees. Workup revealed rheumatoid arthritis with myopathy.

    Impression: Rheumatoid arthritis with inflammatory myopathy

    Code(s):

    ____

18. Inpatient admission: The patient was admitted with known traumatic arthritis and ankylosis of the right hip due to an old fracture of the femoral neck sustained after a fall. The past history revealed arteriosclerotic vascular disease. The patient underwent hip replacement surgery and was released to rehabilitation services.

    Discharge diagnoses: Arthritis and ankylosis of the right hip secondary to old fracture; arteriosclerotic vascular disease

    Code(s):

    ____

19. Chief complaint: Sore right knee

    History of present illness: Patient notes that he was moving some boxes over the weekend. He notes that on 1/28, his right knee became sore and swollen. On 1/30, he had shaking fevers and chills. He now presents for evaluation. When seen in the office, he denied a history of coughing or other illness. There was no history of trauma to the knee.

    The patient's right knee is swollen, which has limited his ability to move. There is no medial or lateral joint line discomfort and no pain on palpitation of the patella. Negative apprehension sign for subluxation. The medial and lateral collateral ligaments are stable. Stress testing of the cruciates was not performed due to the effusion and the lack of reliability of testing with large effusion. There were no tender femoral groin nodes. After suitable prep, while in the office, aspiration was performed on the right knee. Approximately 80 cc of a purulent, turbid-appearing fluid was aspirated. Lab work was done. The cultures showed Staphylococcus aureus with oxacillin sensitivity. The patient was informed of the results and the need for admission to the hospital.

    Hospital course: The patient was admitted on 1/31 after a three-day course of pain in the knee followed by shaking chills. Aspiration in the office indicated the patient had purulent, turbid-appearing fluid. On admission, he was started on IV antibiotics and was seen in consultation by an infectious disease practitioner. The consultant's impression was that the patient had septic arthritis. He was taken to surgery on 2/1, at which time he underwent arthroscopic irrigation and debridement with tube placement. He was maintained on drip-suck irrigation. He was taken back to surgery on 2/4 for repeat irrigation and debridement. Postoperatively, his temperature resolved. The organism was also sensitive to Timentin. He was then discharged on Timentin, on home IVs. He had instructions to return to the office for follow-up.

    Discharge diagnosis: Septic arthritis due to Staph aureus

    Code(s):

    ____

Review Questions

Answer the following questions:

1. How is Lyme disease coded?

2. In category 715, Osteoarthritis and allied disorders, what do the fourth-digit subcategories signify?

3. When is it appropriate to use category 724, Other and unspecified disorders of back?

4. How are pathologic fractures coded?

5. When coding intervertebral disc disorders, what information is necessary for accurate coding?

6. What is the difference between a malunion and a nonunion of a fracture?

Chapter 19

Injury, Poisonings, and Adverse Effects

Objectives

After completing this lesson, the student should be able to do the following:

- Apply knowledge of current, approved ICD-9-CM coding guidelines to assign and sequence accurate codes for diagnoses related to injuries

- Become familiar with the main terms in the Alphabetic Index where codes for the various types of traumatic injuries may be found

- Identify the appropriate uses of category 948, Burns classified according to extent of body surface involved

- Explain the "rule of nines" in estimating the extent of body surface involved with burns

- List the V codes that are appropriately used in conjunction with injury codes

- Apply knowledge of current, approved ICD-9-CM coding guidelines to assign E codes to injuries, poisonings, and adverse effects

- Identify the Alphabetic Index dedicated to the use of E codes

- Apply knowledge of current, approved ICD-9-CM coding guidelines to assign and sequence accurate codes for diagnoses related to poisonings and adverse effects

- Differentiate between poisonings and adverse effects

Introduction

Chapter 17 of the ICD-9-CM codebook covers a wide variety of injuries and includes subsections on poisonings, adverse effects of drugs, and complications of surgical and medical care. Physicians of many specialties use codes from this chapter. Certainly, emergency department physicians and orthopedists use many of the fracture and other injury codes, but general practitioners and internists also use many of the codes from the adverse effects and poisoning sections. In addition, physicians of many specialties may treat patients with burns, including dermatologists, general practitioners, and internists. Chapter 17 contains the following sections:

Categories	Section Titles
800–829	Fractures
830–839	Dislocation
840–848	Sprains and Strains of Joints and Adjacent Muscles
850–854	Intracranial Injury, Excluding Those with Skull Fracture
860–869	Internal Injury of Thorax, Abdomen, and Pelvis
870–879	Open Wound of Head, Neck, and Trunk
880–887	Open Wound of Shoulder and Upper Limb
890–897	Open Wound of Lower Limb
900–904	Injury to Blood Vessels
905–909	Late Effects of Injuries, Poisonings, Toxic Effects, and Other External Causes
910–919	Superficial Injury
920–924	Contusion with Intact Skin Surface
925–929	Crushing Injury
930–939	Effects of Foreign Body Entering through Orifice
940–949	Burns
950–957	Injury to Nerves and Spinal Cord
958–959	Certain Traumatic Complications and Unspecified Injuries
960–979	Poisoning by Drugs, Medicinal, and Biological Substances
980–989	Toxic Effects of Substances Chiefly Nonmedicinal as to Source
990–995	Other and Unspecified Effects of External Causes
996–999	Complications of Surgical and Medical Care, Not Elsewhere Classified

Injuries

Injuries are traumatic in nature and result in damage to body parts. The damage may occur to such an extent that tissues are killed. Various external causes such as a blow, a fall, a gun, a knife, industrial equipment, or a household item may be responsible for an injury. Moreover, traumatic injuries may predispose a person to a nontraumatic disease. For example, bacteria may settle at the site of a bone fracture and cause acute osteomyelitis.

ICD-9-CM classifies injuries to well-defined categories such as fractures, dislocations, sprains, and open wounds, which, in general, may be easier to understand than disease processes. When several injuries are present, the code for the most severe injury should be sequenced first.

Main Terms for Injuries

The Alphabetic Index to Diseases classifies injuries according to the general type of injury, such as a wound, fracture, or dislocation. The subterms under the general type of injury identify the anatomical site.

> **Wound, open** . . .
>   abdomen, abdominal . . . 879.2
>   complicated 879.3
>   wall (anterior) 879.2
>   complicated 879.3
>   lateral 879.4
>   complicated 879.5
>   alveolar (process) 873.62
>   complicated 873.72

Fractures

A break in a bone caused by traumatic injury or a disease process is known as a fracture (codes 800–829). Fractures are coded by the bone involved and the nature of the break. To code fractures accurately and completely, the following questions must be answered:

- Is the fracture traumatic or pathologic? Review the health record for mention of trauma or underlying pathology, such as osteoporosis or bone metastasis. Pathological fractures are not considered traumatic and are not classified to chapter 17 in the ICD-9-CM codebook.

- Where is the fracture located? Review diagnostic studies, such as x-rays, to identify the specific location.

- Is the fracture open or closed?

Closed fractures (with or without delayed healing) include the following terms:

Comminuted	Impacted
Depressed	Linear
Elevated	Simple
Fissured	Slipped epiphysis
Fracture, NOS	Spiral
Greenstick	

Open fractures (with or without delayed healing) are further described as:

Compound	Puncture
Infected	With foreign body
Missile	

A fracture not indicated as closed or open should be classified as closed.

Whenever possible, separate codes should be assigned for multiple fractures unless the Alphabetic Index or the Tabular List provides instructions to the contrary.

> **EXAMPLE:** Closed fracture of the distal radius: 813.42, Other fractures of distal end of radius (alone)
>
> **EXAMPLE:** Closed fracture of the metacarpal bone: 815.00, Closed fracture of unspecified metacarpal bone(s)

Combination categories for multiple injuries are provided for use when the health record contains insufficient detail.

> **EXAMPLE:** Multiple fractures of right upper limb (only information provided in the health record): 818.0, Ill-defined closed fractures of upper limb

Combination categories also may be used when the reporting form limits the number of codes that can be assigned.

> **EXAMPLE:** Patient had many traumatic injuries, including several fractures of the hand bones, which were identified in the health record. Because of all the other, more critical injuries, there was not enough space on the form to code each metacarpal fracture separately. Combination code used: 817.0, Closed multiple fractures of hand bones

Coders are permitted to use an x-ray report to assign a more specific fracture diagnosis code. The physician may not list the specific site of the fracture, but an x-ray report in the health record shows the precise site. It is appropriate for the coder to assign the more specific code from the x-ray report without consulting the physician; however, when there is any question as to the appropriate diagnosis, the coder must contact the physician.

A fifth-digit subclassification often is used in fracture coding to identify the specific site involved.

---

816   **Fracture of one or more phalanges of hand**

     Includes: finger(s)   thumb

The following fifth-digit subclassification is for use with category 816:

     0   **phalanx or phalanges, unspecified**
     1   **middle or proximal phalanx or phalanges**
     2   **distal phalanx or phalanges**
     3   **multiple sites**

816.0   **Closed**

816.1   **Open**

In the preceding example, the fourth digit describes a closed or open fracture of the phalanges, with the fifth digit identifying the specific site.

Dislocations

A dislocation is the displacement of a bone out of its joint. The most common joints affected are the fingers, thumb, and shoulder. Pain and swelling occur, as well as loss of use of the injured part. For healing, the dislocation can be reduced and immobilized with a cast. ICD-9-CM classifies dislocations or displacements to categories 830–839, which also include subluxations (incomplete or partial dislocations). Again, the classification differentiates between open and closed dislocations. Open dislocations are identified with the terms *compound, infected,* or *with foreign body,* whereas closed dislocations are associated with the terms *closed, complete, partial, simple, uncomplicated,* and *dislocation, NOS.*

A dislocation that is not specified as closed or open should be classified as closed. As with fractures, ICD-9-CM uses the fourth-digit subcategory to designate whether the dislocation is open or closed and the fifth digit identifies the specific site of the injury. For example:

---

832   Dislocation of elbow
The following fifth-digit subclassification is for use with category 832:
- **0   elbow unspecified**
- **1   anterior dislocation of elbow**
- **2   posterior dislocation of elbow**
- **3   medial dislocation of elbow**
- **4   lateral dislocation of elbow**
- **9   other**

832.0   Closed dislocation
832.1   Open dislocation

Sprains and Strains

A sprain is a stretching or tearing injury of the supporting ligaments of a joint, which results from the turning or twisting of a body part beyond its normal range of motion. Sprains are characterized by extreme pain, swelling, and discoloration, and they require rest for the injury to heal. Whiplash is a specific type of sprain constituting a compression of the cervical spine that involves the bones, joints, and intervertebral disks, usually due to a sudden throwing of the head forward and then backward.

A strain is a simple overstretching or overexertion of some part of a musculo-tendinous structure (muscle and tendon) that usually responds to rest. ICD-9-CM classifies sprains and strains to categories 840–848, which further subdivide to identify the specific body sites affected.

Codes within the categories 840–848 are current injuries. Patients also may suffer from chronic strains of the neck or back or derangements of different joints. The physician may describe these conditions as chronic, old, or recurrent. Using terms such as *sprain/strain* or *derangement,* the coder should refer to the subterm for the site and another subterm to describe the chronic, old, or recurrent condition. The coder will be referred to codes within the diseases of the musculoskeletal system categories (710–739).

Intracranial Injuries, Excluding Those with Skull Fracture

Intracranial injuries, excluding those with skull fracture, are classified to categories 850–854. At the beginning of this section, the following note appears: "The description 'with open intracranial wound,' used in the fourth-digit subdivisions, includes those specified as open or with mention of infection or foreign body." The note indicates that the fourth-digit subdivision describing an open intracranial wound should be assigned when a diagnostic statement includes the terms *open, infected,* or *foreign body.* In addition, categories 851–854 require the assignment of a fifth digit to indicate the state of consciousness and whether concussion was present. Without further specification, intracranial injury is reported with category 854. Head injury, unspecified, is reported with code 959.01.

Cerebral Concussion

A cerebral concussion is a transient loss of consciousness (less than 24 hours) after a traumatic head injury. Although no intracranial damage occurs, the patient may experience bradycardia, hypotension, and respiratory arrest for a few seconds, as well as retrograde and posttraumatic amnesia. The patient is put under 48-hour observation to check for the development of complications. A computerized axial tomography (CAT) scan may be performed to rule out any intracranial injury. ICD-9-CM classifies concussion to category 850, which further subdivides to identify the level of consciousness and the length of time that a patient has been unconscious.

> **EXAMPLE:** 850.1 With brief loss of consciousness
> 850.11 with loss of consciousness of 30 minutes or less
> 850.12 with loss of consciousness from 31 to 59 minutes

Cerebral Contusion and Laceration

Often caused by a blow to the head, a cerebral contusion is a more severe injury than a concussion. It refers to a bruise of the brain with bleeding into brain tissue, but without disruption of brain continuity. The loss of consciousness that occurs often lasts longer than it does in the case of a concussion. A laceration or fracture often accompanies the contusion. Any type of laceration of the brain results in some destruction of brain tissue and a subsequent scarring that may cause posttraumatic epilepsy. ICD-9-CM classifies cerebral contusion and laceration to category 851, which further subdivides to identify the following:

- The specific part of the brain affected (cortex or cerebellum)

- The type of injury (contusion or laceration, with or without open intracranial wound)

- The level of consciousness, as indicated by a fifth digit

Subdural, Subarachnoid, and Extradural Hemorrhage or Hematoma

A subdural hematoma or hemorrhage is the formation of a hematoma between the dura and the leptomeninges. Often resulting from a tear in the arachnoid, the acute form is associated with a laceration or contusion. Chronic subdural hematomas may result from closed head injuries such as falls. Symptoms include headache, increasing drowsiness, hemiparesis, and seizures. Subarachnoid hematoma or hemorrhage occurs directly underneath the arachnoid. ICD-9-CM classifies these hematomas or hemorrhages to category 852, which further subdivides to identify the following:

- The location of the hematoma or hemorrhage (subdural, subarachnoid, or extradural)

- The associated injury (with or without open intracranial wound)

- The level of consciousness, as indicated by a fifth digit

Internal Injury of Thorax, Abdomen, and Pelvis

Internal injuries of the thorax, abdomen, and pelvis are classified to categories 860–869. The fourth-digit subcategories describe the presence or absence of an open wound, and the fifth-digit subclassification identifies the injury's specific site, type, or severity. For example:

> **861.0**　**Heart, without mention of open wound into thorax**
> 　　**861.00**　**Unspecified injury**
> 　　**861.01**　**Contusion**
> 　　　　Cardiac contusion
> 　　　　Myocardial contusion
> 　　**861.02**　**Laceration without penetration of heart chambers**
> 　　**861.03**　**Laceration with penetration of heart chambers**

Open Wounds

An open wound is an injury of the soft tissue parts associated with rupture of the skin. Wounds may be described as crushed, incised, punctured, penetrating, and so on. A penetrating wound involves the passage of an object through tissue, leaving an entrance and exit wound, as in the case of a knife or gunshot wound. The seriousness of a wound depends on its site and extent. When a major vessel or organ is involved, a wound may be life threatening. For example, the rupture of a large artery or vein may cause blood to accumulate in one of the body cavities. This is referred to as hemothorax, hemopericardium, hemoperitoneum, or hemarthrosis, depending on the body cavity involved. The significance of the hemorrhage depends on the volume and rate of blood loss, and the site of the hemorrhage. Large losses may induce hemorrhagic shock.

In ICD-9-CM, open wounds are classified to categories 870–897. The exclusion note at the beginning of this section identifies other wounds that are classified elsewhere in the ICD-9-CM system. For example:

> OPEN WOUND (870–897)
> Includes:　　animal bite　　　laceration
> 　　　　　　avulsion　　　　puncture wound
> 　　　　　　cut　　　　　　traumatic amputation
> *Excludes:*　*burn (940.0–949.5)*
> 　　　　　*crushing (925–929.9)*
> 　　　　　*puncture of internal organs (860.0–869.1)*
> 　　　　　*superficial injury (910.0–919.9)*
> 　　　　　*that incidental to:*
> 　　　　　　*dislocation (830.0–839.9)*
> 　　　　　　*fracture (800.0–829.1)*
> 　　　　　　*internal injury (860.0–869.1)*
> 　　　　　　*intracranial injury (851.0–854.1)*

The notations included at the beginning of this section should be reviewed. The following definition is provided to describe the term *complicated:* "The description 'complicated' used in the fourth-digit subdivisions includes those with mention of delayed healing, delayed treatment, foreign body, or infection." This definition contains specific criteria that must be documented in the health record before a code is selected to describe a complicated wound. The coder is reminded to "use additional code to identify infection."

EXAMPLE:　　Delayed healing of open wound of foot: 892.1, Complicated open wound of foot except toe(s) alone

Because the diagnostic statement includes the phrase *delayed healing,* the wound is considered complicated and code 892.1 is assigned.

ICD-9-CM uses the fourth-digit subcategories and the fifth-digit subclassification to identify the type of open wound, site of wound, complicated or uncomplicated wounds, and involvement of tendon. For example:

874   Open wound of neck
    874.0   Larynx and trachea, without mention of complication
        874.00   Larynx with trachea
        874.01   Larynx
        874.02   Trachea
    874.1   Larynx and trachea, complicated
        874.10   Larynx with trachea
        874.11   Larynx
        874.12   Trachea

880   Open wound of shoulder and upper arm
    The following fifth-digit subclassification is for use with category 880:
        0   shoulder region
        1   scapular region
        2   axillary region
        3   upper arm
        9   multiple sites
    880.0   Without mention of complication
    880.1   Complicated
    880.2   With tendon involvement

Burns

Burns are assigned to categories 940–949 in ICD-9-CM. These injuries include burns caused by electricity, flame, hot objects, lightning, radiation, chemicals, and scalding.

Current burns also are classified by depth, extent, and, where needed, agent (E code). By depth, burns are classified as first, second, and third degree. A first-degree burn is the least severe and involves damage to the epidermis or outer layer of skin alone. A second-degree burn involves the epidermis and dermis. There is edema and blistering of the skin, which is red and moist. A third-degree burn is the most severe and includes all three layers of skin: epidermis, dermis, and subcutaneous. The skin appears charred, white, and dry.

The following coding guidelines apply to burn injuries:

1. Code all burns with the highest degree of burn sequenced first.

2. Classify burns of the same local site (three-digit category level, 940–947), but of different degrees, to the subcategory identifying the highest degree recorded in the diagnosis.

3. Code nonhealing burns as acute burns. Code necrosis of burned skin as a nonhealed burn.

4. Assign code 958.3, Posttraumatic wound infection, not elsewhere classified, as an additional code for any documented infected burn site. Use an additional code to identify the organism.

5. To code multiple burns, assign separate codes for each site. Use category 946, Burns of multiple specified sites, only when the location of the burns is not documented. Category 949, Burn, unspecified, is extremely vague and should be used only rarely.

6. Assign codes from category 948, Burns classified according to extent of body surface involved, when the site of the burn is not specified or to code the percent of body surface burned. In assigning a code from category 948:

   - Fourth-digit codes are used to identify the percentage of total body surface involved in a burn (all degrees).

   - Fifth digits are assigned to identify the percentage of body surface involved in third-degree burns.

   - Fifth digit zero (0) is assigned when no body surface, or less than 10 percent of the body surface, is involved in a third-degree burn.

   Category 948 is based on the classic "rule of nines" in estimating body surface involved: head and neck are assigned 9 percent; each arm, 9 percent; each leg, 18 percent; anterior trunk, 18 percent; posterior trunk, 18 percent; and genitalia, 1 percent. (See figure 19.1.) Physicians may change these percentage assignments, when necessary, to accommodate infants and children who have proportionately larger heads than adults, as well as patients whose abdomens, buttocks, or thighs are proportionately larger than normal.

7. Code encounters for the treatment of the late effects of burns (that is, scars or joint contractures) to the residual condition (sequelae), followed by the appropriate late effect code (906.5–906.9). A late effect E code also may be used, if desired.

8. When appropriate, both a sequela with a late effect code and a current burn code may be assigned on the same record.

Figure 19.1.   Rule of nines

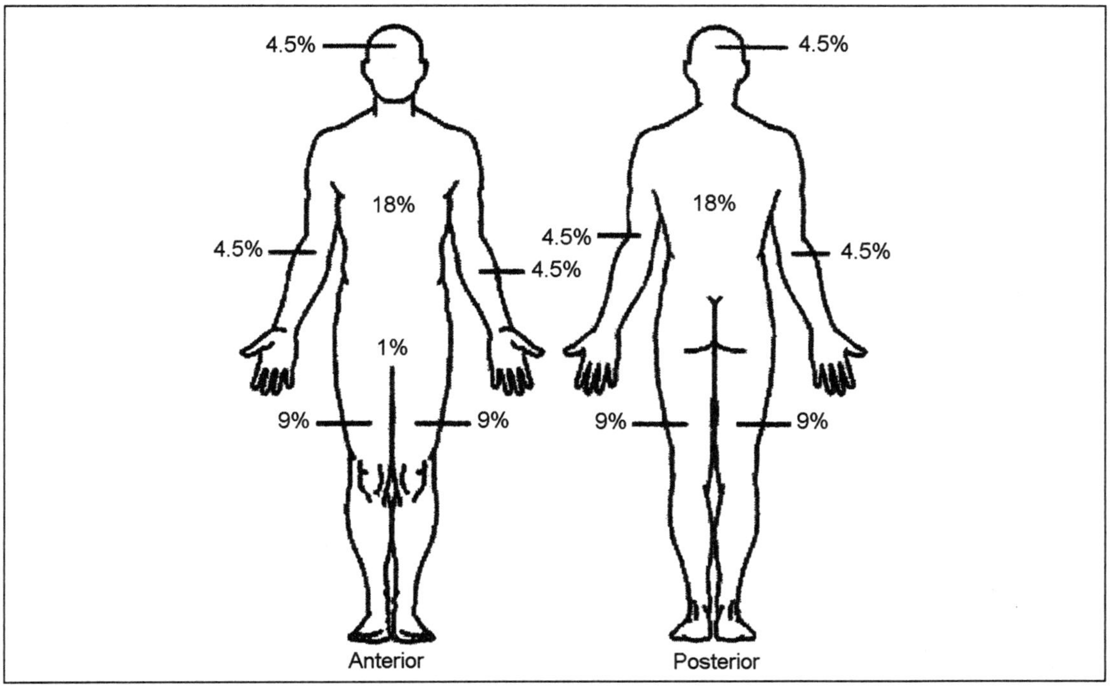

Superficial Injuries

Superficial injuries are classified to categories 910–919. This section of ICD-9-CM includes a variety of superficial injuries from abrasions to splinters. The fourth-digit subcategories specify type of injury and presence or absence of infection. For example:

<table>
<tr><td>910</td><td colspan="2">Superficial injury of face, neck, and scalp, except eye</td></tr>
<tr><td></td><td>910.0</td><td>Abrasion or friction burn without mention of infection</td></tr>
<tr><td></td><td>910.1</td><td>Abrasion or friction burn, infected</td></tr>
<tr><td></td><td>910.2</td><td>Blister without mention of infection</td></tr>
<tr><td></td><td>910.3</td><td>Blister, infected</td></tr>
<tr><td></td><td>910.4</td><td>Insect bite, nonvenomous, without mention of infection</td></tr>
<tr><td></td><td>910.5</td><td>Insect bite, nonvenomous, infected</td></tr>
<tr><td></td><td>910.6</td><td>Superficial foreign body (splinter) without major open wound and without mention of infection</td></tr>
<tr><td></td><td>910.7</td><td>Superficial foreign body (splinter) without major open wound, infected</td></tr>
<tr><td></td><td>910.8</td><td>Other and unspecified superficial injury of face, neck, and scalp without mention of infection</td></tr>
<tr><td></td><td>910.9</td><td>Other and unspecified superficial injury of face, neck, and scalp, infected</td></tr>
</table>

Bites

Bites or stings from venomous animals or insects are reported with code 989.5, Toxic effect of venomous substance. This includes bites from creatures such as snakes, lizards, spiders, bees, and wasps, among others.

Contusions with Intact Skin Surface

Contusions are injuries of the soft tissue. Although the skin is not broken, the small vessels, or capillaries, rupture and bleed into the tissue. When blood becomes trapped in the interstitial spaces, the result is a hematoma.

ICD-9-CM classifies these types of contusions to categories 920–924. The fourth-digit subcategories are further subdivided to identify the specific site involved. However, superficial injuries such as abrasions or contusions are not coded when associated with more severe injuries (such as fractures and open wounds) of the same site.

Crushing Injuries

Crushing injuries (codes 925–929) quite often occur in the industrial setting. Avulsion (tearing away) of skin and fat or a friction burn of the tissues may result. Abrasion burns are often severe, including third degree. Vessels, nerves, and muscles may be avulsed, and bones may be dislocated or fractured. A common complication is secondary congestion, which can lead to paralysis and severe muscle fibrosis and joint stiffness. Often the overall circulation of the extremity is of greater concern than definitive management of specific structures.

Injuries to Blood Vessels

Injuries to blood vessels are included in categories 900–904. Codes in these categories include arterial hematomas, avulsions, cuts, lacerations, ruptures, and traumatic aneurysms and fistulas secondary to other injuries, such as fractures or open wounds. These codes are usually assigned as additional diagnoses, with the underlying injury listed first.

> **EXAMPLE:** Open wound of the forearm with injury to the ulnar blood vessel: 881.00, Open wound of forearm without mention of complication; 903.3, Injury to ulnar blood vessels

Injuries to Nerves and Spinal Cord

Injuries to the nerves and spinal cord are classified to categories 950–957. This section of the ICD-9-CM codebook includes injuries with or without the presence of an open wound.

Category 952, Spinal cord injury without evidence of spinal bone injury, further subdivides at the fourth- and fifth-digit levels to identify the specific site involved.

When the primary injury is to the blood vessels or nerves, the primary injury is listed first. In cases where a primary injury results in minor damage to peripheral nerves or blood vessels, the primary injury is still listed first, with additional code(s) from categories 950–957, Injury to nerves and spinal cord, and/or 900–904, Injury to blood vessels.

Effects of Foreign Bodies Entering through Orifice

Foreign objects often are found in various body openings in the pediatric population. Children may insert small items into the nose or ear or swallow coins or marbles.

Foreign objects also may lodge in the larynx, bronchi, or esophagus, usually during eating. Laryngeal foreign bodies may produce hoarseness, coughing, and gagging, and partially obstruct the airway, causing stridor. Grasping forceps through a direct laryngoscope can remove laryngeal foreign bodies.

Bronchial foreign bodies usually produce an initial episode of coughing followed by an asymptomatic period before obstructive and inflammatory symptoms occur. Bronchial foreign bodies are removed through a bronchoscope.

Esophageal foreign bodies produce immediate symptoms such as difficulty in swallowing and coughing and/or gagging with the sensation of something "stuck in the throat." These can be removed through an esophagoscope.

Intraocular foreign bodies require removal by an ophthalmic surgeon. Examples of foreign materials that can affect the eyes include airborne debris, metal fragments, and dislodged contact lenses.

ICD-9-CM classifies foreign bodies in orifices to categories 930–939. These categories are further subdivided to identify the specific site or orifice. These codes can be found in the Alphabetic Index by referencing the main term **"Foreign body"** and the subterm "entering through orifice." When the foreign body is associated with an open wound, it is coded as open wound, complicated, by site.

A foreign body inadvertently left in an operative wound is considered a complication of the procedure and is coded as 998.4.

Injuries Resulting from Other and Unspecified Effects of External Causes

Categories 990–995 include codes to describe conditions that are the result of external causes, such as radiation sickness, frostbite, heatstroke or sunstroke, mountain sickness, and electric shocks, as well as adverse effects not classified elsewhere. Specific categories are discussed in the following subsections.

Category 991

Category 991 includes codes that describe conditions of reduced temperature, such as:

- 991.0–991.3, Frostbite
- 991.4, Immersion foot (trench foot)
- 991.5, Chilblains
- 991.6, Hypothermia (as a result of environmental temperature)
- 991.8, Other specified effects of reduced temperature
- 991.9, Unspecified effect of reduced temperature

Category 992

Category 992 includes codes that describe the effects of heat and light, such as:

- 992.0, Heatstroke and sunstroke
- 992.1, Heat syncope
- 992.2, Heat cramps
- 992.3, Heat exhaustion, anhydrotic (due to water depletion)
- 992.4, Heat exhaustion due to salt depletion
- 992.5, Heat exhaustion, unspecified
- 992.6, Heat fatigue, transient
- 992.7, Heat edema
- 992.8, Other specified heat effects
- 992.9, Unspecified heat and light effects

Category 995

Category 995 includes codes that describe adverse effects not classified elsewhere in ICD-9-CM. For example, anaphylactic shock (995.0) is a reaction marked by a sudden onset of rapidly progressing urticaria and respiratory distress. This code is appropriate in situations when anaphylactic shock is due to an adverse effect of a correct medicinal substance properly administered or to situations not otherwise specified. Underlying conditions should be coded first, such as poisonings by drugs, medicinals, and biologic substances chiefly nonmedicinal as to the source. E codes may be assigned to identify the external cause. This code excludes anaphylactic reaction due to serum (999.4) and anaphylactic shock due to adverse food reactions (995.6–995.7), a code that specifies shock due to nonpoisonous foods such as peanuts, milk products, and eggs.

Code 995.2, Unspecified adverse effect of drug, medicinal and biological substance, is used to identify an adverse reaction when the specific type of reaction is not documented. This code is used in the outpatient setting and is inappropriate for inpatient reporting.

Allergic reaction without further specification is reported with code 995.3. A review of the health record is warranted to determine the underlying cause of the allergy. When the information is unavailable, code 995.3 may be reported.

Adverse food reactions that cannot be classified to specific body systems (for example, allergic gastroenteritis or allergic rhinitis) are assigned to code 995.7.

Child maltreatment is classified to subcategory 995.5, with the fifth digit identifying the specific type of maltreatment, such as shaken infant syndrome (995.55), nutritional neglect (995.52), or emotional/psychological abuse (995.51) (*Coding Clinic,* 4th Quarter 1996).

Adult abuse is classified to codes 995.80–995.85. As with the child maltreatment codes, the fifth digit identifies the specific abuse—for example, sexual abuse (995.83) or physical abuse (995.81). When reporting child and adult maltreatment codes, the coder also should report codes describing physical injuries, such as fractures, contusions, and burns.

Systemic inflammatory response syndrome (SIRS) is classified to code 995.9, with fifth digits indicating whether it was due to an infectious or noninfectious process and also whether there was organ dysfunction. The coder is instructed to code first the underlying systemic infection. When organ dysfunction is present, the coder should use an additional code to identify the specific organ dysfunction, such as respiratory failure.

V Codes

Several V code categories and subcategory codes are applicable to chapter 17, including:

V51	Aftercare involving the use of plastic surgery
V52.0	Fitting and adjustment of artificial arm
V52.1	Fitting and adjustment of artificial leg
V53.7	Fitting and adjustment of orthopedic devices
V54	Other orthopedic aftercare
V57	Care involving use of rehabilitation procedures
V67.00	Follow-up exam following surgery, unspecified
V67.4	Follow-up exam following treatment of healed fracture

Detailed descriptions of V codes are provided in chapter 2 of this workbook.

External Causes of Injury and Other Adverse Effects (E Codes)

ICD-9-CM includes a supplementary classification to identify external causes of injury and other conditions (commonly referred to as E codes). E codes provide data for injury research and evaluation of prevention strategies. This supplementary classification includes broad categories describing specific causes of injury and other conditions, such as transport accidents, accidental poisonings, suicide attempts, fires, hurricanes, and tornadoes. E codes help to identify the following circumstances:

- How the injury or poisoning occurred (cause—for example, a fall or a flood)

- Why the injury or poisoning occurred (intent—for example, an accident or a suicide)

- Where the injury or poisoning occurred (place—for example, a home or a public building)

The chapter on external causes in ICD-9-CM includes the following sections:

Categories	**Section Titles**
E800–E848	Transport Accidents
E849	Place of Occurrence
E850–E858	Accidental Poisoning by Drugs, Medicinal Substances, and Biologicals
E860–E869	Accidental Poisoning by Other Solid and Liquid Substances, Gases, and Vapors
E870–E876	Misadventures to Patients During Surgical and Medical Care
E878–E879	Surgical and Medical Procedures as the Cause of Abnormal Reaction of Patient or Later Complication, without Mention of Misadventure at the Time of Procedure
E880–E888	Accidental Falls
E890–E899	Accidents Caused by Fire and Flames
E900–E909	Accidents Due to Natural and Environmental Factors
E910–E915	Accidents Caused by Submersion, Suffocation, and Foreign Bodies
E916–E928	Other Accidents
E929	Late Effects of Accidental Injury
E930–E949	Drugs, Medicinal and Biological Substances Causing Adverse Effects in Therapeutic Use
E950–E959	Suicide and Self-inflicted Injury
E960–E969	Homicide and Injury Purposely Inflicted by Other Persons
E970–E978	Legal Intervention
E979	Terrorism
E980–E989	Injury Undetermined Whether Accidentally or Purposely Inflicted
E990–E999	Injury Resulting from Operations of War

E codes from the supplementary classification are used in addition to a code from the main body of the classification and cannot be assigned as solo codes. They provide additional information that may be extremely useful to public health agencies and may help healthcare planners determine the kinds of accidents a particular facility treats.

Fourth-Digit Subdivisions

Fourth digits are provided in many E code categories to identify the injured person. Those categories requiring fourth digits are preceded by a section mark to refer to a footnote at the bottom of the page. Fourth-digit subdivisions for the external cause (E) code appear immediately after the Alphabetic Index to External Causes. The fourth-digit subdivisions also appear in the Tabular List of E codes.

The fourth-digit subdivisions are specific to each of the following E code category groups:

RAILWAY ACCIDENTS (E800–E807)
MOTOR VEHICLE TRAFFIC AND NONTRAFFIC ACCIDENTS (E810–E825)
OTHER ROAD VEHICLE ACCIDENTS (E826–E829)
WATER TRANSPORT ACCIDENTS (E830–E838)
AIR AND SPACE TRANSPORT ACCIDENTS (E840–E845)

Alphabetic Index to External Causes

The Alphabetic Index to External Causes of Injury and Poisoning is a separate index that follows the Table of Drugs and Chemicals (in most codebooks). It is organized by main terms (in boldface type) describing the accident, circumstance, event, or specific agent that caused the injury or other adverse effect, such as collision, earthquake, or dog bite. For example:

Bite
    animal (nonvenomous) NEC E906.5
        other specified (except arthropod) E906.3
        venomous NEC E905.9
    arthropod (nonvenomous) NEC E906.4
        venomous—*see* sting
    black widow spider E905.1
    cat E906.3
    centipede E905.4
    cobra E905.0
    copperhead snake E905.0
    Coral snake E905.0

Use of E Codes

In many healthcare settings, the use of E codes is optional, except for categories E930–E949 in the section titled Drugs, Medicinal, and Biological Substances Causing Adverse Effects in Therapeutic Use. An E code may be used as an additional code in any category when the documentation in the health record supports that use, but it cannot be assigned as a principal diagnosis.

E Codes for Place of Occurrence

Subcategory E849, Place of occurrence, is provided to note the place where an injury or poisoning occurred. Code E849 and its subdivisions are italicized in the Tabular List to indicate that this code is not to be used for primary tabulation. The E code identifying the cause of the accident, event, or adverse effect must be assigned first, followed by the place of occurrence E code, where applicable. Place of occurrence E codes can be located in the Alphabetic Index to External Causes under "**Accident** (to), occurring (at) (in)."

E Codes for Late Effects

When the condition being coded is a late effect of an illness or injury, the E code for the late effect must be assigned rather than a current E code, if the healthcare facility assigns E codes. The E codes for external causes of late effects include:

- E929, Late effects of accidental injury
- E959, Late effects of self-inflicted injury
- E969, Late effects of injury purposely inflicted by other person
- E977, Late effects of injuries due to legal intervention
- E989, Late effects of injury, undetermined whether accidentally or purposely inflicted
- E999, Late effects of injury due to war operations and terrorism

Late effect E codes are found in the Alphabetic Index to External Causes under **"Late effect of."**

Coding Guidelines for E Codes

The general guidelines related to the use of E codes include:

1. An E code may be used with any code in the 001–V83 range to indicate an injury, poisoning, or adverse effect due to an external cause.

2. The appropriate E code should be assigned for all initial treatments of an injury, poisoning, or adverse effect of drugs. If the visit is not for the initial treatment, an E code should not be assigned.

3. A late effect E code should be used for subsequent visits when a late effect of the initial injury or poisoning is being treated. There is no late effect E code for adverse effect of drugs. If the initial injury or poisoning does not result in a residual, a late effect code should not be assigned.

4. The full range of E codes should be used to completely describe the cause, intent, and place of occurrence, if applicable, for all injuries, poisonings, and adverse effects of drugs.

5. As many E codes as necessary should be assigned to fully explain each cause. If only one E code can be reported, the E code most related to the principal diagnosis should be assigned.

6. The selection of the appropriate E code is guided by the Index to External Causes, which follows the Table of Drugs and Chemicals, and by inclusion and exclusion notes in the Tabular List.

7. An E code can never be used as a principal diagnosis.

Child and Adult Abuse Guidelines for E Codes

When the cause of an injury or neglect is intentional child or adult abuse (995.50–995.59, 995.80–995.85), the first E code listed should be assigned from categories E960–E966, E968 or 969, Homicide and Injury Purposely Inflicted by Other Persons. An E code from category E967, Perpetrator of child and adult abuse, should be added as an additional E code to identify the perpetrator, when known. Inclusion terms for codes E967.0 and E967.2 include the partner of the child's parent or guardian. An inclusion term for code E967.3 is added to better explain the relationship between perpetrator and victim. E967.3 is used when the perpetrator is the spouse, ex-spouse, partner, or ex-partner of the victim.

External Cause Code(s) with Systemic Inflammatory Response Syndrome (SIRS) Guidelines for E Codes

An external cause code(s) may be used with codes 995.93, Systemic inflammatory response syndrome due to noninfectious process without organ dysfunction, and 995.94, Systemic inflammatory response syndrome due to noninfectious process with organ dysfunction, if trauma was the initiating insult that precipitated the SIRS. The external cause code(s) should correspond to the most serious injury resulting from the trauma. The external cause code(s) should only be assigned if the trauma necessitated the admission in which the patient also developed SIRS. If a patient is admitted with SIRS but the trauma has been treated previously, the external cause codes should not be used.

In cases of neglect when the intent is determined to be accidental, the first E code listed should be E904.0, Abandonment or neglect of infants and helpless persons.

Poisonings and Adverse Effects of Drugs

ICD-9-CM provides two different sets of code numbers to differentiate between poisonings and adverse effects or reactions to substances. A separate index called the Table of Drugs and Chemicals follows the Alphabetic Index to Diseases and Injuries. It is used to code poisonings and adverse reactions.

The Table of Drugs and Chemicals provides an alphabetic listing of drugs and other agents. The first column identifies the specific substance. The second column is used when a particular case meets the criteria for poisoning (the criteria follow). The remaining five columns describe the circumstance (E code) under which the adverse reaction or poisoning occurred.

Adverse Effects of Drugs

Adverse effects of, or reactions to, drugs can occur in situations where the medication is properly administered and correctly prescribed in both therapeutic and diagnostic procedures. Common causes of adverse effects include:

- Cumulative effects (often documented as drug toxicity in the health record) that result when the inactivation and/or excretion of the drug is slower than the rate at which the drug is being administered

- Hypersensitivities or allergic reactions that occur as qualitatively different responses to a drug, which are acquired only after reexposure to the drug

- Synergistic reactions that enhance the effect of another drug administered prior to, or concurrent with, the drug

- Interactions with another prescribed medication that result in a change in the effectiveness of the drug

- Side effects that have unwanted, predictable pharmacologic effects that occur within therapeutic code ranges

The following instructions should be followed for the coding of adverse effects of drugs:

1. Code the manifestation or the nature of the adverse reaction, such as urticaria, vertigo, gastritis, and so on.

2. Locate the drug in the substance column of the Table of Drugs and Chemicals in the Alphabetic Index.

3. Select the E code for the drug from the therapeutic use column of the Table of Drugs and Chemicals.

> **EXAMPLE:** Atrial tachycardia due to digitalis glycosides toxicity:
> 427.89, Other specified cardiac dysrhythmias (atrial tachycardia);
> E942.1, Cardiotonic glycosides and drugs of similar action causing
> adverse effects in therapeutic use (adverse effect of digitalis)

4. If the adverse effect is the result of the interaction between two or more prescription drugs, assign E codes for both drugs.

> **EXAMPLE:** Premature supraventricular beats due to the interaction of digitalis glycosides and Valium, both correctly prescribed and administered: 427.61, Supraventricular premature beats; E942.1, Cardiotonic glycosides and drugs of similar action causing adverse effects in therapeutic use (adverse effect of digitalis); E939.4, Benzodiazepine-based tranquilizers causing adverse effects in therapeutic use (adverse effect of Valium)

5. Code late effects of an adverse effect of a correct substance properly administered as follows:

    a. Code first the residual or late effect, such as blindness or deafness.

    b. Assign code 909.5, Late effect of adverse effect of drug, medicinal or biological substance, to identify a late effect of an adverse reaction. Look in the Alphabetic Index to Diseases under "**Late,** effect(s) (of), adverse effect of drug, medicinal or biological substance" to locate code 909.5.

    c. Note that a specific E code is not provided to identify the external cause of a late effect of an adverse reaction to a correct substance properly administered. The E code is the same as the original selected from the therapeutic use column of the Table of Drugs and Chemicals.

> **EXAMPLE:** Hearing loss occurring as a result of previously administered streptomycin therapy: 389.9, Unspecified hearing loss; 909.5, Late effect of adverse effect of drug, medicinal or biological substance; E930.6, Antimycobacterial antibiotics causing adverse effects in therapeutic use

The following diagram illustrates the process for coding adverse reactions to correct substances properly administered. **It is important to remember that the use of a code from E930–E949 is mandatory for adverse effects.**

Code current effect (for example, coma)	← *Principal Diagnosis* →	Code late effect (for example, blindness)
		Plus Late effect 909.5
And		**And**
E code from therapeutic use column of Table of Drugs and Chemicals (E930–E949)	← *Other Diagnosis* →	E code from therapeutic use column of Table of Drugs and Chemicals (E930–E949)

Unspecified Adverse Effects of Drugs

Sometimes an adverse effect of a drug is unknown or, more often, not documented in the health record. Unspecified adverse effects of drugs are usually indicated by diagnostic statements, such as:

- Toxic effect of

- Drug toxicity

- Drug intoxication

- Drug allergy/hypersensitivity

The following coding instructions apply to assigning codes for unspecified adverse effects:

1. To indicate an unspecified adverse effect or drug allergy, first assign code 995.2, Unspecified adverse effect of drug, medicinal and biological substance. Code 995.2 is found in the Alphabetic Index under "**Effect, adverse** NEC, drugs and medicinals NEC." When the health record includes phrases such as *drug intoxication* without further specification as to the effect, assign code 796.0, Nonspecific abnormal toxicological findings. Code 995.2 should never be used to report an unspecified adverse effect of a drug or a medicinal or biological substance in the inpatient setting.

2. Assign an E code from the therapeutic use column of the Table of Drugs and Chemicals to describe the drug or medicinal substance causing the unspecified adverse effect.

    > **EXAMPLE:**   Digitalis intoxication: 796.0, Nonspecific abnormal toxicologic findings; E942.1, Cardiotonic glycosides and drugs of similar action causing adverse effects in therapeutic use (adverse effect of digitalis)

    > **EXAMPLE:**   Unspecified drug reaction to Dilantin: 995.2, Unspecified adverse effect of drug, medicinal and biological substance; E936.1, Hydantoin derivatives and drugs of similar action causing adverse effects in therapeutic use

    If the drug causing the unspecified adverse reaction is unknown, assign code E947.9, Unspecified drug or medicinal substance. This code is indexed under "Drug" in the Table of Drugs and Chemicals.

3. A late effect of an unspecified adverse effect is coded in the same manner as late effects of specified adverse effects, as follows:

    a. Code first the residual or late effect, such as blindness or deafness.

    b. Assign code 909.5, Late effect of adverse effect of drug, medicinal or biological substance, to identify a late effect of an unspecified adverse reaction. Look in the Alphabetic Index under "**Late,** effect(s) (of), adverse effect of drug, medicinal or biological substance" to locate code 909.5. If the specific residual is not identified, list code 909.5 first.

    c. Select the appropriate code from the therapeutic use column of the Table of Drugs and Chemicals to identify the drug involved.

EXAMPLE: Residuals of previous severe allergic reaction to chemotherapy (Fluorouracil), which was discontinued six months earlier: 909.5, Late effect of adverse effect of drug, medicinal or biological substance; E933.1, Antineoplastic and immunosuppressive drugs causing adverse effects in therapeutic use (adverse effect of Fluorouracil)

The following diagram is designed to assist in coding unspecified adverse or allergic reactions. Use of a code from E930–E949 is mandatory.

Code 995.2, Unspecified adverse effect of drug, medicinal and biological substance	← *Principal Diagnosis* →	Code effect (if known) (for example, blindness)
Or		**Plus**
796.0, Nonspecific abnormal toxicological finding (angiotoxicity or intoxication)	← *Other Diagnosis* →	Late effect 909.5
And		**And**
E code from therapeutic use column of Table of Drugs and Chemicals (E930–E949)	← *Other Diagnosis* →	E code from therapeutic use column of Table of Drugs and Chemicals (E930–E949)

Poisonings

Poisoning refers to conditions caused by drugs, medicinal substances, and other biological substances only when the substance involved is not used according to a physician's instructions. Poisonings can occur in the following manner:

- Wrong dosage of medication given in error during a diagnostic or therapeutic procedure or during the course of medical care

- Wrong dosage of medication given in error by nonmedical personnel, such as a mother to an infant or a child to an elderly parent

- Medication given to a wrong person by medical or nonmedical personnel

- Medication taken by wrong person

- Wrong dosage of medication taken by self

- Intoxication (other than cumulative effect)

- Overdose

- Medications (prescription or nonprescription) taken in combination with alcoholic beverages

- Over-the-counter medications taken in combination with prescribed medications without consulting a physician

The following instructions apply to the coding of poisonings:

1. Use the Table of Drugs and Chemicals in the Alphabetic Index to locate the drug or other agent.

2. Assign the code from the poisoning column.

3. Code the specified effect of the poisoning, such as coma, vertigo, or drowsiness.

4. Identify the external cause of poisoning from the appropriate column of the Table of Drugs and Chemicals. The external cause is "Accident," unless the health record or coding rule specifies otherwise (that is, suicide attempt, assault). Although the use of E codes is optional for many providers, some states mandate the coding of external causes (E codes).

> **EXAMPLE:** Aspirin (over-the-counter pain medication) overdose resulting in a coma, suicide attempt: 965.1, Poisoning by salicylates (overdose on aspirin); 780.01, Coma; E950.0, Suicide and self-inflicted poisoning by analgesics, antipyretics, and antirheumatics (suicide attempt)

5. A late effect of a poisoning is coded as follows:

   a. Code first the residual (specified effect), such as deafness or blindness.

   b. Assign a code to identify a late effect of poisoning by drugs: 909.0, Late effect of poisoning due to drug, medicinal or biological substance (found in the Alphabetic Index to Diseases under "**Late,** effect(s) (of), poisoning due to drug, medicinal or biological substance"); or 909.1, Late effect of toxic effects of nonmedical substances (found in the Alphabetic Index under "**Late,** effect(s) (of), toxic effect of, nonmedical substance").

   c. Use the Alphabetic Index to External Causes of Injury and Poisoning to assign one of the following E codes to describe the late effect of an external cause:

      - Code E929.2, Late effects of accidental poisoning, which is found under "**Late effect of,** poisoning, accidental"

      - Code E959, Late effects of self-inflicted injury, which is found under "**Late effect of,** suicide, attempt (any means)"

      - Code E969, Late effects of injury purposely inflicted by other person, which is found under "**Late effect of,** assault"

      - Code E977, Late effects of injuries due to legal intervention, which is found under "**Late effect of,** legal intervention"

      - Code E989, Late effects of injury, undetermined whether accidentally or purposely inflicted, which is found under "**Late effect of,** injury undetermined whether accidentally or purposely inflicted"

The following diagram is designed for assistance in coding poisonings. As mentioned earlier, E codes for poisonings are generally optional, but many healthcare facilities do mandate their use. Codes that classify poisonings due to drugs (960–979) are never to be reported with codes that classify the external causes of adverse reactions to drugs taken therapeutically (E930–E949).

Code current injury from 960–979	← *Principal Diagnosis* →	Code specified late effect (for example, deafness)
Plus		**Plus**
Specified effect (for example, tachycardia)	← *Other Diagnosis* →	Late effect 909.0 or 909.1
And		**And**

E code from one of
the following external
cause columns of the
Table of Drugs and
Chemicals:
  accident
  suicide, attempt
  assault
  undetermined
	← *Other Diagnosis* →	E929.2 or E959 or
		E977 or E969 or E989

Chapter 19 Exercises

Review the following statements and assign the appropriate codes:

1. Simple greenstick fracture, shafts of tibia and fibula

    ____

2. Comminuted fracture of humerus

    ____

3. Fracture of femur due to gunshot wound

    ____

4. Compound fracture of lower end of ulna

    ____

5. Fracture of right fibula due to osteogenesis imperfecta

    ____

6. Anterior dislocation of the elbow

    ____

7. Sprain of lateral collateral ligament of knee

    ____

8. Chronic lumbosacral strain

    ____

Chapter 19 Exercises (Continued)

9. Concussion without loss of consciousness

10. Laceration of wrist with tendon involvement

11. Contusion of liver

12. Open frontal fracture with subarachnoid hemorrhage with brief loss of consciousness

13. Tibial shaft fracture

14. Dislocation of the first and second cervical vertebra

15. Cerebral contusion with brief loss of consciousness

16. Traumatic laceration of liver, moderate

17. Avulsion of eye

18. Traumatic below-the-knee amputation with delayed healing

19. Open wound of buttock

20. Nonvenomous insect bite, elbow, infected

21. Contusion of the lower leg and knee

22. Spinal cord injury, C1–C4

23. Crushing injury of left hand and wrist

24. Bean in nose

(Continued on next page)

Chapter 19 Exercises (Continued)

25. Q-tip stuck in ear

26. First- and second-degree burns of the palm

27. First-degree burn of the thigh and second-degree burn of the left arm

28. Splinter in left index finger with infection

29. Third-degree burns of chest and face (25 percent of body surface)

30. Second- and third-degree burn of back involving 20 percent of body surface

31. Ataxia due to interaction of carbamazepine and erythromycin

32. Constipation from Oncovin injected for Hodgkin's disease

33. Excessive drowsiness due to overdose of Periactin

34. Hemiplegia resulting from previous adverse reaction to Enovid

35. Residuals from previous episode of acute hypersensitivity to sulfonamide

36. Allergic reaction to unknown drug

37. Rash due to allergy to penicillin

Assign diagnosis codes and E codes to the following statements and cases, as appropriate:

38. Fracture, humerus (shaft); fell off ladder at home

39. Intracapsular fracture, neck of femur; patient slipped on ice when getting her mail

40. Fracture of second, third, and fourth ribs; patient was gored by a bull

Chapter 19 Exercises (Continued)

41. Headache, dizziness; box fell on the patient's head while she was grocery shopping

42. Compound fracture of right wrist; 13-year-old struck by car while he was delivering news-papers on his bike

43. Osteomyelitis of femur due to an old compound fracture resulting from an automobile accident six months ago in which the patient was the driver

44. Convulsions due to an old skull fracture sustained when the patient fell from a ladder two years ago

45. Scars of arm due to an old burn sustained in a house fire three years ago

46. Inpatient admission: The patient is a 33-year-old construction worker who fell three stories from scaffolding at a construction site. He struck his head and was unconscious for about 10 minutes. An x-ray showed that he had an open skull fracture with cerebral laceration and contusion. Patient complained of severe headache and dizziness.

    Discharge diagnoses: Headache and dizziness due to skull fracture; cerebral laceration and contusions

    Code(s):

47. Outpatient visit: The patient is a 10-year-old male who had just returned from a camping trip at summer camp. Apparently, he ran into a raspberry patch and was punctured by thorns. This morning, he awakened with a swollen, painful area on his calf. On examination, the puncture wounds had healed and required no treatment, but the patient was prescribed antibiotics for cellulitis.

    Impression: Cellulitis due to Streptococcus A

    Code(s):

48. Inpatient admission: The patient was drinking heavily when he slipped on the floor and dislocated his shoulder. He is a known chronic alcoholic with cirrhosis of the liver. Lab tests were performed to monitor the status of the cirrhosis, and the shoulder was replaced to its proper position.

    Discharge diagnoses: Dislocated shoulder; alcoholic cirrhosis of the liver

    Code(s):

49. Outpatient visit: The patient (the driver) was involved in a minor motor vehicle accident and went to his physician complaining about a painful right hand. The physician noticed the hand was swollen and painful to the touch and sent the patient to the local hospital for an x-ray to rule out a fractured hand.

    Impression: Suspected hand fracture

    Code(s):

(Continued on next page)

Chapter 19 Exercises (Continued)

50. Outpatient visit #1: The patient is a three-year-old whose clothing caught fire while she was helping her mother bake at home. She suffered first- and second-degree burns of the abdomen and right arm. The physician dressed the burns and prescribed antibiotics.

    Impression: Burns of the abdomen and right arm

    Code(s): ____

    Outpatient visit #2: The mother brings the child back to the physician because of nonhealing first- and second-degree burns that happened three weeks ago.

    Impression: Nonhealing burns

    Code(s): ____

51. Outpatient visit: A 31-year-old mine worker was severely burned several months ago while at work when a propane tank exploded near his face. At the time, he had second- and third-degree burns of the face and neck. He was seen in consultation by a plastic surgeon for severe fibrosis and scarring of the skin. A grafting procedure was scheduled.

    Impression: Fibrosis and scarring of the face; late effect of second- and third-degree burns of the face and neck

    Code(s): ____

52. Outpatient visit: The patient is a two-month-old female who was seen for a severe rash all over the body. She had been given penicillin last week for a suppurative otitis media. The physician examined her ears, which were still inflamed, and prescribed a sulfa drug for her ears and lotion for her rash.

    Impression: Reaction to penicillin; suppurative otitis media

    Code(s): ____

53. Outpatient visit: During a basketball game three nights ago, the patient fell on his right knee after being pushed by another player. An arthroscopy revealed medial meniscus tear.

    Impression: Medial meniscus tear

    Code(s): ____

54. Inpatient admission: The patient, a type II diabetic, was admitted with a fracture of the hip. X-rays revealed an intertrochanteric fracture, and the patient was taken to surgery for treatment.

    Discharge diagnoses: Fractured hip; type II diabetic

    Code(s): ____

55. Outpatient visit #1: The patient was seen by the physician with acute exacerbation of her asthma. The physician prescribed antibiotics, bronchodilators, and IV steroids.

    Impression: Acute exacerbation of asthma

    Code(s): ____

Chapter 19 Exercises (Continued)

Outpatient visit #2: The patient was seen experiencing jitteriness and anxiety due to an accidental overdose of Solu-Medrol (AHFS 68:04) that had been prescribed for her asthma, which is currently under control. She was cautioned to be careful about dosage amounts.

Impression: Accidental overdose of Solu-Medrol; asthma

Code(s):

---

56. Emergency department visit: A 22-year-old female was brought to emergency services in a semicomatose state. Her fiancé indicated that she had drunk between five and eight beers at dinner and then had taken a Valium to sleep. She was very unresponsive.

Impression: Adverse reaction to alcohol and drugs

Code(s):

---

57. Inpatient admission: History of present illness: This 16-year-old male was involved in a one-car accident at approximately 2 a.m. Apparently, the car skidded on some oil or water on the road and struck a mailbox. The patient was an unrestrained passenger who either struck the windshield or was thrown through it. He was diagnosed with an L-1 fracture, neurologically intact. In addition, he was noted to have a laceration of his left frontal parietal area. The laceration was debrided and repaired.

Pertinent lab and x-ray findings: White blood cell count on admission shows 12.7; hemoglobin and hematocrit 13.2 and 37.1, respectively; sodium 134; potassium 3.9; chloride 100; bicarb 25; glucose 96; creatinine 0.8; and BUN 7. Urinalysis also done on admission shows 3+ blood, 5 to 10 white cells, greater than 50 RBCs, otherwise unremarkable. Admission urine culture and sensitivity showed no growth. Blood flow studies showed the following impression: normal venous Doppler study. Thoracolumbar spine films showed the following: two views demonstrate a fracture of the first lumbar vertebral body. Most of the fracture involves the superior end plate. There is narrowing of the posterior aspect of the L-1/2 disc space, perhaps slight widening anteriorly. There are no other findings.

Pertinent physical findings: Patient is moving all extremities to command. He has no evidence of cyanosis or edema, and there are no palpable bony or joint abnormalities. He is drowsy, but easily arousable. He is oriented times 3. He responds appropriately to questions when asked. His sensation is intact to touch and pinprick throughout. Lower extremities 5/5 in all groups bilaterally. Deep tendon reflexes 2+ and equal bilaterally.

Hospital course: The patient was admitted to assess neurologic integrity and to begin definitive rehabilitation. As previously mentioned, although suffering from an L-1 fracture, the patient was neurologically intact. He was treated symptomatically for pain discomfort and to protect the spine. Then, he was given a lumbosacral orthosis and began sitting gradually. The patient tolerated that well and was ready for discharge. He was discharged home in the care of his mother with a prescription for the following medication: Vicodin, po q-4h prn for pain. At discharge, he was medically stable and on a regular diet. The patient was instructed to keep the brace on at all times except when bathing. He was further instructed to log roll when in bed and not to stretch, bend, or twist back. The patient was told to walk as much as possible, wear tennis shoes when walking, and when riding in the car to wear the seat belt. If he experienced any numbness, tingling, or loss of sensation at any time, he was instructed to call his attending physician immediately.

Discharge diagnoses: Lumbar fracture from motor vehicle accident; no loss of consciousness; laceration of left frontal parietal area

Code(s):

Review Questions

Answer the following questions:

1. How are multiple fractures coded?

2. For categories 850–854, what does the description "with open intracranial wound" mean as it is used in the fourth-digit subdivisions?

3. In relation to open wounds, what constitutes a "complicated" injury?

4. How are burns of the same site, but of different degrees, coded?

5. How are nonhealing burns coded?

6. When is it appropriate to use a code from category 948, Burns classified according to extent of body surface?

7. What categories of E codes are mandatory to use?

8. What are the appropriate E codes to use when a diagnosis of child or adult abuse is made?

9. What are common causes of adverse effects of drugs?

10. What code should be used when the specific adverse effect of drug use is not stated?

11. What types of adverse reactions to drugs are coded as "poisonings"?

12. How is a late effect of an adverse effect to a drug correctly taken coded?

13. How is a late effect of a poisoning coded?

Chapter 20

Complications of Surgical and Medical Care

Objectives

After completing this lesson, the student should be able to do the following:

- Apply knowledge of current, approved ICD-9-CM coding guidelines to assign and sequence accurate codes for diagnoses related to complications of surgical and medical care

- Identify locations in the Alphabetic Index where terms relating to complications of surgical and medical care can be found

- Differentiate between mechanical complications and reactions of the body to foreign bodies such as grafts, implants, and other prosthetic devices

Introduction

Complications of surgical and medical care that are not classified elsewhere in the ICD-9-CM codebook are assigned to categories 996–999, which are subdivided as follows:

Categories	Titles
996	Complications Peculiar to Certain Specified Procedures
997	Complications Affecting Specified Body Systems, Not Elsewhere Classified
998	Other Complications of Procedures, Not Elsewhere Classified
999	Complications of Medical Care, Not Elsewhere Classified

How to Determine Complications of Surgical or Medical Care

To properly classify complications, the coder must be certain that the complicating condition resulted from, or was caused by, the surgical or medical care rendered. When the complication is classified to the 996–999 series, an additional code for the specific complication may be assigned. For example, a patient with an indwelling catheter developed a streptococcal infection due to the catheter. The first code to assign is 996.64, Infection or inflammation due to indwelling urinary catheter. A note under code 996.64 advises the coder to "Use additional code to identify the specified infection." Therefore, code 041.00 also should be assigned to indicate the streptococcal organism.

A time limit has not been designated for using categories 996–999 because some complications may occur during or directly following surgery, during the same hospitalization, or several days, weeks, or months later.

In some cases, the documentation in the health record will clearly state a complication, such as colitis due to radiation therapy. In other cases, it will identify symptoms that may refer to a complication, such as red and warm surgical wound with drainage. Again, the physician should be asked to clarify whether a complication is present.

Complications specific to one anatomical site are classified in that anatomical site's chapter of the ICD-9-CM codebook. All other complications are included in codes 996–999.

EXAMPLE:	519.00	Unspecified tracheostomy complications
	579.2	Blind loop syndrome
	429.4	Functional disturbances following cardiac surgery

In ICD-9-CM, the long exclusion note appearing at the beginning of the complications section should be heeded.

COMPLICATIONS OF SURGICAL AND MEDICAL CARE,
NOT ELSEWHERE CLASSIFIED (996–999)

Excludes: *adverse effects of medicinal agents (001.0–799.9, 995.0–995.8)*
burns from local applications and irradiation (940.0–949.5)
complications of:
    conditions for which the procedure was performed
    surgical procedures during abortion, labor, and delivery
      (630–676.9)
poisoning and toxic effects of drugs and chemicals (960.0–989.9)
postoperative conditions in which no
      complications are present, such as:
    artificial opening status (V44.0–V44.9)
    closure of external stoma (V55.0–V55.9)
    fitting of prosthetic device (V52.0–V52.9)
specified complications classified elsewhere
    anesthetic shock (995.4)
    electrolyte imbalance (276.0–276.9)
    postlaminectomy syndrome (722.80–722.83)
    postmastectomy lymphedema syndrome (457.0)
    postoperative psychosis (293.0–293.9)
    any other condition classified elsewhere in the Alphabetic
      Index when described as due to a procedure

It should be noted that many complications/conditions are not classified to this section. For example, adverse effects of medicinal agents are assigned to codes 001.0–799.9 and 995.0–995.89.

Complications Described as Postoperative Conditions

Often physicians describe a condition that arises after surgery as being postoperative, even though it is not a complication of the surgery. Coders should ask the attending physician for clarification when there is no causal relationship between the postoperative condition and the surgical procedure. For example, a patient's blood pressure dropped to 87/42 postoperatively in the recovery room following repair of a right, recurrent inguinal hernia. The attending physician ordered Atropine 0.5 mg IV at 10:56 a.m. and again at 11:03 a.m. This episode of hypotension was not considered a complication of surgical care but, rather, a postoperative event.

Further, the attending physician should be queried about conditions such as postoperative fever and postoperative atelectasis (collapse of the lung) to determine whether these are "expected" occurrences from surgery or "unexpected" complications of surgical care. For example, an open-heart surgery patient's postoperative chest x-rays may show discoid atelectasis in both posterobasilar segments of the lung without evidence of pneumonia, edema, or failure. The physician should be queried as to whether the atelectasis was expected or unexpected and whether it required additional treatment (such as chest pulmonary toiletry and/or medication).

Coding Guidelines

The following coding guidelines apply to complications of surgical or medical care:

1. Locate the main term for the complication in the Alphabetic Index (for example, **"Malabsorption"**).

2. Check for a subterm indicating that the condition is a result of a complication of medical or surgical care. For example:

Malabsorption 579.9
   postsurgical 579.3

---

3. If a specific code is not identified, look under **"Complications"** to locate an appropriate code by condition or system. For example:

Complications
   aortocoronary (bypass) graft 996.03

---

4. When no appropriate code can be found, assign the following nonspecific complication codes only when documentation in the health record supports their assignment. For example:

Complications
   medical care NEC 999.9
   surgical procedures 998.9

---

5. Assign a second code for greater specificity if the complication code is too general. For example:

997.1   Cardiac complications
   Cardiac:
      arrest
      insufficiency   during or resulting
   Cardiorespiratory failure   from a procedure
   Heart failure

   | *Excludes:* | *the listed conditions as long-term effects of cardiac surgery or due to the presence of cardiac prosthetic device (429.4)*

In this example, a second code would be assigned to further describe the cardiac complication, such as cardiac arrest, heart failure, and so on.

Category 996

The codes in category 996 are used to identify complications resulting from the use of artificial substitutes or natural sources. The large inclusion note at the beginning of this category describes the manner in which the artificial substitutes or natural sources were used.

Codes 996.00–996.59 identify mechanical complications of prosthetic devices, implants, and grafts. Mechanical complications include the mechanical breakdown, displacement, leakage, mechanical obstruction, perforation, or protrusion of the device, implant, or graft. For example:

996.4   Mechanical complication of internal orthopedic device, implant, and graft
Mechanical complications involving:
external (fixation) device utilizing internal screw(s), pin(s), or other methods of fixation
grafts of bone, cartilage, muscle, or tendon
internal (fixation) device such as nail, plate, rod, etc.

Excludes: *complications of external orthopedic device, such as: pressure ulcer due to cast (707.0)*

Subcategory code 996.4 is further subdivided to identify specific types of mechanical complication:

996.41   Mechanical loosening of prosthetic joint

996.42   Dislocation of prosthetic joint

996.43   Prosthetic joint implant failure

996.44   Peri-prosthetic failure around prosthetic joint

996.45   Peri-prosthetic osteolysis

996.46   Articular bearing surface wear of prosthetic joint

996.47   Other mechanical complication of prosthetic joint implant

996.49   Other mechanical complication of other internal orthopedic device, implant, and graft

The coder is also advised to "Use additional code to identify joint replaced by prosthesis (V43.60–V43.69)."

Subcategory 996.6 identifies infection and inflammatory reaction due to an internal prosthetic device, implant, and graft. The fifth-digit subclassification identifies the type of device, implant, or graft, or the organ system involved. For example:

996.61   Due to cardiac device, implant, and graft
Cardiac pacemaker or defibrillator:
electrode(s), lead(s)
pulse generator
subcutaneous pocket
Coronary artery bypass graft
Heart valve prosthesis

Subcategory 996.7 classifies other complications of internal prosthetic device, implant, and graft, such as embolism, fibrosis, hemorrhage, pain, stenosis, thrombus, and complications and occlusion not otherwise specified. Again, the fifth-digit subclassification identifies the specific device or organ system involved.

EXAMPLE: 996.73   Due to renal dialysis device, implant, and graft

Subcategory code 996.8 classifies complications of transplanted organs, including failure or rejection. The specific organ is identified at the fifth-digit subclassification. An additional code should be assigned to identify the nature of the complication, such as cytomegalovirus infection.

EXAMPLE: 996.81 Complications of transplanted kidney
078.5 Cytomegaloviral disease

Subcategory 996.9 classifies complications of a reattached extremity or body part, with the fifth-digit subclassification identifying the specific extremity or body part.

EXAMPLE: 996.92 Complications of reattached hand

Category 997

The codes in category 997 are used to identify complications of specified body systems that are not classified elsewhere in the ICD-9-CM system. The subcategories and subclassifications identify the organ system involved or the specific complication, such as hepatic failure resulting from a surgical procedure (997.4). For example:

997.4　**Digestive system complications**
　　Complications of:
　　　intestinal (internal) anastomosis and bypass, not
　　　　elsewhere classified, except that involving
　　　　urinary tract
　　Hepatic failure
　　Hepatorenal syndrome　}　specified as due to
　　Intestinal obstruction NOS　}　a procedure

　　Excludes:　*gastrostomy complications (536.40–536.49)*
　　　　specified gastrointestinal complications
　　　　　classified elsewhere, such as:
　　　　blind loop syndrome (579.2)
　　　　colostomy and enterostomy complications
　　　　　(569.60–569.69)
　　　　gastrojejunal ulcer (534.0–534.9)
　　　　infection of external stoma (569.61)
　　　　infection of esophagostomy (530.86)
　　　　mechanical complication of esophagostomy (530.87)
　　　　pelvic peritoneal adhesions, female (614.6)
　　　　peritoneal adhesions (568.0)
　　　　peritoneal adhesions with obstruction (560.81)
　　　　postcholecystectomy syndrome (576.0)
　　　　postgastric surgery syndromes (564.2)
　　　　vomiting following gastrointestinal surgery (564.3)

The note at the beginning of category 997 is a reminder that an additional code may be assigned to further identify the specific complication.

EXAMPLE: 997.1 Cardiac complications
427.31 Atrial fibrillation

A cerebrovascular hemorrhage or infarction that occurs as a result of medical intervention is coded to 997.02, Iatrogenic cerebrovascular infarction or hemorrhage. A secondary code from the code range 430–432 or from a code from subcategories 443 or 434 with a fifth digit of "1" should also be used to identify the type of hemorrhage or infarct.

Category 998

The codes in category 998 are used to identify other complications of procedures not classified elsewhere in the ICD-9-CM system. The subcategories and subclassifications identify the type of complication—for example, postoperative shock, hemorrhage, or hematoma; accidental puncture or laceration; disruption of operative wound; foreign body accidentally left in operative wound or body cavity; reaction to foreign body accidentally left in operative wound or body cavity; postoperative infection; postoperative fistula; and so on. Sample codes include:

- 998.11, Hemorrhage complicating a procedure
- 998.12, Hematoma complicating a procedure
- 998.31, Disruption of internal operation wound
- 998.32, Disruption of external operation wound
- 998.59, Other postoperative infection

Category 999

The codes in category 999 are used to identify complications of medical care not elsewhere classified. The inclusion note at the beginning of this category identifies types of complications included in this category. For example:

999   Complications of medical care, not elsewhere classified

Includes: complications, not elsewhere classified, of:

dialysis (hemodialysis) (peritoneal) (renal)
extracorporeal circulation
hyperalimentation therapy
immunization
infusion
inhalation therapy
injection
inoculation
perfusion
transfusion
vaccination
ventilation therapy

The exclusion note identifies the complications classified elsewhere in ICD-9-CM:

Excludes:	*specified complications classified elsewhere, such as:*

complications of implanted device (996.0–996.9)
contact dermatitis due to drugs (692.3)
dementia dialysis (294.8)
    transient (293.9)
dialysis disequilibrium syndrome (276.0–276.9)
poisoning and toxic effects of drugs and chemicals (960.0–989.9)
postvaccinal encephalitis (323.5)
water and electrolyte imbalance (276.0–276.9)

Chapter 20 Exercises

Review the following statements and cases and assign the appropriate codes:

1. Postoperative cellulitis of lower leg

2. Complication of breast implant

3. Infection of colostomy

4. Displacement of intrauterine contraceptive device

5. Urinary retention due to surgery

6. Air embolism due to intravenous infusion

7. Office visit: The patient was seen with persistent knee pain subsequent to insertion of a right knee prosthesis one year ago. X-ray revealed peri-prosthetic fracture around prosthetic joint. A recurrent thrombophlebitis was also noted in the right lower extremity and Coumadin was ordered. The physician ordered physical therapy and antibiotics for the thrombophlebitis. The patient was scheduled for a right knee debridement and revision.

   Impression: Malfunctioning knee prosthesis; thrombophlebitis of right lower leg

   Code(s):

8. Office visit: The patient was seen six weeks post pin insertion for stress fracture of the left femur. The operative wound site revealed an infection. Cultures of the wound grew Methicillin-resistant Staphylococcus aureus. The patient was referred to home health for outpatient IV antibiotic therapy.

   Impression: Postoperative soft tissue infection, left thigh

   Code(s):

9. Office visit: The patient was seen for complaints of shortness of breath and productive cough. The physician ordered an injection of penicillin. The patient went into anaphylactic shock with acute respiratory failure. CPR was administered, and the patient was transported by ambulance to emergency services.

   Impression: Upper respiratory infection; anaphylactic shock due to penicillin

   Code(s):

10. Inpatient admission: The patient was admitted to the hospital because of increased creatinine levels diagnosed during a routine postoperative visit. The patient is six months post kidney transplant. Biopsy results revealed chronic rejection syndrome.

    Discharge diagnosis: Chronic rejection syndrome

    Code(s):

Chapter 20 Exercises (Continued)

11. Inpatient admission: The patient was admitted to the hospital for treatment of a cervical carcinoma. During the hysterectomy procedure, the patient had a cardiac arrest. The patient was resuscitated and the operation continued. Prior to discharge, the patient developed a postoperative wound infection that was drained; IV antibiotics were started. Following aggressive treatment, the patient was discharged.

    Discharge diagnoses: Carcinoma of cervix; cardiac arrest during surgery; postoperative wound infection

    Code(s):

12. Inpatient admission: A 50-year-old male was admitted with severe internal penile prosthesis infection and purulent drainage at the base of the left corpora. He has an 11-year history of type II diabetes mellitus. Blood glucose on admission was 160. The patient is admitted with a temperature of 99.2 and a blood pressure of 138/88.

    Pertinent laboratory results:

    Blood glucose (normal values 65–110)
    12/28   122
    12/28   145
    12/28   128
    12/28   140
    12/31   134
    01/01   162
    01/08   152
    01/11   130

    Hematocrit and hemoglobin:
    Normal values:
       Hemoglobin: 13.5–18 male; 12–16 female
       Hematocrit: 40–54% male; 36–46% female
          12/27   10.5/30.6
          12/28   8.0/23.4
          1/11   8.6/25.9

    Urinalysis
          12/27   WBC = 5–10
          Blood = small
          Sp. Gr. = 1.030
          RBC = 1–5

    C&S = Beta-hemolytic Strep Group B; colony count >10,000

    Hospital course: On 12/28, and after 24 hours of hydration, the patient was taken to the OR, where removal of an inflatable penile prosthesis was performed. The patient tolerated the procedure well and was taken to recovery in good condition. The patient received two weeks of oral antibiotics and was discharged on 1/12. Discharge medications were Cipro 500 mg po bid and Tylenol #3. The patient was discharged with Accu-check machine to monitor his blood glucose levels, which were uncontrolled during the hospitalization even with increased dosages of insulin. The patient's glucose levels will be checked daily on an outpatient basis to try to bring the levels into better control.

    Discharge diagnoses: Infection of internal penile prosthesis due to Strep Group B; type II diabetes mellitus

    Code(s):

Review Questions

Answer the following questions:

1. What are examples of mechanical complications of devices, implants, or grafts?

2. What types of conditions are classified to subcategory 996.7, Other complications of internal (biological) (synthetic) prosthetic device, implant, and graft?

3. How should conditions that occur after surgery be coded?

4. How does the coder know that a complication is coded in the 996–999 series and not in another section of the ICD-9-CM codebook?

5. Under what circumstances might an additional code be necessary to completely code a diagnosis of a complication?

6. What time limit is given for determining a condition to be a complication of a medical or surgical procedure?

Chapter 21

Overview of Reimbursement and Coding Systems

Objectives

After completing this lesson, the student should be able to do the following:

- Identify the various third-party payers such as commercial companies, federal and state governments, and managed care corporations

- Describe the various elements of the federal government's Medicare program

- Define "assignment" as it relates to the Medicare Part B program

- Describe the basic elements of the Resource-based Relative Value System

- Project anticipated changes in the diagnosis and coding systems

Introduction

The custodians of the billing and coding functions in the physician's office are integral parts of the reimbursement puzzle. They face the challenge of remaining current with the latest coding and billing regulations in order to keep the physicians' practices competitive, while staying in compliance with federal and state guidelines.

Correct Coding Procedures

An essential element of the reimbursement picture is the correct coding of diagnoses and procedures. Diagnoses are coded using the ICD-9-CM classification system. Procedures and evaluation and management (E/M) services are assigned Current Procedural Terminology (CPT) codes. Coders are responsible for accurate coding to ensure correct data for statistical and research purposes, as well as for reimbursement purposes. Reimbursement can come from either patients or third-party payers. Third-party payers include commercial insurance companies, managed care organizations, and state or federal entitlement programs such as Medicare, Medicaid, and TRICARE.

Claim forms for reimbursement may be submitted electronically or in hard copy. Electronic claims submission is preferred because it expedites reimbursement. The CMS-1500 or health insurance claim form was approved by the American Medical Association (AMA) in April 1975 as a "universal claim form" that could be used by all insurers. (See appendix A.) The healthcare provider and the patient subsequently receive a statement called an Explanation of Benefits, which explains the services provided, the price of the services, and payments made by the healthcare plan. Medicare now uses a Medicare Summary Notice (MSN) to communicate this information.

Medicare

A major third-party payer is the federal government through the Medicare program. Medicare was established in 1965 as part of the Social Security Act. The secretary of the Department of Health and Human Services (DHHS) has overall responsibility for the program, which is then delegated to the Centers for Medicare and Medicaid Services (CMS). The funding for Medicare comes from payroll taxes paid to the Social Security Administration. In addition to providing healthcare coverage to qualified individuals over 65 years old, Medicare benefits blind and disabled individuals and individuals with end-stage renal disease. Individuals covered under Medicare are called beneficiaries.

The Medicare program consists of two parts—hospital insurance (Part A) and supplemental medical insurance (Part B). Part A pays for costs associated with hospital/healthcare facility care, and Part B pays for physician services and durable medical equipment. Individuals with Part B supplemental insurance pay a monthly premium. Many Medicare beneficiaries supplement their Medicare benefits with private insurance policies, which is referred to as Medigap coverage. As part of the Balanced Budget Act of 1997, Medicare Part C (Medicare Advantage) was established to provide additional options for coverage.

CMS contracts with private insurance companies to carry out the routine operations of the Medicare program. These organizations are known as fiscal intermediaries (Part A) or carriers (Part B). The fiscal intermediary or carrier disburses the Medicare funds to the beneficiaries and providers. Providers include hospitals, physicians, and suppliers of other healthcare services and equipment. Different organizations process the Part A and Part B claims, respectively.

To be covered, all Medicare Part B services must be either medically necessary or one of several approved preventative services. Part B services also are generally subject to a deductible and coinsurance. When a provider believes that Medicare will not pay for some or all of the services rendered, the beneficiary must receive an Advance Beneficiary Notice (ABN). The ABN informs the patient that he or she will be personally and fully responsible for the payment. It must be issued each time the provider determines that Medicare payment will not be made for medical necessity reasons, and it must be issued as soon as this determination is made. When the proper ABN is not provided, the beneficiary cannot be held liable for the expenses. Medicare defines medical necessity as a need for a particular item or service for the diagnosis or treatment of any disease, injury, or defect. Examples of medically necessary services or items include those that are:

- Appropriate for the diagnosis or treatment of a condition, illness, disease, or injury

- In accordance with current standards of good medical care

- Not just for the convenience of the beneficiary or provider

- The most appropriate supply, item, or service that can be provided to the patient

Physicians may choose to sign an agreement to accept "assignment," which means that they accept what Medicare pays and will not bill the beneficiary for anything above the deductible and copayment. Physicians usually are reimbursed at 80 percent of the allowable charge, and the copayment is 20 percent. The payment from Medicare goes directly to the physician under the assignment model. Some of the advantages to accepting assignment include the following:

- Claims are processed faster.

- The fee schedule is 5 percent higher than it is for nonparticipating physicians.

- The physician's name is listed in a participating physician (PAR) directory made available to all Medicare beneficiaries.

A nonparticipating physician (non-PAR) may or may not accept assignment. However, assignment is mandatory for clinical laboratory tests. A non-PAR physician collects the fee from the patient but files the claim for the patient. Participating physicians receive the Medicare Fee Schedule (MFS) amount for services provided, whereas non-PAR physicians receive somewhat less than the MFS. Medicare does limit the amount that a non-PAR physician can charge a beneficiary. This "limiting charge" amount is 15 percent above the allowable amount. The following example shows the difference in payment for a PAR and a non-PAR:

Participating provider

Physician's fee	$180.00
MFS	$105.00
Medicare pays 80% of MFS or	$ 84.00
Patient pays 20% of MFS or	$ 21.00
Physician write-off ($180–$105)	$ 75.00

Nonparticipating provider who accepts assignment

Physician's fee	$180.00
MFS	$105.00
Medicare nonPAR fee (95% of $105)	$ 99.75
Medicare pays 80% of nonPAR fee	$ 79.80
Patient pays 20% of nonPAR fee	$ 19.95
Physician write-off ($180–$99.75)	$ 80.25

Nonparticipating provider who does not accept assignment

Physician's normal fee	$180.00
MFS	$105.00
Medicare nonPAR fee (95% of $105)	$ 99.75
Limiting charge (115% of $ 99.75)	$114.71
Patient billed	$114.71
Medicare pays patient (80% of nonPAR fee)	$ 79.80
Patient out of pocket ($114.71–$79.80)	$ 34.91

Prior to January 1, 1992, physicians were paid the lowest of:

- Physician's actual charge

- Physician's usual charge for the service provided

- Prevailing or customary charge, which is the average fee charged by providers within an area

In 1989, the Omnibus Budget Reconciliation Act (OBRA) was enacted, which mandated that physician fee schedules be established for physician payment for services provided. Thus, the Resource-based Relative Value Scale (RBRVS) system was established. The basis for this system is the Healthcare Common Procedure Coding System (known as HCPCS). There are three levels or groups of HCPCS codes. These are:

- Level I codes, which are composed of the AMA's Current Procedural Terminology (CPT) codes and modifiers.

- Level II codes, or CMS-defined national codes that were developed to code services, materials, drugs, and procedures that are not covered in CPT. These alphanumeric codes range from A000 to V5999.

- Level III codes, which also are alphanumeric codes, are developed by the respective Medicare fiscal carriers. These are known as Local Codes and range from W0000 to Z9999. The use of Local Codes was discontinued on December 31, 2003.

Each HCPCS code has an associated charge determined by the relative value units (RVUs) assigned to it, which is then modified by geographic adjustment factors and converted into a dollar amount using an annual conversion factor. The three component RVUs that make up the final RVU are as follows:

- Work, which is defined as the amount of time needed to complete the service, the intensity or effort expended, and the technical expertise required

- Overhead, which is that part of the cost associated with items such as rent, employees, and supplies

- Malpractice, which is identified as the cost of medical malpractice insurance coverage associated with a particular specialty or service

The sum of these three component RVUs equals the total RVU for a service. The RVU for each CPT code is adjusted for regional overhead and malpractice costs using geographic practice cost indices (GPCIs), referred to as "gypsies." There are specific GPCIs for each of the three components of the RVU.

The final step in the process is to convert the RVU to a dollar amount by multiplying it by the conversion factor, a national dollar amount that is updated annually.

Other Third-Party Payers

There are many other third-party payers, both commercial and governmental. The following subsections examine some of both types.

Government Health Programs

Medicaid is a government-sponsored healthcare insurance program that became effective in 1966 as Title 19 of the Social Security Act. Designed to offer assistance to low-income people, Medicaid is jointly administered by the federal and state governments. Medicaid policies for eligibility, services, and reimbursement vary considerably among the various states, with low income being one of several criteria for eligibility. Some Medicare beneficiaries also are eligible for Medicaid benefits. For beneficiaries with coverage by both programs, Medicaid is considered the payer of last resort.

A new government-sponsored program, the State Children's Health Insurance Program (SCHIP), was initiated as part of the Balanced Budget Act of 1997 and allows states to extend health insurance coverage to children who are uninsured by any other program. The Indian Health Service, part of the Department of Health and Human Services, provides healthcare to American Indians and Alaskan natives.

The Civilian Health and Medical Program of the Uniformed Services (CHAMPUS), the original federal program designed to provide retired military personnel and families of military personnel with health benefits, was established by the U.S. Congress in 1966 and then replaced in 1998 by TRICARE. TRICARE offers three options for care:

- TRICARE Prime: This option provides the most comprehensive healthcare benefits of the three options.

- TRICARE Extra: This is a cost-effective preferred provider network option. Costs for services may be lower because only doctors who have agreed to charge a set amount for services provided treat the patients.

- TRICARE Standard: This is the new name for the formerly named CHAMPUS program. It allows beneficiaries to choose the physician they want to see and the government pays a percentage of the cost.

CHAMPVA, the Civilian Health and Medical Program of the Veterans Administration, offers coverage for spouses and children of veterans who are permanently disabled or deceased due to service-related duties.

Commercial Coverage

Commercial coverage takes many forms, including traditional insurance plans and managed care plans such as preferred provider organizations (PPOs), health maintenance organizations (HMOs), and independent practice associations (IPAs).

Blue Cross and Blue Shield were the first two prepaid or subscription healthcare plans in the United States. Currently, Blue Cross and Blue Shield offer healthcare insurance to individuals, small businesses, seniors, and large corporations in all fifty states, the District of Columbia, and Puerto Rico.

Among the managed care plans, an HMO provides healthcare services to a group of subscribers who pay monthly premiums. Providers, in turn, receive monthly fees for each subscriber and then provide all needed services for the patient. There are four types or models of HMOs:

- The group model provides contracted healthcare services through a privately owned or managed physician practice.

- The IPA provides healthcare services to subscribers through independent physicians who treat the patients in their own offices and receive payment from the HMO, either on a fee-for-service basis or using the capitation method. Under the capitation method, the physician is paid a fixed amount per month per patient, regardless of whether the patient is actually treated.

- The network model contracts with large physician groups to provide services.

- With the staff model, physicians are hired to provide healthcare services to the enrollees and generally have no private patients.

A PPO is a group of providers who contract with an employer to provide healthcare to its employees at a discounted rate.

Tools to Support the Reimbursement Process

Several tools and references are used to support the reimbursement process. One tool is the fee schedule, which is a list of services and procedures (usually CPT and HCPCS codes) and the payment levels allowed by the third-party payer. For example, the physician will need access to Medicare's fee schedule to determine approved fees for Medicare patients. The physician or the practice also should be familiar with the current version of the National Correct Coding Initiative edits, which are rules upon which reimbursement by Medicare is based. Submitted claims are subjected to more than 100,000 edits in order to control improper coding, which results in inflated reimbursement. These edits are designed to prevent "unbundling," which is the process of fragmenting component parts of a service into separately billable services. Examples of unbundling include breaking out bilateral procedures when one code is appropriate, separating a surgical approach from the procedure, downcoding one service to use an additional code, and using E/M codes incorrectly. All of these practices inappropriately increase reimbursement.

Other valuable resources are Medicare's Carrier Manual, Medicare's National Coverage Determinations Manual, and Local Coverage Determinations (LCDs). An LCD (formerly a local medical review policy, or LMRP) provides guidance on whether an item or service is covered, and specifies under what clinical circumstances it is considered medically reasonable and necessary for the diagnosis and treatment of an illness or injury. LCDs assist providers, physicians, and suppliers in submitting correct claims for payment. These policies outline how contractors will review claims to ensure that they meet Medicare coverage requirements.

Future of Coding Systems

Both the diagnosis and procedural coding systems will be undergoing change in the next few years. For example, ICD-9-CM will be replaced by ICD-10-CM, a new version of the international coding system. An exact timetable has not been announced at this point. The uncertainty is partly a result of the Health Insurance Portability and Accountability Act (HIPAA), which mandates that a universal coding system be adopted. ICD-10-CM is expected to be selected for this purpose. The World Health Organization (WHO) published the *International Statistical Classification of Diseases and Related Health Problems, 10th edition,* in 1992. The U.S. modification is in the final stages.

The new system is an alphanumeric coding scheme with expanded code size and restructured chapters and subcategories. ICD-10-CM is divided into 21 chapters, which are further subdivided into homogenous "blocks" of three-character categories. Within each block, some of the three-character categories are for single conditions and others are for groups of diseases. In addition, there are provisions of "other" conditions that do not fit any other category. Most of the three-character categories are further subdivided into more specific subcategories. See figure 21.1 for a brief comparison of ICD-9-CM to ICD-10-CM.

The International Classification of Diseases, 10th Revision, Procedure Classification System (ICD-10-PCS) has been developed as a replacement for volume 3 of the ICD-9-CM. ICD-10-PCS has a multiaxial, seven-character alphanumerical code structure that provides a unique code for each procedure and allows for new procedures to be easily incorporated into the system.

At the same time that the ICD system is being revised, the AMA is in the process of developing the next generation of CPT. CPT-5 will enhance existing features of CPT and correct some of the problem areas. The new revision, which is in part in response to the passage of HIPAA, will be phased in over the course of several years. The AMA is committed to making improvements in the structure of CPT codes to reflect the coding demands of the modern healthcare delivery system and to be selected as the standard for reporting physicians' services.

Several specific issues are being addressed as part of the development of CPT-5. Some of these are:

- The need for a coding system to meet the requirements of managed care organizations

- Identification of CPT improvements relative to the needs of data for research, accreditation, and quality improvement

- Expansion of CPT to include codes for the provision of services by nonphysician healthcare professionals

- Concerns about CPT code adaptability to an electronic medical record or health information system

- Provision of health services at different sites of service

Changes in the coding and reimbursement systems and ongoing changes in the policies of third-party payers will continue to challenge coders, billers, office managers, and other healthcare professionals to stay focused on the goal of appropriate reimbursement based on accurate and ethical coding.

Figure 21.1.   Brief comparison of ICD-9-CM to ICD-10-CM

ICD-10-CM was designed to offer significant advantages over ICD-9-CM. These changes should result in major improvements in both the quality and uses of data for various healthcare settings.

Significant improvements in both the content and the format of the ICD-10-CM include the following:

A.   General Changes and Overall Improvements

- ICD-10-CM codes are alphanumeric and include all letters except "U," thus providing a greater pool of code numbers.

- ICD-9-CM's V and E codes are incorporated into the main classification in ICD-10-CM.

- The length of codes in ICD-10-CM can be a maximum of seven characters as opposed to ICD-9-CM's five digits.

- ICD-10-CM offers the addition of information relative to ambulatory and managed care encounters.

- Conditions that are new or that were not uniquely identified in ICD-9-CM have been assigned code numbers in ICD-10-CM.

- In ICD-10-CM, some three-character categories are not used in order to allow for revisions/future expansion.

- Instead of grouping by categories of injury or type of wound, ICD-10-CM groups injuries by site of the injury and then the type.

- Excludes notes have been expanded to provide guidance on the hierarchy of the chapters and to clarify priority of code assignment.

- Some conditions with a new treatment protocol or perhaps a recently discovered/new etiology are listed in a more appropriate chapter.

- Combination codes are used both for symptom and diagnosis, and for etiology and manifestations.

- Codes for postoperative complications have been expanded, and a distinction has been made between intraoperative complications and postprocedural disorders.

B.   Major Changes from ICD-9-CM to ICD-10-CM

In general, most of the changes were of the following types:

1.   **Grouping of codes:** Conditions have been grouped in a more logical fashion than in ICD-9-CM. This may have been accomplished by means of movement from one chapter to another or one section to another. Many codes have been added to, deleted from, combined, or moved in ICD-10-CM. ICD-10-CM boasts of some chapters that are entirely unique, although these contain codes that were found in other chapters in ICD-9-CM.

2.   **More complete descriptions:** In ICD-10-CM, the subcategory titles are usually complete so that the coder does not have to read previous codes to understand the meaning of the code.

Figure 21.1.   **(Continued)**

3. **Fifth and sixth digits:** Fifth and sixth digits are incorporated into the code listing rather than having common fifth digits listed at the beginning of a chapter, section, or category. In ICD-10-CM, the terminology used is "characters" rather than digits.

4. **Laterality:** ICD-10-CM incorporates laterality of conditions or injuries at the fifth- or sixth-digit level.

5. **Increased specificity:** ICD-10-CM offers greatly expanded detail for the various conditions. Many categories that were limited to three or four digits in ICD-9-CM have fifth, sixth, and even seventh characters/extensions in ICD-10-CM. In some cases, single ICD-9-CM codes were split into several ICD-10-CM codes to provide greater specificity.

6. **Excludes notes:** Two unique kinds of excludes notes are used in ICD-10-CM.

7. **Use of extensions:** Extensions are used in ICD-10-CM to provide additional information. These extensions are most often found in the injury codes but also are found in other chapters.

8. **Combination codes:** Numerous codes in ICD-10-CM group etiology and manifestation. In ICD-9-CM, two codes generally are required to code etiology and manifestation.

9. **Terminology used:** Many of the category code/subcategory code titles have been changed to reflect new technology and more recent medical terminology.

10. **Postprocedural conditions:** Many more codes are added to ICD-10-CM to describe postoperative or postprocedural conditions.

11. **Trimester specificity:** ICD-10-CM codes in the pregnancy, delivery, and puerperium chapter include codes designating the trimester in which the condition occurs.

12. **New codes:** Many new codes are added to ICD-10-CM that were not classified in ICD-9-CM. Notably, codes for blood type and alcohol level are included in ICD-10-CM.

Glossary of Reimbursement Terms

Assignment: An agreement between a physician and CMS whereby a physician or supplier agrees to accept the Medicare-approved amount as payment in full for services or supplies provided under Part B. Medicare pays the physician or supplier 80 percent of the approved amount after the annual $100 deductible has been met; the beneficiary pays the remaining 20 percent.

Beneficiary: The individual who is receiving benefits under Medicare.

Carrier: An organization that has contracted with the federal government to process claims from physicians or suppliers for services covered under Medicare Part B.

CHAMPUS/CHAMPVA: Congressionally funded health benefits plans for retired military personnel or spouses and children of military personnel. CHAMPVA specifically benefits spouses and children of disabled veterans.

Claim: A request to a third-party payer for payment for services provided to the insured.

CMS-1500 form: A universal claim form that is used to submit claims to third-party payers for physician services.

Coinsurance: The portion of the costs of services provided that the beneficiary pays.

Conversion factor: A national dollar amount that Congress designates to convert relative value units to dollars. It is updated annually.

Covered services: Services or suppliers that are reimbursed by Medicare.

Deductible: The amount of money a beneficiary must pay before Medicare begins to cover the cost of services provided.

Durable medical equipment: Equipment such as wheelchairs, walkers, or oxygen that a physician may order for a beneficiary.

Fiscal intermediary: An organization that has contracted with the federal government to handle Medicare claims for services from hospitals, skilled nursing facilities, and hospice programs under Medicare Part A.

Geographic Practice Cost Indices (GPCIs):   Indices that are used to adjust relative value units to take prevailing charges in a particular geographic area into account when determining appropriate reimbursement.

Health maintenance organization (HMO):   A form of healthcare delivery system in which a subscriber is assigned to a primary care physician (PCP) who manages the healthcare needs of the enrollee. Referrals to specialists must come from the PCP.

Individual practice association (IPA):   A group of physicians that provides healthcare services to a defined population for a predetermined fee. HMOs often contract with an IPA to provide services to their members.

Limiting charge: The highest charge that a nonparticipating physician may charge a Medicare patient. The limiting charge is equal to 15 percent above Medicare's approved amount.

Managed care organization: An organization that manages the healthcare needs for an enrolled group of individuals. It is similar to the traditional insurance concept except there is some influence on cost control, such as preauthorizations for tests or procedures.

Nonparticipating physician: A physician who has an option regarding accepting assignment from Medicare.

Out-of-pocket expenses: Expenses that are not reimbursed by a third party.

Part A insurance: The part of Medicare that covers services provided by hospitals, skilled nursing facilities, home health agencies, and hospice programs.

Part B insurance: The part of Medicare that covers services provided by physicians and outpatient facilities.

Participating physician: A physician who agrees to accept assignment for Medicare claims.

Preferred provider organization (PPO):   Physicians or other providers who have agreed to provide healthcare services at a discounted price to enrollees in a healthcare insurance program. Enrollees are allowed to use any provider, but using a network provider generally results in a lower cost.

Resource-based Relative Value System (RBRVS):   Payment method for reimbursing physicians under Medicare Part B. The system uses a relative value unit for the work, expense, and malpractice components of physicians' services.

Chapter 22

Challenges of Compliance and Ethical Coding

Objectives

After completing this lesson, the student should be able to do the following:

- Describe the various federal laws and/or programs that form the basis for healthcare fraud and abuse initiatives
- Differentiate between fraud and abuse and give examples of each
- Outline the steps in the development of a physician compliance plan

Introduction

As the largest third-party payer, the Medicare program is the frequent target of fraud and abuse, which costs the government billions of healthcare dollars. Over the past several years, the government has enacted legislation and committed resources (money and people) to fight this bilking of the Medicare and Medicaid programs.

Legislation Addressing Fraud and Abuse

A number of federal laws and/or programs form the basis for prosecution of healthcare fraud and abuse perpetrators. Some of these are:

- The Federal False Claims Act, enacted in 1863, allows a private citizen to sue an individual or a company it believes to be submitting false bills to the federal government. The original intent of this act was to discourage war profiteers who were committing fraud against the Army in the post–Civil War era. In 1986, the Federal False Claims Amendment Act was signed into law by President Reagan. This amendment strengthened the government's ability to prosecute healthcare providers or suppliers who defraud the government. In the original law, there had to be a specific intent to defraud. The amendment removes the "intent" criterion. It also delineates penalties for each offense that a provider is found guilty of and allows triple damages to be imposed. The act offers financial incentives to informants, or "relators," who report providers to the government. This is known as a *qui tam* action. Furthermore, the law protects the relators from being threatened or harassed in any way by the employer. Relators are awarded between 15 and 30 percent of the total monies recovered.

- The Health Insurance Portability and Accountability Act (HIPAA), enacted in 1996 by President Clinton, has several significant provisions establishing expanded fraud and abuse controls. HIPAA strengthened the jurisdiction of DHHS and increased the investigative powers and funding available to the Office of Inspector General (OIG) and the FBI for healthcare fraud and abuse controls. HIPAA provides for criminal penalties for healthcare professionals who "knowingly and willfully" attempt to defraud any of the healthcare benefit programs. It also provides for imprisonment for violators. Further, this legislation provides that physicians or other providers are accountable for information they "know or should know." This means that if an issue was addressed in an official source, such as *Coding Clinic,* it is expected that the physician should have known it.

- Operation Restore Trust is a DHHS program that involves federal and state government officials as well as private-sector representatives. The project is designed to combat fraud and abuse through various initiatives. Several million dollars of overpayments have been recouped, and numerous criminal convictions and civil judgments have been handed down as a result of Operation Restore Trust.

- The Balanced Budget Act of 1997 includes 15 sections on fraud and abuse and gives government agencies additional tools in the fight to control healthcare costs.

In addition to these federal laws and programs, many states have legislation and programs designed to combat fraud and abuse. States are particularly active in the prosecution of Medicaid false claims.

Agencies Involved in Investigating Fraud and Abuse

Several government agencies actually participate in the war against fraud and abuse. The OIG investigates and prosecutes individuals who overbill Medicare. It also develops an annual "work plan" that delineates the specific target areas that will be monitored in a given year.

The FBI is the principal investigative arm of the Department of Justice that conducts civil and criminal fraud investigations. The Postal Inspection Service has authority to investigate fraudulent schemes involving the U.S. Mail Service. The Defense Criminal Investigative Service (DCIS) is responsible for investigating potential fraud against the government's military healthcare plans. The U.S. attorneys' offices and state attorney generals also are involved in prosecuting violators.

Definitions and Examples of Fraud and Abuse

Medicare defines fraud as an "intentional deception or misrepresentation" that results in an unauthorized benefit to an individual. Fraud may take many forms, including:

- Billing for services or supplies that were not provided, which may include phantom billing or ghost billing for patients who were not seen by the provider

- Altering claim forms or medical records to obtain higher reimbursement than is appropriate

- Receiving kickbacks in exchange for referring patients to specific facilities

- Misrepresenting the types of services provided, dates of services, or even the identity of the patient

- Billing for noncovered services

- Billing for "gang" visits, which is billing for visits to multiple patients (for example, in a nursing home) when no specific services were provided

- Billing for equipment that was never provided

Abuse involves billing practices that are inconsistent with generally acceptable fiscal policies. This usually results from inadvertent coding or billing mistakes and is not considered fraudulent.

Physician Compliance

One way that physicians can prevent or minimize potentially abusive or fraudulent activities is through the development of a compliance plan. The OIG has published a model compliance plan for small and individual physician practices. This document delineates seven basic steps, or program guidelines.

Model Compliance Plan

Step 1. Instigate Auditing and Monitoring

The OIG contends that an audit is an invaluable tool for a physician practice to determine what, if any, problem areas exist. Any problems that are encountered can be addressed with corrective measures. Periodic auditing of billing practices to determine that the documentation in the record supports the services billed, that medical necessity guidelines are followed, and that bills are coded correctly is an essential part of the compliance puzzle. An initial baseline audit should be undertaken to give the practice a benchmark against which to measure future results.

Step 2. Implement Written Policies, Procedures, and Standards of Conduct

In developing policies and procedures, the physician should be aware of the risk areas that the OIG has identified for physician practices. These include:

- Coding and billing: The American Health Information Management Association has established Standards of Ethical Coding that can be used as the basis for a healthcare facility's code of conduct. (See appendix B for a copy of the standards, appendix C for the AHIMA Practice Brief on Data Quality, and appendix D for the AHIMA Position Statement on Data Quality.)

- Certification of need for durable medical equipment and home health services

- Documentation in the medical record

- Billing for noncovered services as if they are covered

- Upcoding (billing for a more expensive service than the one actually performed)

- Unbundling

- Clustering (coding/charging one or two middle levels of service codes exclusively)

Step 3. Designate a Compliance Officer or Contact to Monitor Compliance Efforts

The individual designated to monitor compliance efforts may be the office manager, the practice administrator, the billing supervisor, or an outside consultant or consulting firm. Responsibilities of the position might include:

- Overseeing and monitoring implementation of the compliance program

- Establishing methods such as audits to improve the practice's efficiency and quality of services and to reduce its vulnerability to fraud and abuse charges

- Periodically revising the compliance program in light of changes in government and third-party rules and regulations

- Developing, coordinating, and participating in training programs

- Investigating reports or allegations concerning possible unethical or improper business practices

Step 4. Develop Training and Educational Programs

Training and educational programs may take several forms, including in-house training sessions or outside seminars and workshops, and may be supplemented by written newsletters with coding tips or bulletin boards. Up-to-date coding books, newsletters, and reference materials should be made available for office personnel. Moreover, the physician practice should offer both initial and recurrent training in compliance. The training might address the operation and importance of the compliance program, consequences of violating the practice's standards and procedures, and the employees' role in the program's operation. Training in specific coding guidelines and billing practices also is necessary.

Step 5. Respond Appropriately to Detected Violations

When offenses are discovered, they should be investigated and corrective measures undertaken. Physician practices should develop indicators that would signal a problem. These might include:

- A significant change in the number of claim rejections or reduction in payments
- Changes in the pattern of CPT code usage
- Increased number of challenges to the medical necessity of services provided

Corrective actions may include refunding overpayments from a third-party payer or even self-reporting to the government.

Step 6. Develop Open Lines of Communication to Keep Practice Employees Updated about Compliance Activities

Open lines of communication may be accomplished through suggestion boxes, bulletin boards, hot lines, an established open-door policy between the physician or compliance officer and the employees, and/or discussions at staff meetings.

Step 7. Enforce Disciplinary Standards through Well-Published Guidelines

Disciplinary action may take several forms, including oral warnings, written reprimands, probation or demotion, suspension, termination, or referral for criminal prosecution.

A well-established compliance program can assist a physician practice in developing and implementing controls and procedures that will ensure adherence to federal healthcare programs and other third-party-payer requirements.

Summary

The challenges facing the coding and billing personnel in the physician office setting are numerous. A thorough knowledge of ICD-9-CM coding guidelines as well as access to various coding resources such as *Coding Clinic* are essential to accurate coding and billing. Physicians should be aware of the government and private-sector initiatives to combat fraud and abuse and diligently monitor their reimbursement practices to meet the requirements of third-party payers. Establishment of a compliance program, including requirements for continuing education of the reimbursement personnel, will assist the physician practice in adhering to private-sector and government rules and regulations.

References and Bibliography

American Hospital Association. 1985–2005. *Coding Clinic for ICD-9-CM*. Chicago: American Hospital Association.

American Psychiatric Association. 2000. *Diagnostic and Statistical Manual of Mental Disorders*. 4th ed, Text Revision. Arlington, Va.: American Psychiatric Association.

Anderson, Kenneth, and Lois Anderson. 2003. *Mosby's Pocket Dictionary of Medicine, Nursing and Allied Health*. 4th ed. St. Louis: Mosby, Inc.

Berkow, Robert, Mark Burs, and Mark Beers, eds. 1999. *Merck Manual of Diagnosis and Therapy*. 17th ed. Rahway, N.J.: Merck and Company.

Brown, Faye. 2005. *ICD-9-CM Coding Handbook with Answers*. Chicago: American Hospital Association.

Buck, Carol J. 2004. *Step-by-Step Medical Coding*. 5th ed. Philadelphia: W. B. Saunders.

Holt, John G., ed. 2001. *Bergey's Manual of Systematic Bacteriology*. Volume 1. Baltimore: Lippencott, Williams and Wilkins.

Ingenix. 2005. *Hospital and Payor ICD-9-CM: Volumes 1, 2, and 3*. Salt Lake City: Ingenix.

Johnson, Sandra L. 2000. *Understanding Medical Coding: A Comprehensive Guide*. Albany, N.Y.: Delmar Publishers.

Puckett, Craig D. 2004. *The Educational Annotation of ICD-9-CM*. 5th ed. Reno, Nev.: Channel Publishing.

Rogers, Vickie. 2004. *Applying Inpatient Coding Skills under Prospective Payment*. Chicago: American Health Information Management Association.

Schraffenberger, Lou Ann. 2005. *Basic ICD-9-CM Coding*. Chicago: American Health Information Management Association.

Williams & Wilkins. 2000. *Stedman's Medical Dictionary*. 27th ed. Baltimore: Williams & Wilkins.

Appendix A

CMS-1500 Claim Form

PLEASE
DO NOT
STAPLE
IN THIS
AREA

CARRIER

HEALTH INSURANCE CLAIM FORM

PICA | | | | PICA

1. MEDICARE (Medicare #)   MEDICAID (Medicaid #)   CHAMPUS (Sponsor's SSN)   CHAMPVA (VA File #)   GROUP HEALTH PLAN (SSN or ID)   FECA BLK LUNG (SSN)   OTHER (ID) | 1a. INSURED'S I.D. NUMBER   (FOR PROGRAM IN ITEM 1)

2. PATIENT'S NAME (Last Name, First Name, Middle Initial) | 3. PATIENT'S BIRTH DATE MM DD YY   SEX M F | 4. INSURED'S NAME (Last Name, First Name, Middle Initial)

5. PATIENT'S ADDRESS (No., Street) | 6. PATIENT RELATIONSHIP TO INSURED   Self   Spouse   Child   Other | 7. INSURED'S ADDRESS (No., Street)

CITY   STATE | 8. PATIENT STATUS   Single   Married   Other | CITY   STATE

ZIP CODE   TELEPHONE (Include Area Code) ( ) | Employed   Full-Time Student   Part-Time Student | ZIP CODE   TELEPHONE (INCLUDE AREA CODE) ( )

9. OTHER INSURED'S NAME (Last Name, First Name, Middle Initial) | 10. IS PATIENT'S CONDITION RELATED TO: | 11. INSURED'S POLICY GROUP OR FECA NUMBER

a. OTHER INSURED'S POLICY OR GROUP NUMBER | a. EMPLOYMENT? (CURRENT OR PREVIOUS) YES NO | a. INSURED'S DATE OF BIRTH MM DD YY   SEX M F

b. OTHER INSURED'S DATE OF BIRTH MM DD YY   SEX M F | b. AUTO ACCIDENT?   PLACE (State) YES NO | b. EMPLOYER'S NAME OR SCHOOL NAME

c. EMPLOYER'S NAME OR SCHOOL NAME | c. OTHER ACCIDENT? YES NO | c. INSURANCE PLAN NAME OR PROGRAM NAME

d. INSURANCE PLAN NAME OR PROGRAM NAME | 10d. RESERVED FOR LOCAL USE | d. IS THERE ANOTHER HEALTH BENEFIT PLAN? YES NO *If yes*, return to and complete item 9 a-d.

READ BACK OF FORM BEFORE COMPLETING & SIGNING THIS FORM.

12. PATIENT'S OR AUTHORIZED PERSON'S SIGNATURE I authorize the release of any medical or other information necessary to process this claim. I also request payment of government benefits either to myself or to the party who accepts assignment below.

SIGNED _____________ DATE _____________

13. INSURED'S OR AUTHORIZED PERSON'S SIGNATURE I authorize payment of medical benefits to the undersigned physician or supplier for services described below.

SIGNED _____________

14. DATE OF CURRENT: ILLNESS (First symptom) OR INJURY (Accident) OR PREGNANCY(LMP) MM DD YY | 15. IF PATIENT HAS HAD SAME OR SIMILAR ILLNESS. GIVE FIRST DATE MM DD YY | 16. DATES PATIENT UNABLE TO WORK IN CURRENT OCCUPATION FROM MM DD YY TO MM DD YY

17. NAME OF REFERRING PHYSICIAN OR OTHER SOURCE | 17a. I.D. NUMBER OF REFERRING PHYSICIAN | 18. HOSPITALIZATION DATES RELATED TO CURRENT SERVICES FROM MM DD YY TO MM DD YY

19. RESERVED FOR LOCAL USE | 20. OUTSIDE LAB? YES NO $ CHARGES

21. DIAGNOSIS OR NATURE OF ILLNESS OR INJURY. (RELATE ITEMS 1,2,3 OR 4 TO ITEM 24E BY LINE)

1. |___.___   3. |___.___ | 22. MEDICAID RESUBMISSION CODE   ORIGINAL REF. NO.

2. |___.___   4. |___.___ | 23. PRIOR AUTHORIZATION NUMBER

24. A DATE(S) OF SERVICE						B Place of Service	C Type of Service	D PROCEDURES, SERVICES, OR SUPPLIES (Explain Unusual Circumstances) CPT/HCPCS | MODIFIER	E DIAGNOSIS CODE	F $ CHARGES	G DAYS OR UNITS	H EPSDT Family Plan	I EMG	J COB	K RESERVED FOR LOCAL USE
	From MM	DD	YY	To MM	DD	YY										
1																
2																
3																
4																
5																
6																

25. FEDERAL TAX I.D. NUMBER   SSN EIN | 26. PATIENT'S ACCOUNT NO. | 27. ACCEPT ASSIGNMENT? (For govt. claims, see back) YES NO | 28. TOTAL CHARGE $ | 29. AMOUNT PAID $ | 30. BALANCE DUE $

31. SIGNATURE OF PHYSICIAN OR SUPPLIER INCLUDING DEGREES OR CREDENTIALS (I certify that the statements on the reverse apply to this bill and are made a part thereof.)

SIGNED _____________ DATE _____________

32. NAME AND ADDRESS OF FACILITY WHERE SERVICES WERE RENDERED (If other than home or office)

33. PHYSICIAN'S, SUPPLIER'S BILLING NAME, ADDRESS, ZIP CODE & PHONE #

PIN#   GRP#

PHYSICIAN OR SUPPLIER INFORMATION

PATIENT AND INSURED INFORMATION

(APPROVED BY AMA COUNCIL ON MEDICAL SERVICE 8/88)   ***PLEASE PRINT OR TYPE***   APPROVED OMB-0938-0008 FORM CMS-1500 (12/90), FORM RRB-1500, APPROVED OMB-1215-0055 FORM OWCP-1500, APPROVED OMB-0720-0001 (CHAMPUS)

BECAUSE THIS FORM IS USED BY VARIOUS GOVERNMENT AND PRIVATE HEALTH PROGRAMS, SEE SEPARATE INSTRUCTIONS ISSUED BY APPLICABLE PROGRAMS.

NOTICE: Any person who knowingly files a statement of claim containing any misrepresentation or any false, incomplete or misleading information may be guilty of a criminal act punishable under law and may be subject to civil penalties.

REFERS TO GOVERNMENT PROGRAMS ONLY

MEDICARE AND CHAMPUS PAYMENTS: A patient's signature requests that payment be made and authorizes release of any information necessary to process the claim and certifies that the information provided in Blocks 1 through 12 is true, accurate and complete. In the case of a Medicare claim, the patient's signature authorizes any entity to release to Medicare medical and nonmedical information, including employment status, and whether the person has employer group health insurance, liability, no-fault, worker's compensation or other insurance which is responsible to pay for the services for which the Medicare claim is made. See 42 CFR 411.24(a). If item 9 is completed, the patient's signature authorizes release of the information to the health plan or agency shown. In Medicare assigned or CHAMPUS participation cases, the physician agrees to accept the charge determination of the Medicare carrier or CHAMPUS fiscal intermediary as the full charge, and the patient is responsible only for the deductible, coinsurance and noncovered services. Coinsurance and the deductible are based upon the charge determination of the Medicare carrier or CHAMPUS fiscal intermediary if this is less than the charge submitted. CHAMPUS is not a health insurance program but makes payment for health benefits provided through certain affiliations with the Uniformed Services. Information on the patient's sponsor should be provided in those items captioned in "Insured"; i.e., items 1a, 4, 6, 7, 9, and 11.

BLACK LUNG AND FECA CLAIMS

The provider agrees to accept the amount paid by the Government as payment in full. See Black Lung and FECA instructions regarding required procedure and diagnosis coding systems.

SIGNATURE OF PHYSICIAN OR SUPPLIER (MEDICARE, CHAMPUS, FECA AND BLACK LUNG)

I certify that the services shown on this form were medically indicated and necessary for the health of the patient and were personally furnished by me or were furnished incident to my professional service by my employee under my immediate personal supervision, except as otherwise expressly permitted by Medicare or CHAMPUS regulations.

For services to be considered as "incident" to a physician's professional service, 1) they must be rendered under the physician's immediate personal supervision by his/her employee, 2) they must be an integral, although incidental part of a covered physician's service, 3) they must be of kinds commonly furnished in physician's offices, and 4) the services of nonphysicians must be included on the physician's bills.

For CHAMPUS claims, I further certify that I (or any employee) who rendered services am not an active duty member of the Uniformed Services or a civilian employee of the United States Government or a contract employee of the United States Government, either civilian or military (refer to 5 USC 5536). For Black-Lung claims, I further certify that the services performed were for a Black Lung-related disorder.

No Part B Medicare benefits may be paid unless this form is received as required by existing law and regulations (42 CFR 424.32).

NOTICE: Any one who misrepresents or falsifies essential information to receive payment from Federal funds requested by this form may upon conviction be subject to fine and imprisonment under applicable Federal laws.

NOTICE TO PATIENT ABOUT THE COLLECTION AND USE OF MEDICARE, CHAMPUS, FECA, AND BLACK LUNG INFORMATION
(PRIVACY ACT STATEMENT)

We are authorized by CMS, CHAMPUS and OWCP to ask you for information needed in the administration of the Medicare, CHAMPUS, FECA, and Black Lung programs. Authority to collect information is in section 205(a), 1862, 1872 and 1874 of the Social Security Act as amended, 42 CFR 411.24(a) and 424.5(a) (6), and 44 USC 3101;41 CFR 101 et seq and 10 USC 1079 and 1086; 5 USC 8101 et seq; and 30 USC 901 et seq; 38 USC 613; E.O. 9397.

The information we obtain to complete claims under these programs is used to identify you and to determine your eligibility. It is also used to decide if the services and supplies you received are covered by these programs and to insure that proper payment is made.

The information may also be given to other providers of services, carriers, intermediaries, medical review boards, health plans, and other organizations or Federal agencies, for the effective administration of Federal provisions that require other third parties payers to pay primary to Federal program, and as otherwise necessary to administer these programs. For example, it may be necessary to disclose information about the benefits you have used to a hospital or doctor. Additional disclosures are made through routine uses for information contained in systems of records.

FOR MEDICARE CLAIMS: See the notice modifying system No. 09-70-0501, titled, 'Carrier Medicare Claims Record,' published in the <u>Federal Register</u>, Vol. 55 No. 177, page 37549, Wed. Sept. 12, 1990, or as updated and republished.

FOR OWCP CLAIMS: Department of Labor, Privacy Act of 1974, "Republication of Notice of Systems of Records," <u>Federal Register</u> Vol. 55 No. 40, Wed Feb. 28, 1990, See ESA-5, ESA-6, ESA-12, ESA-13, ESA-30, or as updated and republished.

FOR CHAMPUS CLAIMS: <u>PRINCIPLE PURPOSE(S):</u> To evaluate eligibility for medical care provided by civilian sources and to issue payment upon establishment of eligibility and determination that the services/supplies received are authorized by law.

<u>ROUTINE USE(S):</u> Information from claims and related documents may be given to the Dept. of Veterans Affairs, the Dept. of Health and Human Services and/or the Dept. of Transportation consistent with their statutory administrative responsibilities under CHAMPUS/CHAMPVA; to the Dept. of Justice for representation of the Secretary of Defense in civil actions; to the Internal Revenue Service, private collection agencies, and consumer reporting agencies in connection with recoupment claims; and to Congressional Offices in response to inquiries made at the request of the person to whom a record pertains. Appropriate disclosures may be made to other federal, state, local, foreign government agencies, private business entities, and individual providers of care, on matters relating to entitlement, claims adjudication, fraud, program abuse, utilization review, quality assurance, peer review, program integrity, third-party liability, coordination of benefits, and civil and criminal litigation related to the operation of CHAMPUS.

<u>DISCLOSURES:</u> Voluntary; however, failure to provide information will result in delay in payment or may result in denial of claim. With the one exception discussed below, there are no penalties under these programs for refusing to supply information. However, failure to furnish information regarding the medical services rendered or the amount charged would prevent payment of claims under these programs. Failure to furnish any other information, such as name or claim number, would delay payment of the claim. Failure to provide medical information under FECA could be deemed an obstruction.

It is mandatory that you tell us if you know that another party is responsible for paying for your treatment. Section 1128B of the Social Security Act and 31 USC 3801-3812 provide penalties for withholding this information.

You should be aware that P.L. 100-503, the "Computer Matching and Privacy Protection Act of 1988", permits the government to verify information by way of computer matches.

MEDICAID PAYMENTS (PROVIDER CERTIFICATION)

I hereby agree to keep such records as are necessary to disclose fully the extent of services provided to individuals under the State's Title XIX plan and to furnish information regarding any payments claimed for providing such services as the State Agency or Dept. of Health and Human Services may request.

I further agree to accept, as payment in full, the amount paid by the Medicaid program for those claims submitted for payment under that program, with the exception of authorized deductible, coinsurance, co-payment or similar cost-sharing charge.

SIGNATURE OF PHYSICIAN (OR SUPPLIER): I certify that the services listed above were medically indicated and necessary to the health of this patient and were personally furnished by me or my employee under my personal direction.

NOTICE: This is to certify that the foregoing information is true, accurate and complete. I understand that payment and satisfaction of this claim will be from Federal and State funds, and that any false claims, statements, or documents, or concealment of a material fact, may be prosecuted under applicable Federal or State laws.

Appendix B

Ethics in Coding

Preamble to the American Health Information Management Association Code of Ethics

The ethical obligations of the health information management (HIM) professional include the protection of patient privacy and confidential information; disclosure of information; development, use, and maintenance of health information systems and health records; and the quality of information. Both handwritten and computerized medical records contain many sacred stories—stories that must be protected on behalf of the individual and the aggregate community of persons served in the healthcare system. Healthcare consumers are increasingly concerned about the loss of privacy and the inability to control the dissemination of their protected information. Core health information issues include what information should be collected, how the information should be handled, who should have access to the information, and under what conditions the information should be disclosed.

Ethical obligations are central to the professional's responsibility, regardless of the employment site or the method of collection, storage, and security of health information. Sensitive information (genetic, adoption, drug, alcohol, sexual, and behavioral information) requires special attention to prevent misuse. Entrepreneurial roles require expertise in the protection of the information in the world of business and interactions with consumers.

Professional Values

The mission of the HIM profession is based on core professional values developed since the inception of the Association in 1928. These values and the inherent ethical responsibilities for AHIMA members and credentialed HIM professionals include providing service; protecting medical, social, and financial information; promoting confidentiality; and preserving and securing health information. Values to the healthcare team include promoting the quality and advancement of healthcare, demonstrating HIM expertise and skills, and promoting interdisciplinary cooperation and collaboration. Professional values in relationship to the employer include protecting committee deliberations and complying with laws, regulations, and policies. Professional values related to the public include advocating change, refusing to participate or conceal unethical practices, and reporting violations of practice standards to the proper authorities. Professional values to individual and professional associations include obligations to be honest, bringing honor to self, peers and profession, committing to continuing education and lifelong learning, performing Association duties honorably, strengthening professional membership, representing the profession to the public, and promoting and participating in research.

These professional values will require a complex process of balancing the many conflicts that can result from competing interests and obligations of those who seek access to health information and require an understanding of ethical decision-making.

Purpose of the American Health Information Management Association Code of Ethics

The HIM professional has an obligation to demonstrate actions that reflect values, ethical principles, and ethical guidelines. The American Health Information Management Association (AHIMA) Code of Ethics sets forth these values and principles to guide conduct. The code is relevant to all AHIMA members and credentialed HIM professionals and students, regardless of their professional functions, the settings in which they work, or the populations they serve.

The AHIMA Code of Ethics serves six purposes:

- Identifies core values on which the HIM mission is based.

- Summarizes broad ethical principles that reflect the profession's core values and establishes a set of ethical principles to be used to guide decision-making and actions.

- Helps HIM professionals identify relevant considerations when professional obligations conflict or ethical uncertainties arise.

- Provides ethical principles by which the general public can hold the HIM professional accountable.

- Socializes practitioners new to the field to HIM's mission, values, and ethical principles.

- Articulates a set of guidelines that the HIM professional can use to assess whether they have engaged in unethical conduct.

The code includes principles and guidelines that are both enforceable and aspirational. The extent to which each principle is enforceable is a matter of professional judgment to be exercised by those responsible for reviewing alleged violations of ethical principles.

The Use of the Code

Violation of principles in this code does not automatically imply legal liability or violation of the law. Such determination can only be made in the context of legal and judicial proceedings. Alleged violations of the code would be subject to a peer review process. Such processes are generally separate from legal or administrative procedures and insulated from legal review or proceedings to allow the profession to counsel and discipline its own members although in some situations, violations of the code would constitute unlawful conduct subject to legal process.

Guidelines for ethical and unethical behavior are provided in this code. The terms "shall and shall not" are used as a basis for setting high standards for behavior. This does not imply that everyone "shall or shall not" do everything that is listed. For example, not everyone participates in the recruitment or mentoring of students. A HIM professional is not being unethical if this is not part of his or her professional activities; however, if students are part of one's professional responsibilities, there is an ethical obligation to follow the guidelines stated in the code. This concept is true for the entire code. If someone does the stated activities, ethical behavior is the standard. The guidelines are not a comprehensive list. For example, the statement "protect all confidential information to include personal, health, financial, genetic, and outcome information" can also be interpreted as "shall not fail to protect all confidential information to include personal, health, financial, genetic, and outcome information."

A code of ethics cannot guarantee ethical behavior. Moreover, a code of ethics cannot resolve all ethical issues or disputes or capture the richness and complexity involved in striving to make responsible choices within a moral community. Rather, a code of ethics sets forth values and ethical principles, and offers ethical guidelines to which professionals aspire and by which their actions can be judged. Ethical behaviors result from a personal commitment to engage in ethical practice.

Professional responsibilities often require an individual to move beyond personal values. For example, an individual might demonstrate behaviors that are based on the values of honesty, providing service to others, or demonstrating loyalty. In addition to these, professional values might require promoting confidentiality, facilitating interdisciplinary collaboration, and refusing to participate or conceal unethical practices. Professional values could require a more comprehensive set of values than what an individual needs to be an ethical agent in their personal lives.

The AHIMA Code of Ethics is to be used by AHIMA and individuals, agencies, organizations, and bodies (such as licensing and regulatory boards, insurance providers, courts of law, agency boards of directors, government agencies, and other professional groups) that choose to adopt it or use it as a frame of reference. The AHIMA Code of Ethics reflects the commitment of all to uphold the profession's values and to act ethically. Individuals of good character who discern moral questions and, in good faith, seek to make reliable ethical judgments, must apply ethical principles.

The code does not provide a set of rules that prescribe how to act in all situations. Specific applications of the code must take into account the context in which it is being considered and the possibility of conflicts among the code's values, principles, and guidelines. Ethical responsibilities flow from all human relationships, from the personal and familial to the social and professional. Further, the AHIMA Code of Ethics does not specify which values, principles, and guidelines are the most important and ought to outweigh others in instances when they conflict.

Code of Ethics 2004

Ethical Principles: The following ethical principles are based on the core values of the American Health Information Management Association and apply to all health information management professionals.

Health information management professionals:

> ***I. Advocate, uphold, and defend the individual's right to privacy and the doctrine of confidentiality in the use and disclosure of information.***

> ***II. Put service and the health and welfare of persons before self-interest and conduct themselves in the practice of the profession so as to bring honor to themselves, their peers, and to the health information management profession.***

III. *Preserve, protect, and secure personal health information in any form or medium and hold in the highest regard the contents of the records and other information of a confidential nature, taking into account the applicable statutes and regulations.*

IV. *Refuse to participate in or conceal unethical practices or procedures.*

V. *Advance health information management knowledge and practice through continuing education, research, publications, and presentations.*

VI. *Recruit and mentor students, peers and colleagues to develop and strengthen professional workforce.*

VII. *Represent the profession accurately to the public.*

VIII. *Perform honorably health information management association responsibilities, either appointed or elected, and preserve the confidentiality of any privileged information made known in any official capacity.*

IX. *State truthfully and accurately their credentials, professional education, and experiences.*

X. *Facilitate interdisciplinary collaboration in situations supporting health information practice.*

XI. *Respect the inherent dignity and worth of every person.*

How to Interpret the Code of Ethics

The following ethical principles are based on the core values of the American Health Information Management Association and apply to all health information management professionals. Guidelines included for each ethical principle are a non-inclusive list of behaviors and situations that can help to clarify the principle. They are not to be meant as a comprehensive list of all situations that can occur.

I. Advocate, uphold, and defend the individual's right to privacy and the doctrine of confidentiality in the use and disclosure of information.

Health information management professionals **shall:**

1.1. Protect all confidential information to include personal, health, financial, genetic, and outcome information.

1.2. Engage in social and political action that supports the protection of privacy and confidentiality, and be aware of the impact of the political arena on the health information system. Advocate for changes in policy and legislation to ensure protection of privacy and confidentiality, coding compliance, and other issues that surface as advocacy issues as well as facilitating informed participation by the public on these issues.

1.3. Protect the confidentiality of all information obtained in the course of professional service. Disclose only information that is directly relevant or necessary to achieve the purpose of disclosure. Release information only with valid consent from a patient or a person legally authorized to consent on behalf of a patient or as authorized by federal or state regulations. The need-to-know criterion is essential when releasing health information for initial disclosure and all redisclosure activities.

1.4. Promote the obligation to respect privacy by respecting confidential information shared among colleagues, while responding to requests from the legal profession, the media, or other non-healthcare related individuals, during presentations or teaching and in situations that could cause harm to persons.

II. *Put service and the health and welfare of persons before self-interest and conduct themselves in the practice of the profession so as to bring honor to themselves, their peers, and to the health information management profession.*

Health information management professionals **shall:**

2.1. Act with integrity, behave in a trustworthy manner, elevate service to others above self-interest, and promote high standards of practice in every setting.

2.2. Be aware of the profession's mission, values, and ethical principles, and practice in a manner consistent with them by acting honestly and responsibly.

2.3. Anticipate, clarify, and avoid any conflict of interest, to all parties concerned, when dealing with consumers, consulting with competitors, or in providing services requiring potentially conflicting roles (for example, finding out information about one facility that would help a competitor). The conflicting roles or responsibilities must be clarified and appropriate action must be taken to minimize any conflict of interest.

2.4. Ensure that the working environment is consistent and encourages compliance with the AHIMA Code of Ethics, taking reasonable steps to eliminate any conditions in their organizations that violate, interfere with, or discourage compliance with the code.

2.5. Take responsibility and credit, including authorship credit, only for work they actually perform or to which they contribute. Honestly acknowledge the work of and the contributions made by others verbally or written, such as in publication.

Health information management professionals **shall not:**

2.6. Permit their private conduct to interfere with their ability to fulfill their professional responsibilities.

2.7. Take unfair advantage of any professional relationship or exploit others to further their personal, religious, political, or business interests.

III. *Preserve, protect, and secure personal health information in any form or medium and hold in the highest regard the contents of the records and other information of a confidential nature obtained in the official capacity, taking into account the applicable statutes and regulations.*

Health information management professionals **shall:**

3.1. Protect the confidentiality of patients' written and electronic records and other sensitive information. Take reasonable steps to ensure that patients' records are stored in a secure location and that patients' records are not available to others who are not authorized to have access.

3.2. Take precautions to ensure and maintain the confidentiality of information transmitted, transferred, or disposed of in the event of a termination, incapacitation, or death of a healthcare provider to other parties through the use of any media. Disclosure of identifying information should be avoided whenever possible.

3.3. Inform recipients of the limitations and risks associated with providing services via electronic media (such as computer, telephone, fax, radio, and television).

IV. Refuse to participate in or conceal unethical practices or procedures.

Health information management professionals **shall:**

4.1. Act in a professional and ethical manner at all times.

4.2. Take adequate measures to discourage, prevent, expose, and correct the unethical conduct of colleagues.

4.3. Be knowledgeable about established policies and procedures for handling concerns about colleagues' unethical behavior. These include policies and procedures created by AHIMA, licensing and regulatory bodies, employers, supervisors, agencies, and other professional organizations.

4.4. Seek resolution if there is a belief that a colleague has acted unethically or if there is a belief of incompetence or impairment by discussing their concerns with the colleague when feasible and when such discussion is likely to be productive. Take action through appropriate formal channels, such as contacting an accreditation or regulatory body and/or the AHIMA Professional Ethics Committee.

4.5. Consult with a colleague when feasible and assist the colleague in taking remedial action when there is direct knowledge of a health information management colleague's incompetence or impairment.

Health information management professionals **shall not:**

4.6. Participate in, condone, or be associated with dishonesty, fraud and abuse, or deception. A non-inclusive list of examples includes:

- Allowing patterns of retrospective documentation to avoid suspension or increase reimbursement

- Assigning codes without physician documentation

- Coding when documentation does not justify the procedures that have been billed

- Coding an inappropriate level of service

- Miscoding to avoid conflict with others

- Engaging in negligent coding practices

- Hiding or ignoring review outcomes, such as performance data

- Failing to report licensure status for a physician through the appropriate channels

- Recording inaccurate data for accreditation purposes

- Hiding incomplete medical records

- Allowing inappropriate access to genetic, adoption, or behavioral health information

- Misusing sensitive information about a competitor

- Violating the privacy of individuals

V. Advance health information management knowledge and practice through continuing education, research, publications, and presentations.

Health information management professionals **shall:**

5.1. Develop and enhance continually their professional expertise, knowledge, and skills (including appropriate education, research, training, consultation, and supervision). Contribute to the knowledge base of health information management and share with colleagues their knowledge related to practice, research, and ethics.

5.2. Base practice decisions on recognized knowledge, including empirically based knowledge relevant to health information management and health information management ethics.

5.3. Contribute time and professional expertise to activities that promote respect for the value, integrity, and competence of the health information management profession. These activities may include teaching, research, consultation, service, legislative testimony, presentations in the community, and participation in their professional organizations.

5.4. Engage in evaluation or research that ensures the anonymity or confidentiality of participants and of the data obtained from them by following guidelines developed for the participants in consultation with appropriate institutional review boards. Report evaluation and research findings accurately and take steps to correct any errors later found in published data using standard publication methods.

5.5. Take reasonable steps to provide or arrange for continuing education and staff development, addressing current knowledge and emerging developments related to health information management practice and ethics.

Health information management professionals **shall not:**

5.6. Design or conduct evaluation or research that is in conflict with applicable federal or state laws.

5.7. Participate in, condone, or be associated with fraud or abuse.

VI. Recruit and mentor students, peers and colleagues to develop and strengthen professional workforce.

Health information management professionals **shall:**

6.1. Evaluate students' performance in a manner that is fair and respectful when functioning as educators or clinical internship supervisors.

6.2. Be responsible for setting clear, appropriate, and culturally sensitive boundaries for students.

6.3. Be a mentor for students, peers and new health information management professionals to develop and strengthen skills.

6.4. Provide directed practice opportunities for students.

Health information management professionals **shall not:**

6.5. Engage in any relationship with students in which there is a risk of exploitation or potential harm to the student.

VII. *Accurately represent the profession to the public.*

Health information management professionals **shall:**

7.1 Be an advocate for the profession in all settings and participate in activities that promote and explain the mission, values, and principles of the profession to the public.

VIII. *Perform honorably health information management association responsibilities, either appointed or elected, and preserve the confidentiality of any privileged information made known in any official capacity.*

Health information management professionals **shall:**

8.1. Perform responsibly all duties as assigned by the professional association.

8.2. Resign from an Association position if unable to perform the assigned responsibilities with competence.

8.3. Speak on behalf of professional health information management organizations, accurately representing the official and authorized positions of the organizations.

IX. *State truthfully and accurately their credentials, professional education, and experiences.*

Health information management professionals **shall:**

9.1. Make clear distinctions between statements made and actions engaged in as a private individual and as a representative of the health information management profession, a professional health information organization, or the health information management professional's employer.

9.2. Claim and ensure that their representations to patients, agencies, and the public of professional qualifications, credentials, education, competence, affiliations, services provided, training, certification, consultation received, supervised experience, other relevant professional experience are accurate.

9.3. Claim only those relevant professional credentials actually possessed and correct any inaccuracies occurring regarding credentials.

X. *Facilitate interdisciplinary collaboration in situations supporting health information practice.*

Health information management professionals **shall:**

10.1. Participate in and contribute to decisions that affect the well-being of patients by drawing on the perspectives, values, and experiences of those involved in decisions related to patients. Professional and ethical obligations of the interdisciplinary team as a whole and of its individual members should be clearly established.

XI. Respect the inherent dignity and worth of every person.

Health information management professionals **shall:**

11.1. Treat each person in a respectful fashion, being mindful of individual differences and cultural and ethnic diversity.

11.2. Promote the value of self-determination for each individual.

Adapted with permission from the Code of Ethics of the National Association of Social Workers.

Resources

National Association of Social Workers. "Code of Ethics." 1999. Available at http://www.naswdc.org.

Harman, L.B. (Ed.). *Ethical challenges in the management of health information.* Gaithersburg, MD: Aspen, 2001.

AHIMA Code of Ethics, 1957, 1977, 1988, and 1998.

Appendix C

AHIMA Practice Brief on Data Quality

Managing and Improving Data Quality (Updated)

Complete and accurate diagnostic and procedural coded data is necessary for research, epidemiology, outcomes and statistical analyses, financial and strategic planning, reimbursement, evaluation of quality of care, and communication to support the patient's treatment.

Consistency of coding has been a major AHIMA initiative in the quest to improve data quality management in healthcare service reporting. The Association has also taken a stand on the quality of healthcare data and information.[1]

Data Quality Mandates

Adherence to industry standards and approved coding principles that generate coded data of the highest quality and consistency remains critical to the healthcare industry and the maintenance of information integrity throughout healthcare systems. HIM professionals must continue to meet the challenges of maintaining an accurate and meaningful database reflective of patient mix and resource use. As long as diagnostic and procedural codes serve as the basis for payment methodologies, the ethics of clinical coders and healthcare organization billing processes will be challenged.

Ensuring accuracy of coded data is a shared responsibility between HIM professionals, clinicians, business services staff, and information systems integrity professionals. The HIM professional has the unique responsibility of administration, oversight, analysis, and/or coding clinical data in all healthcare organizations. Care must be taken in organizational structures to ensure that oversight of the coding and data management process falls within the HIM department's responsibility area so data quality mandates are upheld and appropriate HIM principles are applied to business practices.

Clinical Collaboration

The Joint Commission and the Medicare Conditions of Participation as well as other accreditation agencies require final diagnoses and procedures to be recorded in the medical record and authenticated by the responsible practitioner. State laws also provide guidelines concerning the content of the health record as a legal document.

Clinical documentation primarily created by physicians is the cornerstone of accurate coding, supplemented by appropriate policies and procedures developed by facilities to meet patient care requirements. Coded data originates from the collaboration between clinicians and HIM professionals with clinical terminology, classification system, nomenclature, data analysis, and compliance policy expertise.

Thus, the need for collaboration, cooperation, and communication between clinicians and support personnel continues to grow as information gathering and storage embrace new technology. Movement of the coding process into the business processing side of a healthcare organization must not preclude access to and regular communication with clinicians.

Clinical Database Evaluation

Regulatory agencies are beginning to apply data analysis tools to monitor data quality and reliability for reimbursement appropriateness and to identify unusual claims data patterns that may indicate payment errors or health insurance fraud. Examples include the Hospital Payment Monitoring Program tool First Look Analysis Tool for Hospital Outlier Monitoring (FATHOM), used by Quality Improvement Organizations, and the comprehensive error rate testing (CERT) process to be used by Centers for Medicare & Medicaid Services carriers to produce national, contractor, provider type, and benefit category-specific paid claims error rates.

Ongoing evaluation of the clinical database by health information managers facilitates ethical reporting of clinical information and early identification of data accuracy problems for timely and appropriate resolution. Pattern analysis of codes is a useful tool for prevention of compliance problems by identifying and correcting clinical coding errors.

Coding errors have multiple causes, some within the control of HIM processes and others that occur outside the scope of HIM due to inadequacy of the source document or the lack of information integrity resulting from inappropriate computer programming routines or software logic.

Data Quality Management and Improvement Initiatives

The following actions are required in any successful program:

- Evaluation and trending of diagnosis and procedure code selections, the appropriateness of reimbursement group assignment, and other coded data elements such as discharge status are required. This action ensures that clinical concept validity, appropriate code sequencing, specific code use requirements, and clinical pertinence are reflected in the codes reported

- Reporting data quality review results to organizational leadership, compliance staff, and the medical staff. This stresses accountability for data quality to everyone involved and allows the root causes of inconsistency or lack of reliability of data validity to be addressed. If the source for code assignment is inadequate or invalid, the results may reflect correct coding by the coding professional, but still represent a data quality problem because the code assigned does not reflect the actual concept or event as it occurred

- Following up on and monitoring identified problems. HIM professionals must resist the temptation to overlook inadequate documentation and report codes without appropriate clinical foundation within the record just to speed up claims processing, meet a business requirement, or obtain additional reimbursement. There is an ethical duty as members of the healthcare team to educate physicians on appropriate documentation practices and maintain high standards for health information practice. Organizational structures must support these efforts by the enforcement of medical staff rules and regulations and continuous monitoring of clinical pertinence of documentation to meet both business and patient care requirements

HIM clinical data specialists who understand data quality management concepts and the relationship of clinical code assignments to reimbursement and decision support for healthcare will have important roles to play in the healthcare organizations of the future. Continuing education and career boosting specialty advancement programs are expected to be the key to job security and professional growth as automation continues to change healthcare delivery, claims processing, and compliance activities.[2]

Data Quality Recommendations

HIM coding professionals and the organizations that employ them are accountable for data quality that requires the following behaviors.

HIM professionals should:

- Adopt best practices made known in professional resources and follow the code of ethics for the profession or their specific compliance programs.[3] This guidance applies to all settings and all health plans

- Use the entire health record as part of the coding process in order to assign and report the appropriate clinical codes for the standard transactions and codes sets required for external reporting and meeting internal abstracting requirements

- Adhere to all official coding guidelines published in the HIPAA standard transactions and code sets regulation. ICD-9-CM guidelines are available for downloading at www.cdc.gov/nchs/data/icd9/icdguide.pdf. Additional official coding advice is published in the quarterly publication AHA *Coding Clinic for ICD-9-CM*. CPT guidelines are located within the CPT code books and additional information and coding advice is provided in the AMA monthly publication *CPT Assistant*. Modifications to the initial HIPAA standards for electronic transactions or adoption of additional standards are submitted first to the designated standard maintenance organization. For more information, go to http://aspe.os. dhhs.gov/admnsimp/final/dsmo.htm.

- Develop appropriate facility or practice-specific guidelines when available coding guidelines do not address interpretation of the source document or guide code selection in specific circumstances. Facility practice guidelines should not conflict with official coding guidelines

- Maintain a working relationship with clinicians through ongoing communication and documentation improvement programs

- Report root causes of data quality concerns when identified. Problematic issues that arise from individual physicians or groups of clinicians should be referred to medical staff leadership or the compliance office for investigation and resolution

- Query when necessary. Best practices and coding guidelines suggest that when coding professionals encounter conflicting or ambiguous documentation in a source document, the physician must be queried to confirm the appropriate code selection[4]

- Consistently seek out innovative methods to capture pertinent information required for clinical code assignment to minimize unnecessary clinician inquiries. Alternative methods of accessing information necessary for code assignment may prevent the need to wait for completion of the health record, such as electronic access to clinical reports

- Ensure that clinical code sets reported to outside agencies are fully supported by documentation within the health record and clearly reflected in diagnostic statements and procedure reports provided by a physician

- Provide the physician the opportunity to review reported diagnoses and procedures on pre- or post-claim or post-bill submission, via mechanisms such as:

  —providing a copy (via mail, fax, or electronic transmission) of the sequenced codes and their narrative descriptions, taking appropriate care to protect patient privacy and security of the information

  —placing the diagnostic and procedural listing within the record and bringing it to the physician's attention within the appropriate time frame for correction when warranted

- Create a documentation improvement program or offer educational programs concerning the relationship of health record entries and health record management to data quality, information integrity, patient outcomes, and business success of the organization

- Conduct a periodic or ongoing review of any automated billing software (chargemasters, service description masters, practice management systems, claims scrubbers, medical necessity software) used to ensure code appropriateness and validity of clinical codes

- Require a periodic or ongoing review of encounter forms or other resource tools that involve clinical code assignment to ensure validity and appropriateness

- Complete appropriate continuing education and training to keep abreast of clinical advancements in diagnosis and treatment, billing and compliance issues, regulatory requirements, and coding guideline changes, and to maintain professional credentials

HIM coding professionals and the organizations that employ them have the responsibility to not engage in, promote, or tolerate the following behaviors that adversely affect data quality. HIM professionals should not:

- Make assumptions requiring clinical judgment concerning the etiology or context of the condition under consideration for code reporting

- Misrepresent the patient's clinical picture through code assignment for diagnoses/procedures unsupported by the documentation in order to maximize reimbursement, affect insurance policy coverage, or because of other third-party payer requirements. This includes falsification of conditions to meet medical necessity requirements when the patient's condition does not support health plan coverage for the service in question or using a specific code requested by a payer when, according to official coding guidelines, a different code is mandatory

- Omit the reporting of clinical codes that represent actual clinical conditions or services but negatively affect a facility's data profile, negate health plan coverage, or lower the reimbursement potential

- Allow changing of clinical code assignments under any circumstances without consultation with the coding professional involved and the clinician whose services are being reported. Changes are allowed only with subsequent validation of the documentation supporting the need for code revision

- Fail to use the physician query process outlined by professional practice standards or required by quality improvement organizations under contract for federal and state agencies that reimburse for healthcare services

- Assign codes to an incomplete record without organizational policies in place to ensure the codes are reviewed after the records are complete. Failure to confirm the accuracy and completeness of the codes submitted for a reimbursement claim upon completion of the medical record can increase both data quality and compliance risks[5]

- Promote or tolerate the falsification of clinical documentation or misrepresentation of clinical conditions or service provided

Prepared by AHIMA's Coding Products and Services team:

Kathy Brouch, RHIA, CCS
Susan Hull, MPH, RHIA, CCS
Karen Kostick, RHIT, CCS, CCS-P
Rita Scichilone, MHSA, RHIA, CCS, CCS-P
Mary Stanfill, RHIA, CCS, CCS-P
Ann Zeisset, RHIT, CCS, CCS-P

Notes

1. For details, see AHIMA's Position Statements on Consistency of Healthcare Diagnostic and Procedural Coding and on the Quality of Healthcare Data and Information at www.ahima.org/dc/positions.

2. For more information on AHIMA's specialty advancement programs, go to http://campus.ahima.org. Institutes for Healthcare Data Analytics and Clinical Data Management are planned for the 2003 AHIMA National Convention. Visit www.ahima.org/convention for more information.

3. AHIMA's Standards of Ethical Coding are available at www.ahima.org/infocenter/guidelines.

4. Prophet, Sue. "Practice Brief: Developing a Physician Query Process." *Journal of AHIMA* 72, no. 9 (2001): 88I–M.

5. More guidelines for HIM policy and procedure development are available in *Health Information Management Compliance: A Model Program for Healthcare Organizations* by Sue Prophet, AHIMA, 2002. Coding from incomplete records is also discussed in the AHIMA Practice Brief "Developing a Coding Compliance Document" in the July/August 2001 *Journal of AHIMA* (vol. 72, no. 7, prepared by AHIMA's Coding Practice Team).

Reference

AHIMA Coding Products and Services Team. "Managing and Improving Data Quality (Updated) (AHIMA Practice Brief)." *Journal of AHIMA* 74, no.7 (July/August 2003): 64A–C.

Appendix D

AHIMA Position Statement on Data Quality

Quality Healthcare Data and Information

The American Health Information Management Association (AHIMA) advocates quality healthcare data and its transformation into meaningful healthcare information to improve the effectiveness and assess the quality of patient care. AHIMA believes that information is one of the most important resources of a healthcare organization.

In the course of healthcare delivery and management, various information systems deliver data that are used for administrative and patient care decisions. Information can be defined as organized data or knowledge that provides a basis for decision-making. AHIMA represents United States' health information management professionals who have received specialized education and training and are certified as Registered Record Administrators (RRA), Accredited Record Technicians (ART), or Certified Coding Specialists (CCS). The members of AHIMA are specialists in collecting, analyzing, processing, integrating, storing, and securing healthcare data and information. This information serves as a means of communication between physicians and other healthcare professionals to document the course of the patient's illness and treatment during each current and subsequent episode of care. Members receive extensive training in the classification and coding of healthcare information for reimbursement, statistical, and research purposes.

Healthcare information and data serve important functions, including:

- Evaluation of the adequacy and appropriateness of patient care;

- Use in making decisions regarding healthcare policies, delivery systems, funding, expansion, education, and research;

- Support for insurance and benefit claims;

- Assistance in protecting the legal interests of the patients, healthcare professionals, and healthcare facilities;

- Identification of disease incidence to control outbreaks and improve the public health;

- Provision of case studies and epidemiological data for the education of health professionals; and

- Provision of data to expand the body of medical knowledge.

To maintain data integrity and the quality of healthcare information, AHIMA members assume a leadership role in a variety of healthcare settings, including managed care, consulting, information systems development, and education, as well as through professional affiliations. AHIMA publishes educational material and is a resource to its members as well as others involved in the creation and utilization of health information. AHIMA interacts with other organizations in developing criteria and guidelines for documentation of patient care.

AHIMA believes the following are necessary components of healthcare data and information systems to ensure its quality, integrity, and reliability.

1. Collaboration by individuals providing healthcare with those processing and using health information.

2. Provision of complete, accurate, and timely documentation of pertinent facts and observations about an individual's health, including past and present illnesses, tests, treatments, and outcomes.

3. Assurance of the integrity of the data and protection of its unauthorized disclosure, whether it is a paper- or computer-based system.

4. Establishment of clear, standard data collection guidelines for all levels of patient care in all sites of service, e.g., inpatient, outpatient, emergency department, ambulatory clinics, medical practices, and home health.

5. Support for the development and use of coding guidelines and adherence to the highest standards for accurate abstracting and coding of health information throughout the United States by all legitimate users, including healthcare organizations, third-party payers, and federal, state, and local governments.

6. Respect for confidentiality of individually-identifiable health information.

7. Commitment to ethical principles in the collection and dissemination of healthcare information.

The quality of healthcare today and in the future is dependent on the quality of healthcare information.

Approved by AHIMA's Board of Directors: December 1996. (Revision currently being considered.)

Appendix E

ICD-9-CM Official Guidelines
for Coding and Reporting

ICD-9-CM Official Guidelines for Coding and Reporting appear as published on the CMS
Web site: www.cms.gov.

ICD-9-CM Official Guidelines for Coding and Reporting

Effective April 1, 2005
Narrative changes appear in bold text
The guidelines have been updated to include the V Code Table

The Centers for Medicare and Medicaid Services (CMS) and the National Center for Health Statistics (NCHS), two departments within the U. S. Federal Government's Department of Health and Human Services (DHHS) provide the following guidelines for coding and reporting using the International Classification of Diseases, 9th Revision, Clinical Modification (ICD-9-CM). These guidelines should be used as a companion document to the official version of the ICD-9-CM as published on CD-ROM by the U.S. Government Printing Office (GPO).

These guidelines have been approved by the four organizations that make up the Cooperating Parties for the ICD-9-CM: the American Hospital Association (AHA), the American Health Information Management Association (AHIMA), CMS, and NCHS. These guidelines are included on the official government version of the ICD-9-CM, and also appear in *"Coding Clinic for ICD-9-CM"* published by the AHA.

These guidelines are a set of rules that have been developed to accompany and complement the official conventions and instructions provided within the ICD-9-CM itself. These guidelines are based on the coding and sequencing instructions in Volumes I, II and III of ICD-9-CM, but provide additional instruction. **Adherence to these guidelines when assigning ICD-9-CM diagnosis and procedure codes is required under the Health Insurance Portability and Accountability Act (HIPAA). The diagnosis codes (Volumes 1-2) have been adopted under HIPAA for all healthcare settings. Volume 3 procedure codes have been adopted for inpatient procedures reported by hospitals**. A joint effort between the healthcare provider and the coder is essential to achieve complete and accurate documentation, code assignment, and reporting of diagnoses and procedures. These guidelines have been developed to assist both the healthcare provider and the coder in identifying those diagnoses and procedures that are to be reported. The importance of consistent, complete documentation in the medical record cannot be overemphasized. Without such documentation accurate coding cannot be achieved. **The entire record should be reviewed to determine the specific reason for the encounter and the conditions treated.**

The term encounter is used for all settings, including hospital admissions. In the context of these guidelines, the term provider is used throughout the guidelines to mean physician or any qualified health care practitioner who is legally accountable for establishing the patient's diagnosis. Only this set of guidelines, approved by the Cooperating Parties, is official.

The guidelines are organized into sections. Section I includes the structure and conventions of the classification and general guidelines that apply to the entire classification, and chapter-specific guidelines that correspond to the chapters as they are arranged in the classification. Section II includes guidelines for selection of principal diagnosis for non-outpatient settings. Section III includes guidelines for reporting additional diagnoses in non-outpatient settings. Section IV is for outpatient coding and reporting.

ICD-9-CM Official Guidelines for Coding and Reporting 1
Section I.   Conventions, general coding guidelines and chapter specific guidelines 6
    A.   Conventions for the ICD-9-CM 6
        1.   Format: 6
        2.   Abbreviations 6
            a.   **Index abbreviations** 6
            b.   **Tabular abbreviations** 6
        3.   Punctuation 6
        4.   Includes and Excludes Notes and Inclusion terms 7
        5.   Other and Unspecified codes 7
            a.   **"Other" codes** 7
            b.   **"Unspecified" codes** 7
        6.   Etiology/manifestation convention ("code first", "use additional code" and "in diseases
              classified elsewhere" notes) 8
        7.   "And" 8
        8.   "With" 9
        9.   "See" and "See Also" 9
    B.   General Coding Guidelines 9
        1.   Use of Both Alphabetic Index and Tabular List 9
        2.   Locate each term in the Alphabetic Index 9
        3.   Level of Detail in Coding 9
        4.   Code or codes from 001.0 through V83.89 10
        5.   Selection of codes 001.0 through 999.9 10
        6.   Signs and symptoms 10
        7.   Conditions that are an integral part of a disease process 10
        8.   Conditions that are not an integral part of a disease process 10
        9.   Multiple coding for a single condition 10
        10.   Acute and Chronic Conditions 11
        11.   Combination Code 11
        12.   Late Effects 11
        13.   Impending or Threatened Condition 12
    C.   Chapter-Specific Coding Guidelines 12
        1.   Chapter 1: Infectious and Parasitic Diseases (001-139) 12
            a.   **Human Immunodeficiency Virus (HIV) Infections** 12
            b.   **Septicemia, Systemic Inflammatory Response Syndrome (SIRS), Sepsis, Severe
                  Sepsis, and Septic Shock** 14
        2.   Chapter 2: Neoplasms (140-239) 17
            a.   **Treatment directed at the malignancy** 18
            b.   **Treatment of secondary site** 18
            c.   **Coding and sequencing of complications** 18
            d.   **Primary malignancy previously excised** 19
            e.   **Admissions/Encounters involving chemotherapy and radiation therapy** 19
            f.   **Admission/encounter to determine extent of malignancy** 20
            g.   **Symptoms, signs, and ill-defined conditions listed in Chapter 16** 20
            h.   **Encounter for prophylactic organ removal** 20
        3.   Chapter 3: Endocrine, Nutritional, and Metabolic Diseases and Immunity Disorders (240-
              279) 21

    a.   **Diabetes mellitus** **21**
4.   Chapter 4: Diseases of Blood and Blood Forming Organs (280-289)................................. 23
    Reserved for future guideline expansion **23**
5.   Chapter 5: Mental Disorders (290-319).. 23
    Reserved for future guideline expansion **23**
6.   Chapter 6: Diseases of Nervous System and Sense Organs (320-389) 23
    Reserved for future guideline expansion **23**
7.   Chapter 7: Diseases of Circulatory System (390-459) 23
    a.   **Hypertension** **23**
    b.   **Cerebral infarction/stroke/cerebrovascular accident (CVA)** **25**
    c.   **Postoperative cerebrovascular accident** **25**
    d.   **Late Effects of Cerebrovascular Disease** **25**
8.   Chapter 8: Diseases of Respiratory System (460-519).. 26
    a.   **Chronic Obstructive Pulmonary Disease [COPD] and Asthma**............................. **26**
    b.   **Chronic Obstructive Pulmonary Disease [COPD] and Bronchitis** **27**
9.   Chapter 9: Diseases of Digestive System (520-579) 28
    Reserved for future guideline expansion **28**
10.   Chapter 10: Diseases of Genitourinary System (580-629) 28
    Reserved for future guideline expansion **28**
11.   Chapter 11: Complications of Pregnancy, Childbirth, and the Puerperium (630-677) 28
    a.   **General Rules for Obstetric Cases** **28**
    b.   **Selection of OB Principal or First-listed Diagnosis** **28**
    c.   **Fetal Conditions Affecting the Management of the Mother** **29**
    d.   **HIV Infection in Pregnancy, Childbirth and the Puerperium** **30**
    e.   **Current Conditions Complicating Pregnancy**.. **30**
    f.   **Diabetes mellitus in pregnancy**... **30**
    g.   **Gestational diabetes**... **31**
    h.   **Normal Delivery, Code 650** **31**
    i.   **The Postpartum and Peripartum Periods** **31**
    j.   **Code 677, Late effect of complication of pregnancy**... **32**
    k.   **Abortions** **33**
12.   Chapter 12: Diseases Skin and Subcutaneous Tissue (680-709) 34
    Reserved for future guideline expansion **34**
13.   Chapter 13: Diseases of Musculoskeletal and Connective Tissue (710-739)........................ 34
    Reserved for future guideline expansion **34**
14.   Chapter 14: Congenital Anomalies (740-759)... 34
    a.   **Codes in categories 740-759, Congenital Anomalies**.. **34**
15.   Chapter 15: Newborn (Perinatal) Guidelines (760-779)... 34
    a.   **General Perinatal Rules** **34**
    b.   **Use of codes V30-V39**.. **36**
    c.   **Newborn transfers** **36**
    d.   **Use of category V29** **36**
    e.   **Use of other V codes on perinatal records** **36**
    f.   **Maternal Causes of Perinatal Morbidity**... **36**
    g.   **Congenital Anomalies in Newborns** **37**
    h.   **Coding Additional Perinatal Diagnoses**.. **37**
    i.   **Prematurity and Fetal Growth Retardation** **37**

j.   Newborn sepsis 38
16.   Chapter 16: Signs, Symptoms and Ill-Defined Conditions (780-799) 38
17.   Chapter 17: Injury and Poisoning (800-999) 38
    a.   Coding of Injuries 38
    b.   Coding of Fractures 39
    c.   Coding of Burns 39
    d.   Coding of Debridement of Wound, Infection, or Burn 41
    e.   Adverse Effects, Poisoning and Toxic Effects 41
18.   Classification of Factors Influencing Health Status and Contact with Health Service
        (Supplemental V01-V84) 43
    a.   Introduction 43
    b.   V codes use in any healthcare setting 44
    c.   V Codes indicate a reason for an encounter 44
    d.   Categories of V Codes 44
19.   Supplemental Classification of External Causes of Injury and Poisoning (E-codes, E800-
        E999) 58
    a.   General E Code Coding Guidelines 58
    b.   Place of Occurrence Guideline 59
    c.   Adverse Effects of Drugs, Medicinal and Biological Substances Guidelines ... 60
    d.   Multiple Cause E Code Coding Guidelines 61
    e.   Child and Adult Abuse Guideline 61
    f.   Unknown or Suspected Intent Guideline 62
    g.   Undetermined Cause 62
    h.   Late Effects of External Cause Guidelines 62
    i.   Misadventures and Complications of Care Guidelines 63
    j.   Terrorism Guidelines 63
        Selection of Principal Diagnosis 65

Section II.   65
    A.   Codes for symptoms, signs, and ill-defined conditions 65
    B.   Two or more interrelated conditions, each potentially meeting the definition for principal
            diagnosis. 65
    C.   Two or more diagnoses that equally meet the definition for principal diagnosis 65
    D.   Two or more comparative or contrasting conditions. 66
    E.   A symptom(s) followed by contrasting/comparative diagnoses 66
    F.   Original treatment plan not carried out 66
    G.   Complications of surgery and other medical care 66
    H.   Uncertain Diagnosis 66
Section III. Reporting Additional Diagnoses **66**
    A.   Previous conditions 67
    B.   Abnormal findings 67
    C.   Uncertain Diagnosis 68
Section IV. Diagnostic Coding and Reporting Guidelines for Outpatient Services **68**
    A.   Selection of first-listed condition 68
    B.   Codes from 001.0 through V84.8 69
    C.   Accurate reporting of ICD-9-CM diagnosis codes 69
    D.   Selection of codes 001.0 through 999.9 69
    E.   Codes that describe symptoms and signs 69

F.   Encounters for circumstances other than a disease or injury 69
G.   Level of Detail in Coding 69
    1.   ICD-9-CM codes with 3, 4, or 5 digits 69
    2.   Use of full number of digits required for a code 70
H. ICD-9-CM code for the diagnosis, condition, problem, or other reason for encounter/visit 70
I.   "Probable", "suspected", "questionable", "rule out", or "working diagnosis" 70
J.   Chronic diseases 70
K.   Code all documented conditions that coexist 70
L.   Patients receiving diagnostic services only 70
M. Patients receiving therapeutic services only 71
N.   Patients receiving preoperative evaluations only 71
O.   Ambulatory surgery 71
P.   Routine outpatient prenatal visits 71

Section I. Conventions, general coding guidelines and chapter specific guidelines

The conventions, general guidelines and chapter-specific guidelines are applicable to all health care settings unless otherwise indicated.

A. Conventions for the ICD-9-CM

The conventions for the ICD-9-CM are the general rules for use of the classification independent of the guidelines. These conventions are incorporated within the index and tabular of the ICD-9-CM as instructional notes. The conventions are as follows:

1. Format:

The ICD-9-CM uses an indented format for ease in reference

2. Abbreviations

a. Index abbreviations

NEC "Not elsewhere classifiable"
This abbreviation in the index represents "other specified" when a specific code is not available for a condition the index directs the coder to the "other specified" code in the tabular.

b. Tabular abbreviations

NEC "Not elsewhere classifiable"
This abbreviation in the tabular represents "other specified". When a specific code is not available for a condition the tabular includes an NEC entry under a code to identify the code as the "other specified" code (See Section I.A.5.a."Other" codes).

NOS "Not otherwise specified"
This abbreviation is the equivalent of unspecified. (See Section I.A.5.b., "Unspecified" codes)

3. Punctuation

[ ] Brackets are used in the tabular list to enclose synonyms, alternative wording or explanatory phrases. Brackets are used in the index to identify manifestation codes. (See Section I.A.6. "Etiology/manifestations")

( ) Parentheses are used in both the index and tabular to enclose supplementary words that may be present or absent in the statement of a disease or procedure without affecting the code number to which it is assigned. The terms within the parentheses are referred to as nonessential modifiers.

:   Colons are used in the Tabular list after an incomplete term which needs one or more of the modifiers following the colon to make it assignable to a given category.

4.   Includes and Excludes Notes and Inclusion terms

Includes: This note appears immediately under a three-digit code title to further define, or give examples of, the content of the category.

Excludes: An excludes note under a code indicates that the terms excluded from the code are to be coded elsewhere. In some cases the codes for the excluded terms should not be used in conjunction with the code from which it is excluded. An example of this is a congenital condition excluded from an acquired form of the same condition. The congenital and acquired codes should not be used together. In other cases, the excluded terms may be used together with an excluded code. An example of this is when fractures of different bones are coded to different codes. Both codes may be used together if both types of fractures are present.

Inclusion terms: List of terms are included under certain four and five digit codes. These terms are the conditions for which that code number is to be used. The terms may be synonyms of the code title, or, in the case of "other specified" codes, the terms are a list of the various conditions assigned to that code. The inclusion terms are not necessarily exhaustive. Additional terms found only in the index may also be assigned to a code.

5.   Other and Unspecified codes

a.   "Other" codes

Codes titled "other" or "other specified" (usually a code with a 4th digit 8 or fifth-digit 9 for diagnosis codes) are for use when the information in the medical record provides detail for which a specific code does not exist. Index entries with NEC in the line designate "other" codes in the tabular. These index entries represent specific disease entities for which no specific code exists so the term is included within an "other" code.

b.   "Unspecified" codes

Codes (usually a code with a 4th digit 9 or 5th digit 0 for diagnosis codes) titled "unspecified" are for use when the information in the medical record is insufficient to assign a more specific code.

6. Etiology/manifestation convention ("code first", "use additional code" and "in diseases classified elsewhere" notes)

Certain conditions have both an underlying etiology and multiple body system manifestations due to the underlying etiology. For such conditions, the ICD-9-CM has a coding convention that requires the underlying condition be sequenced first followed by the manifestation. Wherever such a combination exists, there is a "use additional code" note at the etiology code, and a "code first" note at the manifestation code. These instructional notes indicate the proper sequencing order of the codes, etiology followed by manifestation.

In most cases the manifestation codes will have in the code title, "in diseases classified elsewhere." Codes with this title are a component of the etiology/manifestation convention. The code title indicates that it is a manifestation code. "In diseases classified elsewhere" codes are never permitted to be used as first listed or principal diagnosis codes. They must be used in conjunction with an underlying condition code and they must be listed following the underlying condition.

There are manifestation codes that do not have "in diseases classified elsewhere" in the title. For such codes a "use additional code" note will still be present and the rules for sequencing apply.

In addition to the notes in the tabular, these conditions also have a specific index entry structure. In the index both conditions are listed together with the etiology code first followed by the manifestation codes in brackets. The code in brackets is always to be sequenced second.

The most commonly used etiology/manifestation combinations are the codes for Diabetes mellitus, category 250. For each code under category 250 there is a use additional code note for the manifestation that is specific for that particular diabetic manifestation. Should a patient have more than one manifestation of diabetes, more than one code from category 250 may be used with as many manifestation codes as are needed to fully describe the patient's complete diabetic condition. The **category** 250 diabetes codes should be sequenced first, followed by the manifestation codes.

"Code first" and "Use additional code" notes are also used as sequencing rules in the classification for certain codes that are not part of an etiology/manifestation combination. See - Section I.B.9. "Multiple coding for a single condition".

7. "And"
The word "and" should be interpreted to mean either "and" or "or" when it appears in a title.

8. "With"

The word "with" in the alphabetic index is sequenced immediately following the main term, not in alphabetical order.

9. "See" and "See Also"

The "see" instruction following a main term in the index indicates that another term should be referenced. It is necessary to go to the main term referenced with the "see" note to locate the correct code.

A "see also" instruction following a main term in the index instructs that there is another main term that may also be referenced that may provide additional index entries that may be useful. It is not necessary to follow the "see also" note when the original main term provides the necessary code.

B. General Coding Guidelines

1. Use of Both Alphabetic Index and Tabular List

Use both the Alphabetic Index and the Tabular List when locating and assigning a code. Reliance on only the Alphabetic Index or the Tabular List leads to errors in code assignments and less specificity in code selection.

2. Locate each term in the Alphabetic Index

Locate each term in the Alphabetic Index and verify the code selected in the Tabular List. Read and be guided by instructional notations that appear in both the Alphabetic Index and the Tabular List.

3. Level of Detail in Coding

Diagnosis and procedure codes are to be used at their highest number of digits available.

ICD-9-CM diagnosis codes are composed of codes with either 3, 4, or 5 digits. Codes with three digits are included in ICD-9-CM as the heading of a category of codes that may be further subdivided by the use of fourth and/or fifth digits, which provide greater detail.

A three-digit code is to be used only if it is not further subdivided. Where fourth-digit subcategories and/or fifth-digit subclassifications are provided, they must be assigned. A code is invalid if it has not been coded to the full number of digits required for that code. For example, Acute myocardial infarction, code 410, has fourth digits that describe the location of the infarction (e.g., 410.2, Of inferolateral wall), and fifth digits that identify the episode of care. It would be incorrect to report a code in category 410 without a fourth and fifth digit.

ICD-9-CM Volume 3 procedure codes are composed of codes with either 3 or 4 digits. Codes with two digits are included in ICD-9-CM as the heading of a category of codes that may be further subdivided by the use of third and/or fourth digits, which provide greater detail.

4. Code or codes from 001.0 through V84.8

The appropriate code or codes from 001.0 through V84.8 must be used to identify diagnoses, symptoms, conditions, problems, complaints or other reason(s) for the encounter/visit.

5. Selection of codes 001.0 through 999.9

The selection of codes 001.0 through 999.9 will frequently be used to describe the reason for the admission/encounter. These codes are from the section of ICD-9-CM for the classification of diseases and injuries (e.g., infectious and parasitic diseases; neoplasms; symptoms, signs, and ill-defined conditions, etc.).

6. Signs and symptoms

Codes that describe symptoms and signs, as opposed to diagnoses, are acceptable for reporting purposes when a related definitive diagnosis has not been established (confirmed) by the provider. Chapter 16 of ICD-9-CM, Symptoms, Signs, and Ill-defined conditions (codes 780.0 - 799.9) contain many, but not all codes for symptoms.

7. Conditions that are an integral part of a disease process

Signs and symptoms that are integral to the disease process should not be assigned as additional codes.

8. Conditions that are not an integral part of a disease process

Additional signs and symptoms that may not be associated routinely with a disease process should be coded when present.

9. Multiple coding for a single condition

In addition to the etiology/manifestation convention that requires two codes to fully describe a single condition that affects multiple body systems, there are other single conditions that also require more than one code. "Use additional code" notes are found in the tabular at codes that are not part of an etiology/manifestation pair where a secondary code is useful to fully describe a condition. The sequencing rule is the same as the etiology/manifestation pair - , "use additional code" indicates that a secondary code should be added.

For example, for infections that are not included in chapter 1, a secondary code from category 041, Bacterial infection in conditions classified elsewhere and of unspecified site, may be required to identify the bacterial organism causing the infection. A "use additional code" note will normally be found at the infectious disease code, indicating a need for the organism code to be added as a secondary code.

"Code first" notes are also under certain codes that are not specifically manifestation codes but may be due to an underlying cause. When a "code first" note is present and an underlying condition is present the underlying condition should be sequenced first.

"Code, if applicable, any causal condition first", notes indicate that this code may be assigned as a principal diagnosis when the causal condition is unknown or not applicable. If a causal condition is known, then the code for that condition should be sequenced as the principal or first-listed diagnosis.

Multiple codes may be needed for late effects, complication codes and obstetric codes to more fully describe a condition. See the specific guidelines for these conditions for further instruction.

10. Acute and Chronic Conditions

If the same condition is described as both acute (subacute) and chronic, and separate subentries exist in the Alphabetic Index at the same indentation level, code both and sequence the acute (subacute) code first.

11. Combination Code

A combination code is a single code used to classify:
Two diagnoses, or
A diagnosis with an associated secondary process (manifestation)
A diagnosis with an associated complication

Combination codes are identified by referring to subterm entries in the Alphabetic Index and by reading the inclusion and exclusion notes in the Tabular List.

Assign only the combination code when that code fully identifies the diagnostic conditions involved or when the Alphabetic Index so directs. Multiple coding should not be used when the classification provides a combination code that clearly identifies all of the elements documented in the diagnosis. When the combination code lacks necessary specificity in describing the manifestation or complication, an additional code should be used as a secondary code.

12. Late Effects

A late effect is the residual effect (condition produced) after the acute phase of an illness or injury has terminated. There is no time limit on when a late effect code can be used. The residual may be apparent early, such as in cerebrovascular accident cases, or it may occur months or years later, such as that due to a previous injury. Coding of late effects generally requires two codes sequenced in the following order: The condition or nature of the late effect is sequenced first.   The late effect code is sequenced second.

An exception to the above guidelines are those instances where the code for late effect is followed by a manifestation code identified in the Tabular List and title, or the late effect code has been expanded (at the fourth and fifth-digit levels) to include the manifestation(s). The code for the acute phase of an illness or injury that led to the late effect is never used with a code for the late effect.

13.   Impending or Threatened Condition

Code any condition described at the time of discharge as "impending" or "threatened" as follows:

> If it did occur, code as confirmed diagnosis.
> If it did not occur, reference the Alphabetic Index to determine if the condition has a subentry term for "impending" or "threatened" and also reference main term entries for "Impending" and for "Threatened."
> If the subterms are listed, assign the given code.
> If the subterms are not listed, code the existing underlying condition(s) and not the condition described as impending or threatened.

C. Chapter-Specific Coding Guidelines

In addition to general coding guidelines, there are guidelines for specific diagnoses and/or conditions in the classification. Unless otherwise indicated, these guidelines apply to all health care settings. Please refer to Section II for guidelines on the selection of principal diagnosis.

1.   Chapter 1: Infectious and Parasitic Diseases (001-139)

a.   Human Immunodeficiency Virus (HIV) Infections

1)   Code only confirmed cases

Code only confirmed cases of HIV infection/illness. This is an exception to the hospital inpatient guideline Section II, H.

In this context, "confirmation" does not require documentation of positive serology or culture for HIV; the provider's diagnostic statement that the patient is HIV positive, or has an HIV-related illness is sufficient.

2)   Selection and sequencing of HIV codes

(a)   Patient admitted for HIV-related condition

If a patient is admitted for an HIV-related condition, the principal diagnosis should be 042, followed by additional diagnosis codes for all reported HIV-related conditions.

(b)   **Patient with HIV disease admitted for unrelated condition**

If a patient with HIV disease is admitted for an unrelated condition (such as a traumatic injury), the code for the unrelated condition (e.g., the nature of injury code) should be the principal diagnosis. Other diagnoses would be 042 followed by additional diagnosis codes for all reported HIV-related conditions.

(c)   **Whether the patient is newly diagnosed**

Whether the patient is newly diagnosed or has had previous admissions/encounters for HIV conditions is irrelevant to the sequencing decision.

(d)   **Asymptomatic human immunodeficiency virus**

V08 Asymptomatic human immunodeficiency virus [HIV] infection, is to be applied when the patient without any documentation of symptoms is listed as being "HIV positive," "known HIV," "HIV test positive," or similar terminology. Do not use this code if the term "AIDS" is used or if the patient is treated for any HIV-related illness or is described as having any condition(s) resulting from his/her HIV positive status; use 042 in these cases.

(e)   **Patients with inconclusive HIV serology**

Patients with inconclusive HIV serology, but no definitive diagnosis or manifestations of the illness, may be assigned code 795.71, Inconclusive serologic test for Human Immunodeficiency Virus [HIV].

(f)   **Previously diagnosed HIV-related illness**

Patients with any known prior diagnosis of an HIV-related illness should be coded to 042. Once a patient has developed an HIV-related illness, the patient should always be assigned code 042 on every subsequent admission/encounter. Patients previously diagnosed with any HIV illness (042) should never be assigned to 795.71 or V08.

(g)   **HIV Infection in Pregnancy, Childbirth and the Puerperium**

During pregnancy, childbirth or the puerperium, a patient admitted (or presenting for a health care encounter) because of an HIV-related illness should receive a principal diagnosis code of 647.6X, Other specified infectious and parasitic diseases in the mother classifiable elsewhere, but complicating the pregnancy, childbirth or the puerperium, followed by 042 and the code(s) for the HIV-related illness(es). Codes from Chapter 15 always take sequencing priority.

Patients with asymptomatic HIV infection status admitted (or presenting for a health care encounter) during pregnancy, childbirth, or the puerperium should receive codes of 647.6X and V08.

(h)   **Encounters for testing for HIV**

If a patient is being seen to determine his/her HIV status, use code V73.89, Screening for other specified viral disease. Use code V69.8, Other problems related to lifestyle, as a secondary code if an asymptomatic patient is in a known high risk group for HIV. Should a patient with signs or symptoms or illness, or a confirmed HIV related diagnosis be tested for HIV, code the signs and symptoms or the diagnosis. An additional counseling code V65.44 may be used if counseling is provided during the encounter for the test.

When a patient returns to be informed of his/her HIV test results use code V65.44, HIV counseling, if the results of the test are negative.

If the results are positive but the patient is asymptomatic use code V08, Asymptomatic HIV infection. If the results are positive and the patient is symptomatic use code 042, HIV infection, with codes for the HIV related symptoms or diagnosis. The HIV counseling code may also be used if counseling is provided for patients with positive test results.

b.   **Septicemia, Systemic Inflammatory Response Syndrome (SIRS), Sepsis, Severe Sepsis, and Septic Shock**

1)   **Sepsis as principal diagnosis or secondary diagnosis**

(a) **Sepsis as principal diagnosis**

If sepsis is present on admission, and meets the definition of principal diagnosis, the underlying systemic infection code (e.g., 038.xx, 112.5, etc) should be assigned as the principal diagnosis, followed by code 995.91, Systemic inflammatory response syndrome due to infectious process without organ dysfunction, as required by the sequencing rules in the Tabular List. Codes from subcategory 995.9 can never be assigned as a principal diagnosis.

(b) **Sepsis as secondary diagnoses**

When sepsis develops during the encounter (it was not present on admission), the sepsis codes may be assigned as secondary diagnoses, following the sequencing rules provided in the Tabular List.

(c) **Documentation unclear as to whether sepsis present on admission**

If the documentation is not clear whether the sepsis was present on admission, the provider should be queried. After provider query, if sepsis is determined at that point to have met the definition of principal diagnosis, the underlying systemic infection (038.xx, 112.5, etc) may be used as principal diagnosis along with code 995.91, Systemic inflammatory response syndrome due to infectious process without organ dysfunction.

2) **Septicemia/Sepsis**

In most cases, it will be a code from category 038, Septicemia, that will be used in conjunction with a code from subcategory 995.9 such as the following:

(a) **Streptococcal sepsis**

If the documentation in the record states streptococcal sepsis, codes 038.0 and code 995.91 should be used, in that sequence.

(b) **Streptococcal septicemia**

If the documentation states streptococcal septicemia, only code 038.0 should be assigned, however, the provider should be queried whether the patient has sepsis, an infection with SIRS.

(c)   Sepsis or SIRS must be documented

Either the term sepsis or SIRS must be documented, to assign a code from subcategory 995.9.

3)   Terms sepsis, severe sepsis, or SIRS

If the terms sepsis, severe sepsis, or SIRS are used with an underlying infection other than septicemia, such as pneumonia, cellulitis or a nonspecified urinary tract infection, a code from category 038 should be assigned first, then code 995.91, followed by the code for the initial infection. The use of the terms sepsis or SIRS indicates that the patient's infection has advanced to the point of a systemic infection so the systemic infection should be sequenced before the localized infection. The instructional note under subcategory 995.9 instructs to assign the underlying systemic infection first.

Note: The term urosepsis is a nonspecific term. If that is the only term documented then only code 599.0 should be assigned based on the default for the term in the ICD-9-CM index, in addition to the code for the causal organism if known.

4)   Severe sepsis

For patients with severe sepsis, the code for the systemic infection (e.g., 038.xx, 112.5, etc) or trauma should be sequenced first, followed by either code 995.92, Systemic inflammatory response syndrome due to infectious process with organ dysfunction, or code 995.94, Systemic inflammatory response syndrome due to noninfectious process with organ dysfunction. Codes for the specific organ dysfunctions should also be assigned.

5)   Septic shock

(a)   Sequencing of septic shock

Septic shock is a form of organ dysfunction associated with severe sepsis. A code for the initiating underlying systemic infection followed by a code for SIRS (code 995.92) must be assigned before the code for septic shock. As noted in the sequencing instructions in the Tabular List, the code for septic shock cannot be assigned as a principal diagnosis.

(b)   Septic Shock without documentation of severe sepsis

> **Septic shock cannot occur in the absence of severe sepsis. A code from subcategory 995.9 must be sequenced before the code for septic shock. The use additional code notes and the code first note provide sequencing instructions.**

6)   Sepsis and septic shock associated with abortion

Sepsis and septic shock associated with abortion, ectopic pregnancy, and molar pregnancy are classified to category codes in Chapter 11 (630-639).

7)   Negative or inconclusive blood cultures

Negative or inconclusive blood cultures do not preclude a diagnosis of septicemia or sepsis in patients with clinical evidence of the condition, however, the provider should be queried.

8)   Newborn sepsis

See Section I.C.15.j for information on the coding of newborn sepsis.

9)   Sepsis due to a Postprocedural Infection

Sepsis resulting from a postprocedural infection is a complication of care. For such cases code 998.59, Other postoperative infections, should be coded first followed by the appropriate codes for the sepsis. The other guidelines for coding sepsis should then be followed for the assignment of additional codes.

10)   External cause of injury codes with SIRS

An external cause code is not needed with codes 995.91, Systemic inflammatory response syndrome due to infectious process without organ dysfunction, or code 995.92, Systemic inflammatory response syndrome due to infectious process with organ dysfunction.

Refer to Section I.C.19.a.7   for instruction on the use of external cause of injury codes with codes for SIRS resulting from trauma.

2.   Chapter 2: Neoplasms (140-239)

<u>**General guidelines**</u>

Chapter 2 of the ICD-9-CM contains the codes for most benign and all malignant neoplasms. Certain benign neoplasms, such as prostatic adenomas, may be found in the specific body system chapters. To properly code a neoplasm it is necessary to determine from the record if the neoplasm is benign, in-situ, malignant, or of uncertain histologic behavior. If malignant, any secondary (metastatic) sites should also be determined.

The neoplasm table in the Alphabetic Index should be referenced first. However, if the histological term is documented, that term should be referenced first, rather than going immediately to the Neoplasm Table, in order to determine which column in the Neoplasm Table is appropriate. For example, if the documentation indicates "adenoma," refer to the term in the Alphabetic Index to review the entries under this term and the instructional note to "see also neoplasm, by site, benign." The table provides the proper code based on the type of neoplasm and the site. It is important to select the proper column in the table that corresponds to the type of neoplasm. The tabular should then be referenced to verify that the correct code has been selected from the table and that a more specific site code does not exist.

See Section I. C. 18.d.4. for information regarding V codes for genetic susceptibility to cancer.

a. Treatment directed at the malignancy

If the treatment is directed at the malignancy, designate the malignancy as the principal diagnosis.

b. Treatment of secondary site

When a patient is admitted because of a primary neoplasm with metastasis and treatment is directed toward the secondary site only, the secondary neoplasm is designated as the principal diagnosis even though the primary malignancy is still present.

c. Coding and sequencing of complications

Coding and sequencing of complications associated with the malignancies or with the therapy thereof are subject to the following guidelines:

1) Anemia associated with malignancy

When admission/encounter is for management of an anemia associated with the malignancy, and the treatment is only for anemia, the anemia is designated at the principal diagnosis and is followed by the appropriate code(s) for the malignancy.

2) Anemia associated with chemotherapy

When the admission/encounter is for management of an anemia associated with chemotherapy or radiotherapy and the only treatment is for the anemia, the anemia is sequenced first followed by the appropriate code(s) for the malignancy.

3) Management of dehydration due to the malignancy

When the admission/encounter is for management of dehydration due to the malignancy or the therapy, or a combination of both, and only the dehydration is being treated (intravenous rehydration), the dehydration is sequenced first, followed by the code(s) for the malignancy.

4) Treatment of a complication resulting from a surgical procedure

When the admission/encounter is for treatment of a complication resulting from a surgical procedure, designate the complication as the principal or first-listed diagnosis if treatment is directed at resolving the complication.

d. Primary malignancy previously excised

When a primary malignancy has been previously excised or eradicated from its site and there is no further treatment directed to that site and there is no evidence of any existing primary malignancy, a code from category V10, Personal history of malignant neoplasm, should be used to indicate the former site of the malignancy. Any mention of extension, invasion, or metastasis to another site is coded as a secondary malignant neoplasm to that site. The secondary site may be the principal or first-listed with the V10 code used as a secondary code.

e. Admissions/Encounters involving chemotherapy and radiation therapy

1) Episode of care involves surgical removal of neoplasm

When an episode of care involves the surgical removal of a neoplasm, primary or secondary site, followed by adjunct chemotherapy or radiation treatment, the neoplasm code should be assigned as principal or first-listed diagnosis, using codes in the 140-198 series or where appropriate in the 200-203 series.

2) Patient admission/encounter solely for administration of chemotherapy

If a patient admission/encounter is solely for the administration of chemotherapy or radiation therapy code V58.0, Encounter for radiation therapy, or V58.1, Encounter for chemotherapy, should be the first-listed or principal diagnosis. If a patient receives both chemotherapy and radiation therapy both codes should be listed, in either order of sequence.

3) Patient admitted for radiotherapy/chemotherapy and develops complications

When a patient is admitted for the purpose of radiotherapy or chemotherapy and develops complications such as uncontrolled nausea and vomiting or dehydration, the principal or first-listed diagnosis is V58.0, Encounter for radiotherapy, or V58.1, Encounter for chemotherapy, followed by any codes for the complications.

See Section I.C.18.d.8. for additional information regarding aftercare V codes.

f. Admission/encounter to determine extent of malignancy

When the reason for admission/encounter is to determine the extent of the malignancy, or for a procedure such as paracentesis or thoracentesis, the primary malignancy or appropriate metastatic site is designated as the principal or first-listed diagnosis, even though chemotherapy or radiotherapy is administered.

g. Symptoms, signs, and ill-defined conditions listed in Chapter 16

Symptoms, signs, and ill-defined conditions listed in Chapter 16 characteristic of, or associated with, an existing primary or secondary site malignancy cannot be used to replace the malignancy as principal or first-listed diagnosis, regardless of the number of admissions or encounters for treatment and care of the neoplasm.

h. Encounter for prophylactic organ removal

For encounters specifically for prophylactic removal of breasts, ovaries, or another organ due to a genetic susceptibility to cancer or a family history of cancer, the principal or first listed code should be a code from subcategory V50.4, Prophylactic organ removal, followed by the appropriate genetic susceptibility code and the appropriate family history code.

If the patient has a malignancy of one site and is having prophylactic removal of another site to prevent either a new primary malignancy or metastatic disease, a code for the malignancy should also be assigned in addition to a code from subcategory V50.4. A V50.4 code should not be assigned if the patient is having organ removal for treatment of a malignancy, such as the removal of the testes for the treatment of prostate cancer.

3. **Chapter 3: Endocrine, Nutritional, and Metabolic Diseases and Immunity Disorders (240-279)**

    a. **Diabetes mellitus**

    Codes under category 250, Diabetes mellitus, identify complications/manifestations associated with diabetes mellitus. A fifth-digit is required for all category 250 codes to identify the type of diabetes mellitus and whether the diabetes is controlled or uncontrolled.

    1) **Fifth-digits for category 250:**

        The following are the fifth-digits for the codes under category 250:

        0   type II or unspecified type, not stated as uncontrolled
        1   type I, [juvenile type], not stated as uncontrolled
        2   type II or unspecified type, uncontrolled
        3   type I, [juvenile type], uncontrolled

        The age of a patient is not the sole determining factor, though most type I diabetics develop the condition before reaching puberty. For this reason type I diabetes mellitus is also referred to as juvenile diabetes.

    2) **Type of diabetes mellitus not documented**

        If the type of diabetes mellitus is not documented in the medical record the default is type II.

    3) **Diabetes mellitus and the use of insulin**

        All type I diabetics must use insulin to replace what their bodies do not produce. However, the use of insulin does not mean that a patient is a type I diabetic. Some patients with type II diabetes mellitus are unable to control their blood sugar through diet and oral medication alone and do require insulin.   If the documentation in a medical record does not indicate the type of diabetes but does indicate that the patient uses insulin, the appropriate fifth-digit for type II must be used. For type II patients who routinely use insulin, code V58.67, Long-term (current) use of insulin, should also be assigned to indicate that the patient uses insulin. Code V58.67 should not be assigned if insulin is given temporarily to bring a type II patient's blood sugar under control during an encounter.

4) **Assigning and sequencing diabetes codes and associated conditions**

When assigning codes for diabetes and its associated conditions, the code(s) from category 250 must be sequenced before the codes for the associated conditions. The diabetes codes and the secondary codes that correspond to them are paired codes that follow the etiology/manifestation convention of the classification (See Section I.A.6., Etiology/manifestation convention). Assign as many codes from category 250 as needed to identify all of the associated conditions that the patient has. The corresponding secondary codes are listed under each of the diabetes codes.

5) **Diabetes mellitus in pregnancy and gestational diabetes**

(a) For diabetes mellitus complicating pregnancy, see Section I.C.11.f., Diabetes mellitus in pregnancy.

(b) For gestational diabetes, see Section I.C.11, g., Gestational diabetes.

6) **Insulin pump malfunction**

(a) Underdose of insulin due insulin pump failure

An underdose of insulin due to an insulin pump failure should be assigned 996.57, Mechanical complication due to insulin pump, as the principal or first listed code, followed by the appropriate diabetes mellitus code based on documentation.

(b) Overdose of insulin due to insulin pump failure

The principal or first listed code for an encounter due to an insulin pump malfunction resulting in an overdose of insulin, should also be 996.57, Mechanical complication due to insulin pump, followed by code 962.3, Poisoning by insulins and antidiabetic agents, and the appropriate diabetes mellitus code based on documentation.

4. **Chapter 4: Diseases of Blood and Blood Forming Organs (280-289)**

Reserved for future guideline expansion

5. **Chapter 5: Mental Disorders (290-319)**

Reserved for future guideline expansion

6. **Chapter 6: Diseases of Nervous System and Sense Organs (320-389)**

Reserved for future guideline expansion

7. **Chapter 7: Diseases of Circulatory System (390-459)**

   a. **Hypertension**

   <u>**Hypertension Table**</u>
   The Hypertension Table, found under the main term, "Hypertension", in the Alphabetic Index, contains a complete listing of all conditions due to or associated with hypertension and classifies them according to malignant, benign, and unspecified.

   1) **Hypertension, Essential, or NOS**

      Assign hypertension (arterial) (essential) (primary) (systemic) (NOS) to category code 401 with the appropriate fourth digit to indicate malignant (.0), benign (.1), or unspecified (.9). Do not use either .0 malignant or .1 benign unless medical record documentation supports such a designation.

   2) **Hypertension with Heart Disease**

      Heart conditions (425.8, 429.0-429.3, 429.8, 429.9) are assigned to a code from category 402 when a causal relationship is stated (due to hypertension) or implied (hypertensive). Use an additional code from category 428 to identify the type of heart failure in those patients with heart failure. More than one code from category 428 may be assigned if the patient has systolic or diastolic failure and congestive heart failure.

      The same heart conditions (425.8, 429.0-429.3, 429.8, 429.9) with hypertension, but without a stated casual relationship, are coded separately. Sequence according to the circumstances of the admission/encounter.

3) Hypertensive Renal Disease with Chronic Renal Failure

Assign codes from category 403, Hypertensive renal disease, when conditions classified to categories 585-587 are present. Unlike hypertension with heart disease, ICD-9-CM presumes a cause-and-effect relationship and classifies renal failure with hypertension as hypertensive renal disease.

4) Hypertensive Heart and Renal Disease

Assign codes from combination category 404, Hypertensive heart and renal disease, when both hypertensive renal disease and hypertensive heart disease are stated in the diagnosis. Assume a relationship between the hypertension and the renal disease, whether or not the condition is so designated. Assign an additional code from category 428, to identify the type of heart failure. More than one code from category 428 may be assigned if the patient has systolic or diastolic failure and congestive heart failure.

5) Hypertensive Cerebrovascular Disease

First assign codes from 430-438, Cerebrovascular disease, then the appropriate hypertension code from categories 401-405.

6) Hypertensive Retinopathy

Two codes are necessary to identify the condition. First assign the code from subcategory 362.11, Hypertensive retinopathy, then the appropriate code from categories 401-405 to indicate the type of hypertension.

7) Hypertension, Secondary

Two codes are required: one to identify the underlying etiology and one from category 405 to identify the hypertension. Sequencing of codes is determined by the reason for admission/encounter.

8) Hypertension, Transient

Assign code 796.2, Elevated blood pressure reading without diagnosis of hypertension, unless patient has an established diagnosis of hypertension. Assign code 642.3x for transient hypertension of pregnancy.

9) Hypertension, Controlled

Assign appropriate code from categories 401-405. This diagnostic statement usually refers to an existing state of hypertension under control by therapy.

10)   **Hypertension, Uncontrolled**

Uncontrolled hypertension may refer to untreated hypertension or hypertension not responding to current therapeutic regimen. In either case, assign the appropriate code from categories 401-405 to designate the stage and type of hypertension. Code to the type of hypertension.

11)   **Elevated Blood Pressure**

For a statement of elevated blood pressure without further specificity, assign code 796.2, Elevated blood pressure reading without diagnosis of hypertension, rather than a code from category 401.

b.   **Cerebral infarction/stroke/cerebrovascular accident (CVA)**

The terms stroke and CVA are often used interchangeably to refer to a cerebral infarction. The terms stroke, CVA, and cerebral infarction NOS are all indexed to the default code 434.91, Cerebral artery occlusion, unspecified, with infarction. Code 436, Acute, but ill-defined, cerebrovascular disease, should not be used when the documentation states stroke or CVA.

c.   **Postoperative cerebrovascular accident**

A cerebrovascular hemorrhage or infarction that occurs as a result of medical intervention is coded to 997.02, Iatrogenic cerebrovascular infarction or hemorrhage. Medical record documentation should clearly specify the cause- and-effect relationship between the medical intervention and the cerebrovascular accident in order to assign this code. A secondary code from the code range 430-432 or from a code from subcategories 433 or 434 with a fifth digit of "1" should also be used to identify the type of hemorrhage or infarct.

This guideline conforms to the use additional code note instruction at category 997. Code 436, Acute, but ill-defined, cerebrovascular disease, should not be used as a secondary code with code 997.02.

d.   **Late Effects of Cerebrovascular Disease**

1)   **Category 438, Late Effects of Cerebrovascular disease**

Category 438 is used to indicate conditions classifiable to categories 430-437 as the causes of late effects (neurologic deficits), themselves classified elsewhere. These "late effects" include neurologic deficits that persist after initial onset of conditions classifiable to 430-437. The neurologic deficits caused by cerebrovascular disease may be present from the onset or may arise at any time after the onset of the condition classifiable to 430-437.

2) **Codes from category 438 with codes from 430-437**

Codes from category 438 may be assigned on a health care record with codes from 430-437, if the patient has a current cerebrovascular accident (CVA) and deficits from an old CVA.

3) **Code V12.59**

Assign code V12.59 (and not a code from category 438) as an additional code for history of cerebrovascular disease when no neurologic deficits are present.

Chapter 8: Diseases of Respiratory System (460-519)

a. **Chronic Obstructive Pulmonary Disease [COPD] and Asthma**

1) **Conditions that comprise COPD and Asthma**

The conditions that comprise COPD are obstructive chronic bronchitis, subcategory 491.2, and emphysema, category 492. All asthma codes are under category 493, Asthma. Code 496, Chronic airway obstruction, not elsewhere classified, is a nonspecific code that should only be used when the documentation in a medical record does not specify the type of COPD being treated.

2) **Acute exacerbation of chronic obstructive bronchitis and asthma**

The codes for chronic obstructive bronchitis and asthma distinguish between uncomplicated cases and those in acute exacerbation. An acute exacerbation is a worsening or a decompensation of a chronic condition. An acute exacerbation is not equivalent to an infection superimposed on a chronic condition, though an exacerbation may be triggered by an infection.

3) **Overlapping nature of the conditions that comprise COPD and asthma**

Due to the overlapping nature of the conditions that make up COPD and asthma, there are many variations in the way these conditions are documented. Code selection must be based on the terms as documented. When selecting the correct code for the documented type of COPD and asthma, it is essential to first review the index, and then verify the code in the tabular list. There are many instructional notes under the different COPD subcategories and codes. It is important that all such notes be reviewed to assure correct code assignment.

4) **Acute exacerbation of asthma and status asthmaticus**

An acute exacerbation of asthma is an increased severity of the asthma symptoms, such as wheezing and shortness of breath. Status asthmaticus refers to a patient's failure to respond to therapy administered during an asthmatic episode and is a life threatening complication that requires emergency care. If status asthmaticus is documented by the provider with any type of COPD or with acute bronchitis, the status asthmaticus should be sequenced first. It supersedes any type of COPD including that with acute exacerbation or acute bronchitis. It is inappropriate to assign an asthma code with 5th digit 2, with acute exacerbation, together with an asthma code with 5th digit 1, with status asthmatics. Only the 5th digit 1 should be assigned.

b. **Chronic Obstructive Pulmonary Disease [COPD] and Bronchitis**

1) **Acute bronchitis with COPD**

Acute bronchitis, code 466.0, is due to an infectious organism. When acute bronchitis is documented with COPD, code 491.22, Obstructive chronic bronchitis with acute bronchitis, should be assigned. It is not necessary to also assign code 466.0. If a medical record documents acute bronchitis with COPD with acute exacerbation, only code 491.22 should be assigned. The acute bronchitis included in code 491.22 supersedes the acute exacerbation. If a medical record documents COPD with acute exacerbation without mention of acute bronchitis, only code 491.21 should be assigned.

9.   Chapter 9: Diseases of Digestive System (520-579)

Reserved for future guideline expansion

10.   Chapter 10: Diseases of Genitourinary System (580-629)

Reserved for future guideline expansion

11.   Chapter 11: Complications of Pregnancy, Childbirth, and the Puerperium (630-677)

a.   General Rules for Obstetric Cases

1)   Codes from chapter 11 and sequencing priority

Obstetric cases require codes from chapter 11, codes in the range 630-677, Complications of Pregnancy, Childbirth, and the Puerperium. Chapter 11 codes have sequencing priority over codes from other chapters. Additional codes from other chapters may be used in conjunction with chapter 11 codes to further specify conditions. Should the provider document that the pregnancy is incidental to the encounter, then code V22.2 should be used in place of any chapter 11 codes. It is the provider's responsibility to state that the condition being treated is not affecting the pregnancy.

2)   Chapter 11 codes used only on the maternal record

Chapter 11 codes are to be used only on the maternal record, never on the record of the newborn.

3)   Chapter 11 fifth-digits

Categories 640-648, 651-676 have required fifth-digits, which indicate whether the encounter is antepartum, postpartum and whether a delivery has also occurred.

4)   Fifth-digits, appropriate for each code

The fifth-digits, which are appropriate for each code number, are listed in brackets under each code. The fifth-digits on each code should all be consistent with each other. That is, should a delivery occur all of the fifth-digits should indicate the delivery.

b.   Selection of OB Principal or First-listed Diagnosis

1)   Routine outpatient prenatal visits

For routine outpatient prenatal visits when no complications are present codes V22.0, Supervision of normal first pregnancy, and V22.1, Supervision of other normal pregnancy, should be used as the first-listed diagnoses. These codes should not be used in conjunction with chapter 11 codes.

2)   Prenatal outpatient visits for high-risk patients

For prenatal outpatient visits for patients with high-risk pregnancies, a code from category V23, Supervision of high-risk pregnancy, should be used as the principal or first-listed diagnosis. Secondary chapter 11 codes may be used in conjunction with these codes if appropriate.

3)   Episodes when no delivery occurs

In episodes when no delivery occurs, the principal diagnosis should correspond to the principal complication of the pregnancy, which necessitated the encounter. Should more than one complication exist, all of which are treated or monitored, any of the complications codes may be sequenced first.

4)   When a delivery occurs

When a delivery occurs, the principal diagnosis should correspond to the main circumstances or complication of the delivery. In cases of cesarean delivery, the selection of the principal diagnosis should correspond to the reason the cesarean delivery was performed unless the reason for admission/encounter was unrelated to the condition resulting in the cesarean delivery.

5)   Outcome of delivery

An outcome of delivery code, V27.0-V27.9, should be included on every maternal record when a delivery has occurred. These codes are not to be used on subsequent records or on the newborn record.

c.   Fetal Conditions Affecting the Management of the Mother

1)   Codes from category 655

Known or suspected fetal abnormality affecting management of the mother, and category 656, Other fetal and placental problems affecting the management of the mother, are assigned only when the fetal condition is actually responsible for modifying the management of the mother, i.e., by requiring diagnostic studies, additional observation, special care, or termination of pregnancy. The fact that the fetal condition exists does not justify assigning a code from this series to the mother's record.

2) In utero surgery

In cases when surgery is performed on the fetus, a diagnosis code from category 655, Known or suspected fetal abnormalities affecting management of the mother, should be assigned identifying the fetal condition. Procedure code 75.36, Correction of fetal defect, should be assigned on the hospital inpatient record.

No code from Chapter 15, the perinatal codes, should be used on the mother's record to identify fetal conditions. Surgery performed in utero on a fetus is still to be coded as an obstetric encounter.

d. HIV Infection in Pregnancy, Childbirth and the Puerperium

During pregnancy, childbirth or the puerperium, a patient admitted because of an HIV-related illness should receive a principal diagnosis of 647.6X, Other specified infectious and parasitic diseases in the mother classifiable elsewhere, but complicating the pregnancy, childbirth or the puerperium, followed by 042 and the code(s) for the HIV-related illness(es).

Patients with asymptomatic HIV infection status admitted during pregnancy, childbirth, or the puerperium should receive codes of 647.6X and V08.

e. Current Conditions Complicating Pregnancy

Assign a code from subcategory 648.x for patients that have current conditions when the condition affects the management of the pregnancy, childbirth, or the puerperium. Use additional secondary codes from other chapters to identify the conditions, as appropriate.

f. Diabetes mellitus in pregnancy

Diabetes mellitus is a significant complicating factor in pregnancy. Pregnant women who are diabetic should be assigned code 648.0x, Diabetes mellitus complicating pregnancy, and a secondary code from category 250, Diabetes mellitus, to identify the type of diabetes.

Code V58.67, Long-term (current) use of insulin, should also be assigned if the diabetes mellitus is being treated with insulin.

g.   **Gestational diabetes**

Gestational diabetes can occur during the second and third trimester of pregnancy in women who were not diabetic prior to pregnancy. Gestational diabetes can cause complications in the pregnancy similar to those of pre-existing diabetes mellitus. It also puts the woman at greater risk of developing diabetes after the pregnancy. Gestational diabetes is coded to 648.8x, Abnormal glucose tolerance. Codes 648.0x and 648.8x should never be used together on the same record.

Code V58.67, Long-term (current) use of insulin, should also be assigned if the gestational diabetes is being treated with insulin.

h.   **Normal Delivery, Code 650**

1)   **Normal delivery**

Code 650 is for use in cases when a woman is admitted for a full-term normal delivery and delivers a single, healthy infant without any complications antepartum, during the delivery, or postpartum during the delivery episode. **Code 650 is always a principal diagnosis. It is not to be used if any other code from chapter 11 is needed to describe a current complication of the antenatal, delivery, or perinatal period. Additional codes from other chapters may be used with code 650 if they are not related to or are in any way complicating the pregnancy.**

2)   **Normal delivery with resolved antepartum complication**

Code 650 may be used if the patient had a complication at some point during her pregnancy, but the complication is not present at the time of the admission for delivery.

3)   **V27.0, Single liveborn, outcome of delivery**

V27.0, Single liveborn, is the only outcome of delivery code appropriate for use with 650.

i.   **The Postpartum and Peripartum Periods**

1)   **Postpartum and peripartum periods**

The postpartum period begins immediately after delivery and continues for six weeks following delivery. The peripartum period is defined as the last month of pregnancy to five months postpartum.

2) Postpartum complication

A postpartum complication is any complication occurring within the six-week period.

3) Pregnancy-related complications after 6 week period

Chapter 11 codes may also be used to describe pregnancy-related complications after the six-week period should the provider document that a condition is pregnancy related.

4) Postpartum complications occurring during the same admission as delivery

Postpartum complications that occur during the same admission as the delivery are identified with a fifth digit of "2." Subsequent admissions/encounters for postpartum complications should be identified with a fifth digit of "4."

5) Admission for routine postpartum care following delivery outside hospital

When the mother delivers outside the hospital prior to admission and is admitted for routine postpartum care and no complications are noted, code V24.0, Postpartum care and examination immediately after delivery, should be assigned as the principal diagnosis.

6) Admission following delivery outside hospital with postpartum conditions

A delivery diagnosis code should not be used for a woman who has delivered prior to admission to the hospital. Any postpartum conditions and/or postpartum procedures should be coded.

j.   Code 677, Late effect of complication of pregnancy

1) Code 677

Code 677, Late effect of complication of pregnancy, childbirth, and the puerperium is for use in those cases when an initial complication of a pregnancy develops a sequelae requiring care or treatment at a future date.

2) After the initial postpartum period

This code may be used at any time after the initial postpartum period.

3) Sequencing of Code 677

This code, like all late effect codes, is to be sequenced following the code describing the sequelae of the complication.

k. Abortions

1) Fifth-digits required for abortion categories

Fifth-digits are required for abortion categories 634-637. Fifth-digit 1, incomplete, indicates that all of the products of conception have not been expelled from the uterus. Fifth-digit 2, complete, indicates that all products of conception have been expelled from the uterus prior to the episode of care.

2) Code from categories 640-648 and 651-659

A code from categories 640-648 and 651-659 may be used as additional codes with an abortion code to indicate the complication leading to the abortion.

Fifth digit 3 is assigned with codes from these categories when used with an abortion code because the other fifth digits will not apply. Codes from the 660-669 series are not to be used for complications of abortion.

3) Code 639 for complications

Code 639 is to be used for all complications following abortion. Code 639 cannot be assigned with codes from categories 634-638.

4) Abortion with Liveborn Fetus

When an attempted termination of pregnancy results in a liveborn fetus assign code 644.21, Early onset of delivery, with an appropriate code from category V27, Outcome of Delivery. The procedure code for the attempted termination of pregnancy should also be assigned.

5) Retained Products of Conception following an abortion

Subsequent admissions for retained products of conception following a spontaneous or legally induced abortion are assigned the appropriate code from category 634, Spontaneous abortion, or 635 Legally induced abortion, with a fifth digit of "1" (incomplete). This advice is appropriate even when the patient was discharged previously with a discharge diagnosis of complete abortion.

12. Chapter 12: Diseases Skin and Subcutaneous Tissue (680-709)

Reserved for future guideline expansion

13. Chapter 13: Diseases of Musculoskeletal and Connective Tissue (710-739)

Reserved for future guideline expansion

14. Chapter 14: Congenital Anomalies (740-759)

a. Codes in categories 740-759, Congenital Anomalies

Assign an appropriate code(s) from categories 740-759, Congenital Anomalies, when an anomaly is documented. A congenital anomaly may be the principal/first listed diagnosis on a record or a secondary diagnosis. Use additional secondary codes from other chapters to specify conditions associated with the anomaly, if applicable. Codes from Chapter 14 may be used throughout the life of the patient. If a congenital anomaly has been corrected, a personal history code should be used to identify the history of the anomaly.

For the birth admission, the appropriate code from category V30, Liveborn infants, according to type of birth should be sequenced as the principal diagnosis, followed by any congenital anomaly codes, 740-759.

15. Chapter 15: Newborn (Perinatal) Guidelines (760-779)

For coding and reporting purposes the perinatal period is defined as birth through the 28th day following birth. The following guidelines are provided for reporting purposes. Hospitals may record other diagnoses as needed for internal data use.

a. General Perinatal Rules

1) Chapter 15 Codes

They are <u>never</u> for use on the maternal record. Codes from Chapter 11, the obstetric chapter, are never permitted on

the newborn record. Chapter 15 code may be used throughout the life of the patient if the condition is still present.

2)   Sequencing of perinatal codes

Generally, codes from Chapter 15 should be sequenced as the principal/first-listed diagnosis on the newborn record, with the exception of the appropriate V30 code for the birth episode, followed by codes from any other chapter that provide additional detail. The "use additional code" note at the beginning of the chapter supports this guideline. If the index does not provide a specific code for a perinatal condition, assign code 779.89, Other specified conditions originating in the perinatal period, followed by the code from another chapter that specifies the condition. Codes for signs and symptoms may be assigned when a definitive diagnosis has not been established.

3)   Birth process or community acquired conditions

If a newborn has a condition that may be either due to the birth process or community acquired and the documentation does not indicate which it is, the default is due to the birth process and the code from Chapter 15 should be used.   If the condition is community-acquired, a code from Chapter 15 should not be assigned.

4)   Code all clinically significant conditions

All clinically significant conditions noted on routine newborn examination should be coded. A condition is clinically significant if it requires:

- clinical evaluation; or
- therapeutic treatment; or
- diagnostic procedures; or
- extended length of hospital stay; or
- increased nursing care and/or monitoring; or
- has implications for future health care needs

Note: The perinatal guidelines listed above are the same as the general coding guidelines for "additional diagnoses", except for the final point regarding implications for future health care needs. **Codes should be assigned for conditions that have been specified by the provider as having implications for future health care needs. Codes from the perinatal chapter should not be assigned unless the provider has established a definitive diagnosis.**

b.   Use of codes V30-V39

When coding the birth of an infant, assign a code from categories V30-V39, according to the type of birth. A code from this series is assigned as a principal diagnosis, and assigned only once to a newborn at the time of birth.

c.   Newborn transfers

If the newborn is transferred to another institution, the V30 series is not used at the receiving hospital.

d.   Use of category V29

1)   Assigning a code from category V29

Assign a code from category V29, Observation and evaluation of newborns and infants for suspected conditions not found, to identify those instances when a healthy newborn is evaluated for a suspected condition that is determined after study not to be present. Do not use a code from category V29 when the patient has identified signs or symptoms of a suspected problem; in such cases, code the sign or symptom.

A code from category V29 may also be assigned as a principal code for readmissions or encounters when the V30 code no longer applies. Codes from category V29 are for use only for healthy newborns and infants for which no condition after study is found to be present.

2)   V29 code on a birth record

A V29 code is to be used as a secondary code after the V30, Outcome of delivery, code.

e.   Use of other V codes on perinatal records

V codes other than V30 and V29 may be assigned on a perinatal or newborn record code. The codes may be used as a principal or first-listed diagnosis for specific types of encounters or for readmissions or encounters when the V30 code no longer applies.

See Section I.C.18 for information regarding the assignment of V codes.

f.   Maternal Causes of Perinatal Morbidity

Codes from categories 760-763, Maternal causes of perinatal morbidity and mortality, are assigned only when the maternal condition has actually affected the fetus or newborn. The fact that the mother has an associated medical condition or experiences some complication of pregnancy, labor or delivery does not justify the routine assignment of codes from these categories to the newborn record.

g. Congenital Anomalies in Newborns

For the birth admission, the appropriate code from category V30, Liveborn infants according to type of birth, should be used, followed by any congenital anomaly codes, categories 740-759. **Use additional secondary codes from other chapters to specify conditions associated with the anomaly, if applicable.**

Also, see Section I.C.14 for information on the coding of congenital anomalies.

h. Coding Additional Perinatal Diagnoses

1) Assigning codes for conditions that require treatment

Assign codes for conditions that require treatment or further investigation, prolong the length of stay, or require resource utilization.

2) Codes for conditions specified as having implications for future health care needs

Assign codes for conditions that have been specified by the provider as having implications for future health care needs.

Note: This guideline should not be used for adult patients.

3) Codes for newborn conditions originating in the perinatal period

Assign a code for newborn conditions originating in the perinatal period (categories 760-779), as well as complications arising during the current episode of care classified in other chapters, only if the diagnoses have been documented by the responsible provider at the time of transfer or discharge as having affected the fetus or newborn.

i. Prematurity and Fetal Growth Retardation

Providers utilize different criteria in determining prematurity. A code for prematurity should not be assigned unless it is documented. The 5th digit assignment for codes from category 764 and subcategories 765.0 and 765.1 should be based on the recorded birth weight and estimated gestational age.

A code from subcategory 765.2, Weeks of gestation, should be assigned as an additional code with category 764 and codes from 765.0 and 765.1 to specify weeks of gestation as documented by the provider in the record.

j. Newborn sepsis

Code 771.81, Septicemia [sepsis] of newborn, should be assigned with a secondary code from category 041, Bacterial infections in conditions classified elsewhere and of unspecified site, to identify the organism. It is not necessary to use a code from subcategory 995.9, Systemic inflammatory response syndrome (SIRS), on a newborn record. A code from category 038, Septicemia, should not be used on a newborn record. Code 771.81 describes the sepsis.

16.   Chapter 16: Signs, Symptoms and Ill-Defined Conditions (780-799)

Reserved for future guideline expansion

17.   Chapter 17: Injury and Poisoning (800-999)

a. Coding of Injuries

When coding injuries, assign separate codes for each injury unless a combination code is provided, in which case the combination code is assigned. Multiple injury codes are provided in ICD-9-CM, but should not be assigned unless information for a more specific code is not available. These codes are not to be used for normal, healing surgical wounds or to identify complications of surgical wounds.

The code for the most serious injury, as determined by the provider and the focus of treatment, is sequenced first.

1) Superficial injuries

Superficial injuries such as abrasions or contusions are not coded when associated with more severe injuries of the same site.

2) Primary injury with damage to nerves/blood vessels

When a primary injury results in minor damage to peripheral nerves or blood vessels, the primary injury is sequenced first with additional code(s) from categories 950-957, Injury to nerves and spinal cord, and/or 900-904, Injury to blood vessels. When the primary injury is to the blood vessels or nerves, that injury should be sequenced first.

b. **Coding of Fractures**

The principles of multiple coding of injuries should be followed in coding fractures. Fractures of specified sites are coded individually by site in accordance with both the provisions within categories 800-829 and the level of detail furnished by medical record content. Combination categories for multiple fractures are provided for use when there is insufficient detail in the medical record (such as trauma cases transferred to another hospital), when the reporting form limits the number of codes that can be used in reporting pertinent clinical data, or when there is insufficient specificity at the fourth-digit or fifth-digit level. More specific guidelines are as follows:

1) **Multiple fractures of same limb**

Multiple fractures of same limb classifiable to the same three-digit or four-digit category are coded to that category.

2) **Multiple unilateral or bilateral fractures of same bone**

Multiple unilateral or bilateral fractures of same bone(s) but classified to different fourth-digit subdivisions (bone part) within the same three-digit category are coded individually by site.

3) **Multiple fracture categories 819 and 828**

Multiple fracture categories 819 and 828 classify bilateral fractures of both upper limbs (819) and both lower limbs (828), but without any detail at the fourth-digit level other than open and closed type of fractures.

4) **Multiple fractures sequencing**

Multiple fractures are sequenced in accordance with the severity of the fracture. The provider should be asked to list the fracture diagnoses in the order of severity.

c. **Coding of Burns**

Current burns (940-948) are classified by depth, extent and by agent (E code). Burns are classified by depth as first degree (erythema), second degree (blistering), and third degree (full-thickness involvement).

1) **Sequencing of burn codes**

Sequence first the code that reflects the highest degree of burn when more than one burn is present.

2) **Burns of the same local site**

Classify burns of the same local site (three-digit category level, 940-947) but of different degrees to the subcategory identifying the highest degree recorded in the diagnosis.

3) Non-healing burns

Non-healing burns are coded as acute burns.
Necrosis of burned skin should be coded as a non-healed burn.

4) Code 958.3, Posttraumatic wound infection

Assign code 958.3, Posttraumatic wound infection, not elsewhere classified, as an additional code for any documented infected burn site.

5) Assign separate codes for each burn site

When coding burns, assign separate codes for each burn site. Category 946 Burns of Multiple specified sites, should only be used if the location of the burns are not documented. Category 949, Burn, unspecified, is extremely vague and should rarely be used.

6) Assign codes from category 948, Burns

Burns classified according to extent of body surface involved, when the site of the burn is not specified or when there is a need for additional data. It is advisable to use category 948 as additional coding when needed to provide data for evaluating burn mortality, such as that needed by burn units. It is also advisable to use category 948 as an additional code for reporting purposes when there is mention of a third-degree burn involving 20 percent or more of the body surface.

In assigning a code from category 948:

Fourth-digit codes are used to identify the percentage of total body surface involved in a burn (all degree).

Fifth-digits are assigned to identify the percentage of body surface involved in third-degree burn.

Fifth-digit zero (0) is assigned when less than 10 percent or when no body surface is involved in a third-degree burn.

Category 948 is based on the classic "rule of nines" in estimating body surface involved: head and neck are assigned nine percent, each arm nine percent, each leg

18 percent, the anterior trunk 18 percent, posterior trunk 18 percent, and genitalia one percent. Providers may change these percentage assignments where necessary to accommodate infants and children who have proportionately larger heads than adults and patients who have large buttocks, thighs, or abdomen that involve burns.

7) Encounters for treatment of late effects of burns

Encounters for the treatment of the late effects of burns (i.e., scars or joint contractures) should be coded to the residual condition (sequelae) followed by the appropriate late effect code (906.5-906.9). A late effect E code may also be used, if desired.

8) Sequelae with a late effect code and current burn

When appropriate, both a sequelae with a late effect code, and a current burn code may be assigned on the same record **(when both a current burn and sequelae of an old burn exist).**

d. Coding of Debridement of Wound, Infection, or Burn

Excisional debridement involves an excisional debridement (surgical removal or cutting away), as opposed to a mechanical (brushing, scrubbing, washing) debridement.

For coding purposes, excisional debridement **is assigned to code** 86.22.

Nonexcisional debridement is assigned to **code 86.28.**

e. Adverse Effects, Poisoning and Toxic Effects

The properties of certain drugs, medicinal and biological substances or combinations of such substances, may cause toxic reactions. The occurrence of drug toxicity is classified in ICD-9-CM as follows:

1) Adverse Effect

When the drug was correctly prescribed and properly administered, code the reaction plus the appropriate code from the E930-E949 series. Codes from the E930-E949 series must be used to identify the causative substance for an adverse effect of drug, medicinal and biological substances, correctly prescribed and properly administered. The effect, such as tachycardia, delirium, gastrointestinal hemorrhaging, vomiting, hypokalemia, hepatitis, renal failure, or respiratory failure, is coded and followed by the appropriate code from the E930-E949 series.

Adverse effects of therapeutic substances correctly prescribed and properly administered (toxicity, synergistic reaction, side effect, and idiosyncratic reaction) may be due to (1) differences among patients, such as age, sex, disease, and genetic factors, and (2) drug-related factors, such as type of drug, route of administration, duration of therapy, dosage, and bioavailability.

2) Poisoning

(a) Error was made in drug prescription

Errors made in drug prescription or in the administration of the drug by provider, nurse, patient, or other person, use the appropriate poisoning code from the 960-979 series.

(b) Overdose of a drug intentionally taken

If an overdose of a drug was intentionally taken or administered and resulted in drug toxicity, it would be coded as a poisoning (960-979 series).

(c) Nonprescribed drug taken with correctly prescribed and properly administered drug

If a nonprescribed drug or medicinal agent was taken in combination with a correctly prescribed and properly administered drug, any drug toxicity or other reaction resulting from the interaction of the two drugs would be classified as a poisoning.

(d) Sequencing of poisoning

When coding a poisoning or reaction to the improper use of a medication (e.g., wrong dose, wrong substance, wrong route of administration) the poisoning code is sequenced first, followed by a code for the manifestation. If there is also a diagnosis of drug abuse or dependence to the substance, the abuse or dependence is coded as an additional code.

See Section I.C.3.a.6.b. if poisoning is the result of insulin pump malfunctions and Section I.C.19 for general use of E-codes.

3) Toxic Effects

(a) **Toxic effect codes**

When a harmful substance is ingested or comes in contact with a person, this is classified as a toxic effect.   The toxic effect codes are in categories 980-989.

(b) **Sequencing toxic effect codes**

A toxic effect code should be sequenced first, followed by the code(s) that identify the result of the toxic effect.

(c) **External cause codes for toxic effects**

An external cause code from categories E860-E869 for accidental exposure, codes E950.6 or E950.7 for intentional self-harm, category E962 for assault, or categories E980-E982, for undetermined, should also be assigned to indicate intent.

18. Classification of Factors Influencing Health Status and Contact with Health Service (Supplemental V01-V84)

Note: The chapter specific guidelines provide additional information about the use of V codes for specified encounters.

a. Introduction

ICD-9-CM provides codes to deal with encounters for circumstances other than a disease or injury. The Supplementary Classification of Factors Influencing Health Status and Contact with Health Services (V01.0 - V84.8) is provided to deal with occasions when circumstances other than a disease or injury (codes 001-999) are recorded as a diagnosis or problem.

There are four primary circumstances for the use of V codes:

1) A person who is not currently sick encounters the health services for some specific reason, such as to act as an organ donor, to receive prophylactic care, such as inoculations or health screenings, or to receive counseling on health related issues.

2) A person with a resolving disease or injury, or a chronic, long-term condition requiring continuous care, encounters the health care system for specific aftercare of that disease or injury (e.g., dialysis for renal disease; chemotherapy for malignancy; cast change). A diagnosis/symptom code should be used whenever

a current, acute, diagnosis is being treated or a sign or symptom is being studied.

3) Circumstances or problems influence a person's health status but are not in themselves a current illness or injury.

4) Newborns, to indicate birth status

b. V codes use in any healthcare setting

V codes are for use in any healthcare setting. V codes may be used as either a first listed (principal diagnosis code in the inpatient setting) or secondary code, depending on the circumstances of the encounter. Certain V codes may only be used as first listed, others only as secondary codes. See Section I.C.18.e, **V Code Table.**

c. V Codes indicate a reason for an encounter

They are not procedure codes. A corresponding procedure code must accompany a V code to describe the procedure performed.

d. Categories of V Codes

1) Contact/Exposure

Category V01 indicates contact with or exposure to communicable diseases. These codes are for patients who do not show any sign or symptom of a disease but have been exposed to it by close personal contact with an infected individual or are in an area where a disease is epidemic. These codes may be used as a first listed code to explain an encounter for testing, or, more commonly, as a secondary code to identify a potential risk.

2) Inoculations and vaccinations

Categories V03-V06 are for encounters for inoculations and vaccinations. They indicate that a patient is being seen to receive a prophylactic inoculation against a disease. The injection itself must be represented by the appropriate procedure code. A code from V03-V06 may be used as a secondary code if the inoculation is given as a routine part of preventive health care, such as a well-baby visit.

3) Status

Status codes indicate that a patient is either a carrier of a disease or has the sequelae or residual of a past disease or condition. This includes such things as the presence of prosthetic or mechanical devices resulting from past treatment.

A status code is informative, because the status may affect the course of treatment and its outcome. A status code is distinct from a history code. The history code indicates that the patient no longer has the condition.

A status code should not be used with a diagnosis code from one of the body system chapters, if the diagnosis code includes the information provided by the status code. For example, code V42.1, Heart transplant status, should not be used with code 996.83, Complications of transplanted heart. The status code does not provide additional information. The complication code indicates that the patient is a heart transplant patient.

The status V codes/categories are:

V02	Carrier or suspected carrier of infectious diseases Carrier status indicates that a person harbors the specific organisms of a disease without manifest symptoms and is capable of transmitting the infection.
V08	Asymptomatic HIV infection status This code indicates that a patient has tested positive for HIV but has manifested no signs or symptoms of the disease.
V09	Infection with drug-resistant microorganisms This category indicates that a patient has an infection that is resistant to drug treatment. Sequence the infection code first.
V21	Constitutional states in development
V22.2	Pregnant state, incidental This code is a secondary code only for use when the pregnancy is in no way complicating the reason for visit. Otherwise, a code from the obstetric chapter is required.
V26.5x	Sterilization status
V42	Organ or tissue replaced by transplant
V43	Organ or tissue replaced by other means
V44	Artificial opening status
V45	Other postsurgical states
V46	Other dependence on machines
V49.6	Upper limb amputation status
V49.7	Lower limb amputation status
V49.81	Postmenopausal status
V49.82	Dental sealant status
V49.83	**Awaiting organ transplant status**
V58.6	Long-term (current) drug use

This subcategory indicates a patient's continuous use of a prescribed drug (including such things as aspirin therapy) for the long-term treatment of a condition or for prophylactic use. It is not for use for patients who have addictions to drugs.

V83   Genetic carrier status

Genetic carrier status indicates that a person carries a gene, associated with a particular disease, which may be passed to offspring who may develop that disease. The person does not have the disease and is not at risk of developing the disease.

V84   Genetic susceptibility status

Genetic susceptibility indicates that a person has a gene that increases the risk of that person developing the disease.

Note: Categories V42-V46, and subcategories V49.6, V49.7 are for use only if there are no complications or malfunctions of the organ or tissue replaced, the amputation site or the equipment on which the patient is dependent. These are always secondary codes.

4)   **History (of)**

There are two types of history V codes, personal and family. Personal history codes explain a patient's past medical condition that no longer exists and is not receiving any treatment, but that has the potential for recurrence, and therefore may require continued monitoring. The exceptions to this general rule are category V14, Personal history of allergy to medicinal agents, and subcategory V15.0, Allergy, other than to medicinal agents. A person who has had an allergic episode to a substance or food in the past should always be considered allergic to the substance.

Family history codes are for use when a patient has a family member(s) who has had a particular disease that causes the patient to be at higher risk of also contracting the disease.

Personal history codes may be used in conjunction with follow-up codes and family history codes may be used in conjunction with screening codes to explain the need for a test or procedure. History codes are also acceptable on any medical record regardless of the reason for visit. A history of an illness, even if no longer present, is important information that may alter the type of treatment ordered.

The history V code categories are:

V10	Personal history of malignant neoplasm
V12	Personal history of certain other diseases
V13	Personal history of other diseases
	Except: V13.4, Personal history of arthritis, and V13.6, Personal history of congenital malformations. These conditions are life-long so are not true history codes.
V14	Personal history of allergy to medicinal agents
V15	Other personal history presenting hazards to health
	Except: V15.7, Personal history of contraception.
V16	Family history of malignant neoplasm
V17	Family history of certain chronic disabling diseases
V18	Family history of certain other specific diseases
V19	Family history of other conditions

5)   Screening

Screening is the testing for disease or disease precursors in seemingly well individuals so that early detection and treatment can be provided for those who test positive for the disease.   Screenings that are recommended for many subgroups in a population include: routine mammograms for women over 40, a fecal occult blood test for everyone over 50, an amniocentesis to rule out a fetal anomaly for pregnant women over 35, because the incidence of breast cancer and colon cancer in these subgroups is higher than in the general population, as is the incidence of Down's syndrome in older mothers.

The testing of a person to rule out or confirm a suspected diagnosis because the patient has some sign or symptom is a diagnostic examination, not a screening. In these cases, the sign or symptom is used to explain the reason for the test.

A screening code may be a first listed code if the reason for the visit is specifically the screening exam. It may also be used as an additional code if the screening is done during an office visit for other health problems. A screening code is not necessary if the screening is inherent to a routine examination, such as a pap smear done during a routine pelvic examination.

Should a condition be discovered during the screening then the code for the condition may be assigned as an additional diagnosis.

The V code indicates that a screening exam is planned. A procedure code is required to confirm that the screening was performed.

The screening V code categories:
V28   Antenatal screening
V73-V82   Special screening examinations

6)   Observation

There are two observation V code categories. They are for use in very limited circumstances when a person is being observed for a suspected condition that is ruled out. The observation codes are not for use if an injury or illness or any signs or symptoms related to the suspected condition are present. In such cases the diagnosis/symptom code is used with the corresponding E code to identify any external cause.

The observation codes are to be used as principal diagnosis only. The only exception to this is when the principal diagnosis is required to be a code from the V30, Live born infant, category. Then the V29 observation code is sequenced after the V30 code. Additional codes may be used in addition to the observation code but only if they are unrelated to the suspected condition being observed.

The observation V code categories:
V29   Observation and evaluation of newborns for suspected condition not found
           For the birth encounter, a code from category V30 should be sequenced before the V29 code.
V71   Observation and evaluation for suspected condition not found

7)   Aftercare

Aftercare visit codes cover situations when the initial treatment of a disease or injury has been performed and the patient requires continued care during the healing or recovery phase, or for the long-term consequences of the disease. The aftercare V code should not be used if treatment is directed at a current, acute disease or injury, the diagnosis code is to be used in these cases. Exceptions to this rule are codes V58.0, Radiotherapy, and V58.1, Chemotherapy. These codes are to be first listed, followed by the diagnosis code when a patient's encounter is solely to receive radiation therapy or chemotherapy for the treatment of a neoplasm. Should a patient receive both chemotherapy and radiation therapy during the same encounter code V58.0 and V58.1 may be used together on a record with either one being sequenced first.

The aftercare codes are generally first listed to explain the specific reason for the encounter. An aftercare code may be used as an additional code when some type of aftercare is provided in addition to the reason for admission and no diagnosis code is applicable. An example of this would be the closure of a colostomy during an encounter for treatment of another condition.

Certain aftercare V code categories need a secondary diagnosis code to describe the resolving condition or sequelae, for others, the condition is inherent in the code title.

Additional V code aftercare category terms include, fitting and adjustment, and attention to artificial openings.

Status V codes may be used with aftercare V codes to indicate the nature of the aftercare. For example code V45.81, Aortocoronary bypass status, may be used with code V58.73, Aftercare following surgery of the circulatory system, NEC, to indicate the surgery for which the aftercare is being performed. Also, a transplant status code may be used following code V58.44, Aftercare following organ transplant, to identify the organ transplanted. A status code should not be used when the aftercare code indicates the type of status, such as using V55.0, Attention to tracheostomy with V44.0, Tracheostomy status.

The aftercare V category/codes:

V52	Fitting and adjustment of prosthetic device and implant
V53	Fitting and adjustment of other device
V54	Other orthopedic aftercare
V55	Attention to artificial openings
V56	Encounter for dialysis and dialysis catheter care
V57	Care involving the use of rehabilitation procedures
V58.0	Radiotherapy
V58.1	Chemotherapy
V58.3	Attention to surgical dressings and sutures
V58.41	Encounter for planned post-operative wound closure

V58.42	Aftercare, surgery, neoplasm
V58.43	Aftercare, surgery, trauma
V58.44	**Aftercare involving organ transplant**
V58.49	Other specified aftercare following surgery
V58.7x	Aftercare following surgery
V58.81	Fitting and adjustment of vascular catheter
V58.82	Fitting and adjustment of non-vascular catheter
V58.83	Monitoring therapeutic drug
V58.89	Other specified aftercare

8)   Follow-up

The follow-up codes are used to explain continuing surveillance following completed treatment of a disease, condition, or injury. They imply that the condition has been fully treated and no longer exists. They should not be confused with aftercare codes that explain current treatment for a healing condition or its sequelae. Follow-up codes may be used in conjunction with history codes to provide the full picture of the healed condition and its treatment. The follow-up code is sequenced first, followed by the history code.

A follow-up code may be used to explain repeated visits. Should a condition be found to have recurred on the follow-up visit, then the diagnosis code should be used in place of the follow-up code.

The follow-up V code categories:

V24	Postpartum care and evaluation
V67	Follow-up examination

9)   Donor

Category V59 is the donor codes. They are used for living individuals who are donating blood or other body tissue. These codes are only for individuals donating for others, not for self donations. They are not for use to identify cadaveric donations.

10)   Counseling

Counseling V codes are used when a patient or family member receives assistance in the aftermath of an illness or injury, or when support is required in coping with family or social problems. They are not necessary for use in conjunction with a diagnosis code when the counseling component of care is considered integral to standard treatment.

The counseling V categories/codes:

V25.0	General counseling and advice for contraceptive management
V26.3	Genetic counseling
V26.4	General counseling and advice for procreative management
V61	Other family circumstances
V65.1	Person consulted on behalf of another person
V65.3	Dietary surveillance and counseling
V65.4	Other counseling, not elsewhere classified

11) Obstetrics and related conditions

See Section I.C.11., the Obstetrics guidelines for further instruction on the use of these codes.

V codes for pregnancy are for use in those circumstances when none of the problems or complications included in the codes from the Obstetrics chapter exist (a routine prenatal visit or postpartum care). Codes V22.0, Supervision of normal first pregnancy, and V22.1, Supervision of other normal pregnancy, are always first listed and are not to be used with any other code from the OB chapter.

The outcome of delivery, category V27, should be included on all maternal delivery records. It is always a secondary code.

V codes for family planning (contraceptive) or procreative management and counseling should be included on an obstetric record either during the pregnancy or the postpartum stage, if applicable.

Obstetrics and related conditions V code categories:

V22	Normal pregnancy
V23	Supervision of high-risk pregnancy Except: V23.2, Pregnancy with history of abortion. Code 646.3, Habitual aborter, from the OB chapter is required to indicate a history of abortion during a pregnancy.
V24	Postpartum care and evaluation
V25	Encounter for contraceptive management Except V25.0x (See Section I.C.18.d.11, Counseling)
V26	Procreative management Except V26.5x, Sterilization status, V26.3 and V26.4 (See Section I.C.18.d.11., Counseling)
V27	Outcome of delivery

V28   Antenatal screening
                (See Section I.C.18.d.6., Screening)

12)   Newborn, infant and child

See Section I.C.15, the Newborn guidelines for further instruction on the use of these codes.

Newborn V code categories:
V20   Health supervision of infant or child
V29   Observation and evaluation of newborns for suspected condition not found (See Section I.C.18.d.7, Observation).
V30-V39 Liveborn infant according to type of birth

13)   Routine and administrative examinations

The V codes allow for the description of encounters for routine examinations, such as, a general check-up, or, examinations for administrative purposes, such as, a pre-employment physical. The codes are for use as first listed codes only, and are not to be used if the examination is for diagnosis of a suspected condition or for treatment purposes. In such cases the diagnosis code is used. During a routine exam, should a diagnosis or condition be discovered, it should be coded as an additional code. Pre-existing and chronic conditions and history codes may also be included as additional codes as long as the examination is for administrative purposes and not focused on any particular condition.

Pre-operative examination V codes are for use only in those situations when a patient is being cleared for surgery and no treatment is given.

The V codes categories/code for routine and administrative examinations:

V20.2   Routine infant or child health check
           Any injections given should have a corresponding procedure code.
V70   General medical examination
V72   Special investigations and examinations
           Except V72.5 and V72.6

14)   Miscellaneous V codes

The miscellaneous V codes capture a number of other health care encounters that do not fall into one of the other categories.

Certain of these codes identify the reason for the encounter, others are for use as additional codes that provide useful information on circumstances that may affect a patient's care and treatment.

Miscellaneous V code categories/codes:

V07	Need for isolation and other prophylactic measures
V50	Elective surgery for purposes other than remedying health states
V58.5	Orthodontics
V60	Housing, household, and economic circumstances
V62	Other psychosocial circumstances
V63	Unavailability of other medical facilities for care
V64	Persons encountering health services for specific procedures, not carried out
V66	Convalescence and Palliative Care
V68	Encounters for administrative purposes
V69	Problems related to lifestyle

15)   Nonspecific V codes

Certain V codes are so non-specific, or potentially redundant with other codes in the classification, that there can be little justification for their use in the inpatient setting. Their use in the outpatient setting should be limited to those instances when there is no further documentation to permit more precise coding. Otherwise, any sign or symptom or any other reason for visit that is captured in another code should be used.

Nonspecific V code categories/codes:

V11	Personal history of mental disorder A code from the mental disorders chapter, with an in remission fifth-digit, should be used.
V13.4	Personal history of arthritis
V13.6	Personal history of congenital malformations
V15.7	Personal history of contraception
V23.2	Pregnancy with history of abortion
V40	Mental and behavioral problems
V41	Problems with special senses and other special functions
V47	Other problems with internal organs
V48	Problems with head, neck, and trunk
V49	Problems with limbs and other problems

Exceptions:

V49.6	Upper limb amputation status
V49.7	Lower limb amputation status
V49.81	Postmenopausal status

V49.82	Dental sealant status
V49.83	**Awaiting organ transplant status**
V51	Aftercare involving the use of plastic surgery
V58.2	Blood transfusion, without reported diagnosis
V58.9	Unspecified aftercare
V72.5	Radiological examination, NEC
V72.6	Laboratory examination

Codes V72.5 and V72.6 are not to be used if any sign or symptoms, or reason for a test is documented. See Section IV.K. and Section IV.L. of the Outpatient guidelines.

<u>V Code Table</u>
<u>Items in bold indicate a change from the October 2003 table</u>
<u>Items underlined have been moved within the table since October 2003</u>

FIRST LISTED: V codes/categories/subcategories which are only acceptable as principal/first listed.

Codes:

V22.0	Supervision of normal first pregnancy
V22.1	Supervision of other normal pregnancy
V46.12	**Encounter for respirator dependence during power failure**
V56.0	<u>Extracorporeal dialysis</u>
V58.0	Radiotherapy
V58.1	Chemotherapy

V58.0 and V58.1 may be used together on a record with either one being sequenced first, when a patient receives both chemotherapy and radiation therapy during the same encounter code.

Categories/Subcategories:

V20	Health supervision of infant or child
V24	Postpartum care and examination
V29	Observation and evaluation of newborns for suspected condition not found

Exception: A code from the V30-V39 may be sequenced before the V29 if it is the newborn record.

V30-V39	Liveborn infants according to type of birth
V59	Donors
V66	Convalescence and palliative care

Exception: V66.7 Palliative care

V68	Encounters for administrative purposes
V70	General medical examination

Exception: V70.7 Examination of participant in clinical trial

V71	Observation and evaluation for suspected conditions not found
V72	Special investigations and examinations

Exceptions:
V72.5 Radiological examination, NEC
V72.6 Laboratory examination

FIRST OR ADDITIONAL: V code categories/subcategories which may be either principal/first listed or additional codes

Codes:

V43.22	Fully implantable artificial heart status
V49.81	Asymptomatic postmenopausal status (age-related) (natural)
V70.7	Examination of participant in clinical trial

Categories/Subcategories:

V01	Contact with or exposure to communicable diseases
V02	Carrier or suspected carrier of infectious diseases
V03-06	Need for prophylactic vaccination and inoculations
V07	Need for isolation and other prophylactic measures
V08	Asymptomatic HIV infection status

V10	Personal history of malignant neoplasm
V12	Personal history of certain other diseases
V13	Personal history of other diseases
	Exception:
	V13.4 Personal history of arthritis
	V13.69 Personal history of other congenital malformations
V16-V19	Family history of disease
V23	Supervision of high-risk pregnancy
V25	Encounter for contraceptive management
V26	Procreative management
	Exception: V26.5 Sterilization status
V28	Antenatal screening
V45.7	Acquired absence of organ
V50	Elective surgery for purposes other than remedying health states
V52	Fitting and adjustment of prosthetic device and implant
V53	Fitting and adjustment of other device
V54	Other orthopedic aftercare
V55	Attention to artificial openings
V56	Encounter for dialysis and dialysis catheter care
	Exception: V56.0 Extracorporeal dialysis
V57	Care involving use of rehabilitation procedures
V58.3	Attention to surgical dressings and sutures
V58.4	Other aftercare following surgery
<u>V58.6</u>	<u>Long-term (current) drug use</u>
V58.7	Aftercare following surgery to specified body systems, not elsewhere classified
V58.8	Other specified procedures and aftercare
V61	Other family circumstances
V63	Unavailability of other medical facilities for care
V65	Other persons seeking consultation without complaint or sickness
V67	Follow-up examination
V69	Problems related to lifestyle
V73-V82	Special screening examinations
V83	Genetic carrier status

ADDITIONAL ONLY: V code categories/subcategories which may only be used as additional codes, not principal/first listed

Codes:

V13.61	Personal history of hypospadias
V22.2	Pregnancy state, incidental
V49.82	Dental sealant status
V49.83	**Awaiting organ transplant status**
V66.7	Palliative care

Categories/Subcategories:

V09	Infection with drug-resistant microorganisms

V14	Personal history of allergy to medicinal agents
V15	Other personal history presenting hazards to health
	Exception: V15.7 Personal history of contraception
V21	Constitutional states in development
V26.5	Sterilization status
V27	Outcome of delivery
V42	Organ or tissue replaced by transplant
V43	Organ or tissue replaced by other means
	Exception: V43.22 Fully implantable artificial heart status
V44	Artificial opening status
V45	Other postsurgical states
	Exception: Subcategory V45.7 Acquired absence of organ
V46	Other dependence on machines

Exception: V46.12 Encounter for respirator dependence during power failure

V49.6x	Upper limb amputation status
V49.7x	Lower limb amputation status
V60	Housing, household, and economic circumstances
V62	Other psychosocial circumstances
V64	Persons encountering health services for specified procedure, not carried out
V84	**Genetic susceptibility to disease**

NONSPECIFIC CODES AND CATEGORIES:

V11	Personal history of mental disorder
V13.4	Personal history of arthritis
V13.69	Personal history of congenital malformations
V15.7	Personal history of contraception
V40	Mental and behavioral problems
V41	Problems with special senses and other special functions
V47	Other problems with internal organs
V48	Problems with head, neck, and trunk
V49	Problems with limbs and other problems
	Exceptions:
	V49.6 Upper limb amputation status
	V49.7 Lower limb amputation status
	V49.81 Postmenopausal status (age-related) (natural)
	V49.82 Dental sealant status
	V49.83 Awaiting organ transplant status
V51	Aftercare involving the use of plastic surgery
V58.2	Blood transfusion, without reported diagnosis
V58.5	Orthodontics
V58.9	Unspecified aftercare
V72.5	Radiological examination, NEC
V72.6	Laboratory examination

19. Supplemental Classification of External Causes of Injury and Poisoning (E-codes, E800-E999)

Introduction: These guidelines are provided for those who are currently collecting E codes in order that there will be standardization in the process. If your institution plans to begin collecting E codes, these guidelines are to be applied. The use of E codes is supplemental to the application of ICD-9-CM diagnosis codes. E codes are never to be recorded as principal diagnoses (first-listed in non-inpatient setting) and are not required for reporting to CMS.

External causes of injury and poisoning codes (E codes) are intended to provide data for injury research and evaluation of injury prevention strategies. E codes capture how the injury or poisoning happened (cause), the intent (unintentional or accidental; or intentional, such as suicide or assault), and the place where the event occurred.

Some major categories of E codes include:
>   transport accidents
>   poisoning and adverse effects of drugs, medicinal substances and biologicals
>   accidental falls
>   accidents caused by fire and flames
>   accidents due to natural and environmental factors
>   late effects of accidents, assaults or self injury
>   assaults or purposely inflicted injury
>   suicide or self inflicted injury

These guidelines apply for the coding and collection of E codes from records in hospitals, outpatient clinics, emergency departments, other ambulatory care settings and provider offices, and nonacute care settings, except when other specific guidelines apply.

a. General E Code Coding Guidelines

1) Used with any code in the range of 001-V84.8

An E code may be used with any code in the range of 001-V84.8, which indicates an injury, poisoning, or adverse effect due to an external cause.

2) Assign the appropriate E code for all initial treatments

Assign the appropriate E code for the initial encounter of an injury, poisoning, or adverse effect of drugs, **not for subsequent treatment.**

3) Use the full range of E codes

Use the full range of E codes to completely describe the cause, the intent and the place of occurrence, if applicable, for all injuries, poisonings, and adverse effects of drugs.

4)   **Assign as many E codes as necessary**

Assign as many E codes as necessary to fully explain each cause. If only one E code can be recorded, assign the E code most related to the principal diagnosis.

5)   **The selection of the appropriate E code**

The selection of the appropriate E code is guided by the Index to External Causes, which is located after the alphabetical index to diseases and by Inclusion and Exclusion notes in the Tabular List.

6)   **E code can never be a principal diagnosis**

An E code can never be a principal (first listed) diagnosis.

7)   **External cause code(s) with systemic inflammatory response syndrome (SIRS)**

An external cause code(s) may be used with codes 995.93, Systemic inflammatory response syndrome due to noninfectious process without organ dysfunction, and 995.94, Systemic inflammatory response syndrome due to noninfectious process with organ dysfunction, if trauma was the initiating insult that precipitated the SIRS. The external cause(s) code should correspond to the most serious injury resulting from the trauma. The external cause code(s) should only be assigned if the trauma necessitated the admission in which the patient also developed SIRS. If a patient is admitted with SIRS but the trauma has been treated previously, the external cause codes should not be used.

b.   Place of Occurrence Guideline

Use an additional code from category E849 to indicate the Place of Occurrence for injuries and poisonings. The Place of Occurrence describes the place where the event occurred and not the patient's activity at the time of the event.

Do not use E849.9 if the place of occurrence is not stated.

c.   Adverse Effects of Drugs, Medicinal and Biological Substances Guidelines

1)   Do not code directly from the Table of Drugs

Do not code directly from the Table of Drugs and Chemicals. Always refer back to the Tabular List.

2)   Use as many codes as necessary to describe

Use as many codes as necessary to describe completely all drugs, medicinal or biological substances.

3)   If the same E code would describe the causative agent

If the same E code would describe the causative agent for more than one adverse reaction, assign the code only once.

4)   If two or more drugs, medicinal or biological substances

If two or more drugs, medicinal or biological substances are reported, code each individually unless the combination code is listed in the Table of Drugs and Chemicals. In that case, assign the E code for the combination.

5)   When a reaction results from the interaction of a drug(s)

When a reaction results from the interaction of a drug(s) and alcohol, use poisoning codes and E codes for both.

6)   If the reporting format limits the number of E codes

If the reporting format limits the number of E codes that can be used in reporting clinical data, code the one most related to the principal diagnosis. Include at least one from each category (cause, intent, place) if possible.

If there are different fourth digit codes in the same three digit category, use the code for "Other specified" of that category. If there is no "Other specified" code in that category, use the appropriate "Unspecified" code in that category.

If the codes are in different three digit categories, assign the appropriate E code for other multiple drugs and medicinal substances.

7)   Codes from the E930-E949 series

Codes from the E930-E949 series must be used to identify the causative substance for an adverse effect of drug, medicinal and biological substances, correctly prescribed and properly administered. The effect, such as tachycardia, delirium, gastrointestinal hemorrhaging, vomiting, hypokalemia, hepatitis, renal failure, or respiratory failure, is coded and followed by the appropriate code from the E930-E949 series.

d.   Multiple Cause E Code Coding Guidelines

If two or more events cause separate injuries, an E code should be assigned for each cause. The first listed E code will be selected in the following order:

E codes for child and adult abuse take priority over all other E codes. See Section I.C.19.e., Child and Adult abuse guidelines

E codes for terrorism events take priority over all other E codes except child and adult abuse

E codes for cataclysmic events take priority over all other E codes except child and adult abuse and terrorism.

E codes for transport accidents take priority over all other E codes except cataclysmic events and child and adult abuse and terrorism.

The first-listed E code should correspond to the cause of the most serious diagnosis due to an assault, accident, or self-harm, following the order of hierarchy listed above.

e.   Child and Adult Abuse Guideline

1)   Intentional injury

When the cause of an injury or neglect is intentional child or adult abuse, the first listed E code should be assigned from categories E960-E968, Homicide and injury purposely inflicted by other persons, (except category E967). An E code from category E967, Child and adult battering and other maltreatment, should be added as an additional code to identify the perpetrator, if known.

2)   Accidental intent

In cases of neglect when the intent is determined to be accidental E code E904.0, Abandonment or neglect of infant and helpless person, should be the first listed E code.

f. Unknown or Suspected Intent Guideline

1) If the intent (accident, self-harm, assault) of the cause of an injury or poisoning is unknown

If the intent (accident, self-harm, assault) of the cause of an injury or poisoning is unknown or unspecified, code the intent as undetermined E980-E989.

2) If the intent (accident, self-harm, assault) of the cause of an injury or poisoning is questionable

If the intent (accident, self-harm, assault) of the cause of an injury or poisoning is questionable, probable or suspected, code the intent as undetermined E980-E989.

g. Undetermined Cause

When the intent of an injury or poisoning is known, but the cause is unknown, use codes: E928.9, Unspecified accident, E958.9, Suicide and self-inflicted injury by unspecified means, and E968.9, Assault by unspecified means.

These E codes should rarely be used, as the documentation in the medical record, in both the inpatient outpatient and other settings, should normally provide sufficient detail to determine the cause of the injury.

h. Late Effects of External Cause Guidelines

1) Late effect E codes

Late effect E codes exist for injuries and poisonings but not for adverse effects of drugs, misadventures and surgical complications.

2) Late effect E codes (E929, E959, E969, E977, E989, or E999.1)

A late effect E code (E929, E959, E969, E977, E989, or E999.1) should be used with any report of a late effect or sequela resulting from a previous injury or poisoning (905-909).

3) Late effect E code with a related current injury

A late effect E code should never be used with a related current nature of injury code.

4) Use of late effect E codes for subsequent visits

Use a late effect E code for subsequent visits when a late effect of the initial injury or poisoning is being treated. There is no late effect E code for adverse effects of drugs. Do not use a late effect E code for subsequent visits for follow-up care (e.g., to assess healing, to receive rehabilitative therapy) of the injury or poisoning when no late effect of the injury has been documented.

i. Misadventures and Complications of Care Guidelines

1) Code range E870-E876

Assign a code in the range of E870-E876 if misadventures are stated by the provider.

2) Code range E878-E879

Assign a code in the range of E878-E879 if the provider attributes an abnormal reaction or later complication to a surgical or medical procedure, but does not mention misadventure at the time of the procedure as the cause of the reaction.

j. Terrorism Guidelines

1) Cause of injury identified by the Federal Government (FBI) as terrorism

When the cause of an injury is identified by the Federal Government (FBI) as terrorism, the first-listed E-code should be a code from category E979, Terrorism. The definition of terrorism employed by the FBI is found at the inclusion note at E979. The terrorism E-code is the only E-code that should be assigned. Additional E codes from the assault categories should not be assigned.

2) Cause of an injury is suspected to be the result of terrorism

When the cause of an injury is suspected to be the result of terrorism a code from category E979 should not be assigned. Assign a code in the range of E codes based circumstances on the documentation of intent and mechanism.

3) Code E979.9, Terrorism, secondary effects

Assign code E979.9, Terrorism, secondary effects, for conditions occurring subsequent to the terrorist event. This code should not be assigned for conditions that are due to the initial terrorist act.

4)   Statistical tabulation of terrorism codes

For statistical purposes these codes will be tabulated within the category for assault, expanding the current category from E960-E969 to include E979 and E999.1.

Section II. Selection of Principal Diagnosis

The circumstances of inpatient admission always govern the selection of principal diagnosis. The principal diagnosis is defined in the Uniform Hospital Discharge Data Set (UHDDS) as "that condition established after study to be chiefly responsible for occasioning the admission of the patient to the hospital for care."

The UHDDS definitions are used by hospitals to report inpatient data elements in a standardized manner. These data elements and their definitions can be found in the July 31, 1985, Federal Register (Vol. 50, No, 147), pp. 31038-40.

Since that time the application of the UHDDS definitions has been expanded to include all non-outpatient settings (acute care, short term, long term care and psychiatric hospitals; home health agencies; rehab facilities; nursing homes, etc).

In determining principal diagnosis the coding conventions in the ICD-9-CM, Volumes I and II take precedence over these official coding guidelines. (See Section I.A., Conventions for the ICD-9-CM).

The importance of consistent, complete documentation in the medical record cannot be overemphasized. Without such documentation the application of all coding guidelines is a difficult, if not impossible, task.

A. Codes for symptoms, signs, and ill-defined conditions

Codes for symptoms, signs, and ill-defined conditions from Chapter 16 are not to be used as principal diagnosis when a related definitive diagnosis has been established.

B. Two or more interrelated conditions, each potentially meeting the definition for principal diagnosis.

When there are two or more interrelated conditions (such as diseases in the same ICD-9-CM chapter or manifestations characteristically associated with a certain disease) potentially meeting the definition of principal diagnosis, either condition may be sequenced first, unless the circumstances of the admission, the therapy provided, the Tabular List, or the Alphabetic Index indicate otherwise.

C. Two or more diagnoses that equally meet the definition for principal diagnosis

In the unusual instance when two or more diagnoses equally meet the criteria for principal diagnosis as determined by the circumstances of admission, diagnostic workup and/or therapy provided, and the Alphabetic Index, Tabular List, or another coding guidelines does not provide sequencing direction, any one of the diagnoses may be sequenced first.

D. Two or more comparative or contrasting conditions.

In those rare instances when two or more contrasting or comparative diagnoses are documented as "either/or" (or similar terminology), they are coded as if the diagnoses were confirmed and the diagnoses are sequenced according to the circumstances of the admission. If no further determination can be made as to which diagnosis should be principal, either diagnosis may be sequenced first.

E. A symptom(s) followed by contrasting/comparative diagnoses

When a symptom(s) is followed by contrasting/comparative diagnoses, the symptom code is sequenced first. All the contrasting/comparative diagnoses should be coded as additional diagnoses.

F. Original treatment plan not carried out

Sequence as the principal diagnosis the condition, which after study occasioned the admission to the hospital, even though treatment may not have been carried out due to unforeseen circumstances.

G. Complications of surgery and other medical care

When the admission is for treatment of a complication resulting from surgery or other medical care, the complication code is sequenced as the principal diagnosis. If the complication is classified to the 996-999 series and the code lacks the necessary specificity in describing the complication, an additional code for the specific complication should be assigned.

H. Uncertain Diagnosis

If the diagnosis documented at the time of discharge is qualified as "probable", "suspected", "likely", "questionable", "possible", or "still to be ruled out", code the condition as if it existed or was established. The bases for these guidelines are the diagnostic workup, arrangements for further workup or observation, and initial therapeutic approach that correspond most closely with the established diagnosis.

Note: This guideline is applicable only to short-term, acute, long-term care and psychiatric hospitals.

Section III. Reporting Additional Diagnoses

GENERAL RULES FOR OTHER (ADDITIONAL) DIAGNOSES

For reporting purposes the definition for "other diagnoses" is interpreted as additional conditions that affect patient care in terms of requiring:

clinical evaluation; or
therapeutic treatment; or

diagnostic procedures; or
extended length of hospital stay; or
increased nursing care and/or monitoring.

The UHDDS item #11-b defines Other Diagnoses as "all conditions that coexist at the time of admission, that develop subsequently, or that affect the treatment received and/or the length of stay. Diagnoses that relate to an earlier episode which have no bearing on the current hospital stay are to be excluded." UHDDS definitions apply to inpatients in acute care, short-term, long term care and psychiatric hospital setting. The UHDDS definitions are used by acute care short-term hospitals to report inpatient data elements in a standardized manner. These data elements and their definitions can be found in the July 31, 1985, Federal Register (Vol. 50, No, 147), pp. 31038-40.

Since that time the application of the UHDDS definitions has been expanded to include all non—outpatient settings (acute care, short term, long term care and psychiatric hospitals; home health agencies; rehab facilities; nursing homes, etc).

The following guidelines are to be applied in designating "other diagnoses" when neither the Alphabetic Index nor the Tabular List in ICD-9-CM provide direction. The listing of the diagnoses in the patient record is the responsibility of the attending provider.

A. Previous conditions

If the provider has included a diagnosis in the final diagnostic statement, such as the discharge summary or the face sheet, it should ordinarily be coded. Some providers include in the diagnostic statement resolved conditions or diagnoses and status-post procedures from previous admission that have no bearing on the current stay. Such conditions are not to be reported and are coded only if required by hospital policy.

However, history codes (V10-V19) may be used as secondary codes if the historical condition or family history has an impact on current care or influences treatment.

B. Abnormal findings

Abnormal findings (laboratory, x-ray, pathologic, and other diagnostic results) are not coded and reported unless the provider indicates their clinical significance. If the findings are outside the normal range and the **attending** provider has ordered other tests to evaluate the condition or prescribed treatment, it is appropriate to ask the provider whether the abnormal finding should be added.

Please note: This differs from the coding practices in the outpatient setting for coding encounters for diagnostic tests that have been interpreted by a provider.

C. Uncertain Diagnosis

If the diagnosis documented at the time of discharge is qualified as "probable", "suspected", "likely", "questionable", "possible", or "still to be ruled out", code the condition as if it existed or was established. The bases for these guidelines are the diagnostic workup, arrangements for further workup or observation, and initial therapeutic approach that correspond most closely with the established diagnosis. **Note: This guideline is applicable only to short-term, acute, long-term care and psychiatric hospitals.**

Section IV. Diagnostic Coding and Reporting Guidelines for Outpatient Services

These coding guidelines for outpatient diagnoses have been approved for use by hospitals/ providers in coding and reporting hospital-based outpatient services and provider-based office visits.

Information about the use of certain abbreviations, punctuation, symbols, and other conventions used in the ICD-9-CM Tabular List (code numbers and titles), can be found in Section IA of these guidelines, under "Conventions Used in the Tabular List." Information about the correct sequence to use in finding a code is also described in Section I.

The terms encounter and visit are often used interchangeably in describing outpatient service contacts and, therefore, appear together in these guidelines without distinguishing one from the other.

Though the conventions and general guidelines apply to all settings, coding guidelines for outpatient and provider reporting of diagnoses will vary in a number of instances from those for inpatient diagnoses, recognizing that:

The Uniform Hospital Discharge Data Set (UHDDS) definition of principal diagnosis applies only to inpatients in acute, short-term, long-term care **and psychiatric** hospitals.

Coding guidelines for inconclusive diagnoses (probable, suspected, rule out, etc.) were developed for inpatient reporting and do not apply to outpatients.

A. Selection of first-listed condition

In the outpatient setting, the term first-listed diagnosis is used in lieu of principal diagnosis.

In determining the first-listed diagnosis the coding conventions of ICD-9-CM, as well as the general and disease specific guidelines take precedence over the outpatient guidelines.

Diagnoses often are not established at the time of the initial encounter/visit. It may take two or more visits before the diagnosis is confirmed.

The most critical rule involves beginning the search for the correct code assignment through the Alphabetic Index. Never begin searching initially in the Tabular List as this will lead to coding errors.

B. Codes from 001.0 through V84.8

The appropriate code or codes from 001.0 through V84.8 must be used to identify diagnoses, symptoms, conditions, problems, complaints, or other reason(s) for the encounter/visit.

C. Accurate reporting of ICD-9-CM diagnosis codes

For accurate reporting of ICD-9-CM diagnosis codes, the documentation should describe the patient's condition, using terminology which includes specific diagnoses as well as symptoms, problems, or reasons for the encounter. There are ICD-9-CM codes to describe all of these.

D. Selection of codes 001.0 through 999.9

The selection of codes 001.0 through 999.9 will frequently be used to describe the reason for the encounter. These codes are from the section of ICD-9-CM for the classification of diseases and injuries (e.g. infectious and parasitic diseases; neoplasms; symptoms, signs, and ill-defined conditions, etc.).

E. Codes that describe symptoms and signs

Codes that describe symptoms and signs, as opposed to diagnoses, are acceptable for reporting purposes when a diagnosis has not been established (confirmed) by the provider. Chapter 16 of ICD-9-CM, Symptoms, Signs, and Ill-defined conditions (codes 780.0 - 799.9) contain many, but not all codes for symptoms.

F. Encounters for circumstances other than a disease or injury

ICD-9-CM provides codes to deal with encounters for circumstances other than a disease or injury. The Supplementary Classification of factors Influencing Health Status and Contact with Health Services (V01.0- V84.8) is provided to deal with occasions when circumstances other than a disease or injury are recorded as diagnosis or problems.

G. Level of Detail in Coding

1. ICD-9-CM codes with 3, 4, or 5 digits

ICD-9-CM is composed of codes with either 3, 4, or 5 digits. Codes with three digits are included in ICD-9-CM as the heading of a category of codes that may be further subdivided by the use of fourth and/or fifth digits, which provide greater specificity.

2. Use of full number of digits required for a code

A three-digit code is to be used only if it is not further subdivided. Where fourth-digit subcategories and/or fifth-digit subclassifications are provided, they must be assigned. A code is invalid if it has not been coded to the full number of digits required for that code. See also discussion under Section I.b.3., General Coding Guidelines, Level of Detail in Coding.

H. ICD-9-CM code for the diagnosis, condition, problem, or other reason for encounter/visit

List first the ICD-9-CM code for the diagnosis, condition, problem, or other reason for encounter/visit shown in the medical record to be chiefly responsible for the services provided. List additional codes that describe any coexisting conditions. **In some cases the first-listed diagnosis may be a symptom when a diagnosis has not been established (confirmed) by the physician.**

I. "Probable", "suspected", "questionable", "rule out", or "working diagnosis"

Do not code diagnoses documented as "probable", "suspected," "questionable," "rule out," or "working diagnosis". Rather, code the condition(s) to the highest degree of certainty for that encounter/visit, such as symptoms, signs, abnormal test results, or other reason for the visit. **Please note:** This differs from the coding practices used by **short-term, acute care, long-term care and psychiatric** hospitals.

J. Chronic diseases

Chronic diseases treated on an ongoing basis may be coded and reported as many times as the patient receives treatment and care for the condition(s)

K. Code all documented conditions that coexist

Code all documented conditions that coexist at the time of the encounter/visit, and require or affect patient care treatment or management. Do not code conditions that were previously treated and no longer exist. However, history codes (V10-V19) may be used as secondary codes if the historical condition or family history has an impact on current care or influences treatment.

L. Patients receiving diagnostic services only

For patients receiving diagnostic services only during an encounter/visit, sequence first the diagnosis, condition, problem, or other reason for encounter/visit shown in the medical record to be chiefly responsible for the outpatient services provided during the encounter/visit. Codes for other diagnoses (e.g., chronic conditions) may be sequenced as additional diagnoses.

For outpatient encounters for diagnostic tests that have been interpreted by a physician, and the final report is available at the time of coding, code any confirmed or definitive diagnosis(es) documented in the interpretation. Do not code related signs and symptoms as additional diagnoses.

Please note: This differs from the coding practice in the hospital inpatient setting regarding abnormal findings on test results.

M. Patients receiving therapeutic services only

For patients receiving therapeutic services only during an encounter/visit, sequence first the diagnosis, condition, problem, or other reason for encounter/visit shown in the medical record to be chiefly responsible for the outpatient services provided during the encounter/visit. Codes for other diagnoses (e.g., chronic conditions) may be sequenced as additional diagnoses.

The only exception to this rule is that when the primary reason for the admission/encounter is chemotherapy, radiation therapy, or rehabilitation, the appropriate V code for the service is listed first, and the diagnosis or problem for which the service is being performed listed second.

N. Patients receiving preoperative evaluations only

For patients receiving preoperative evaluations only, sequence **first** a code from category V72.8, Other specified examinations, to describe the pre-op consultations. Assign a code for the condition to describe the reason for the surgery as an additional diagnosis. Code also any findings related to the pre-op evaluation.

O. Ambulatory surgery

For ambulatory surgery, code the diagnosis for which the surgery was performed. If the postoperative diagnosis is known to be different from the preoperative diagnosis at the time the diagnosis is confirmed, select the postoperative diagnosis for coding, since it is the most definitive.

P. Routine outpatient prenatal visits

For routine outpatient prenatal visits when no complications are present, codes V22.0, Supervision of normal first pregnancy, **or** V22.1, Supervision of other normal pregnancy, should be used as **the** principal diagnosis. These codes should not be used in conjunction with chapter 11 codes.

Appendix F

ICD-10-CM and ICD-10-PCS

Destination 10: Healthcare Organization Preparation for ICD-10-CM and ICD-10-PCS (AHIMA Practice Brief)

Editor's note: This update supplants the September 1998 practice brief "Preparing Your Organization for a New Coding System."

In November 2003 the National Committee on Vital and Health Statistics (NCVHS) submitted a letter to Health and Human Services Secretary Tommy Thompson recommending that the regulatory process be initiated for the adoption of ICD-10-CM and ICD-10-PCS as replacements for the current uses of ICD-9-CM. In this letter, NCVHS stated that the updated ICD systems can better accommodate advances in medicine, reduce the number of rejected claims, and improve reimbursement, care quality, safety, and disease management.

Exactly how will ICD-10-CM and ICD-10-PCS be adopted? Here's what will happen:

1. The secretary accepts the NCVHS recommendation.

2. The federal government publishes a notice of proposed rule making (NPRM) calling for public comment on their policy plus the published ICD-10-CM and ICD-10-PCS materials incorporated by reference.

3. The public at large has at least 30, but more likely 60, days to submit comments on the NPRM and its incorporated materials.

4. The federal government analyzes the public comments. Based on this analysis, any necessary changes are made.

5. The federal government publishes a final rule containing its updated policy, explanations thereof, plus the implementation date.

6. The standard HIPAA compliance clock for new transactions begins—two years for all but small health plans, who get three years.

While the HIPAA-mandated process will take time, experience with the transactions and code sets final rule has shown that careful planning and preparation are required for effective implementation. In addition, transitioning to ICD-10-CM and ICD-10-PCS is more complex than implementation of new code sets in the past because the uses of coded data today are more complex than those for which ICD-9-CM was designed. (See Figure F.1, Uses of Coded Data.)

Figure F.1.   Uses of coded data

Today, coded data are used for:

- Measuring the quality, safety (or medical errors), and efficacy of care
- Making clinical decisions based on output from multiple systems
- Designing payment systems and processing claims for reimbursement
- Conducting research, epidemiological studies, and clinical trials
- Setting health policy
- Designing healthcare delivery systems
- Monitoring resource utilization
- Improving clinical, financial, and administrative performance
- Identifying fraudulent or abusive practices
- Managing care and disease processes
- Tracking public health and risks
- Providing data to consumers regarding costs and outcomes of treatment options

Source: "Testimony of the American Health Information Management Association to the National Committee on Vital and Health Statistics on ICD-10-CM." May 29, 2002. Available at www.ahima.org.

AHIMA believes an implementation plan established well in advance of the scheduled implementation date within the requirements of HIPAA is necessary to ensure a successful transition to ICD-10-CM and ICD-10-PCS. While this practice brief is not a comprehensive document of everything that needs to be done to prepare, the three major stages for the process outlined below illustrate the journey ahead for specific travelers working in healthcare organizations. Additional details for each phase will be available through the FORE Library: HIM Body of Knowledge.

So what should your healthcare organization do to set priorities for the various stages of the transition? And what should HIM professionals be doing to prepare?

Three Years Out

The first stage involves two major tasks: creating an implementation planning team and starting the initial education process. Together, these actions demonstrate a clear direction on the healthcare organization's road map.

Team Design

As in any other major undertaking, putting together a team to oversee the implementation is key to success. Members of the planning team should at least include senior management, medical staff, financial management, HIM, and information systems (IS) management. This group would develop the organization's plan and identify the actions, persons responsible, and deadlines for the various tasks required to complete the process. In addition, this plan should include estimated budget needs for each year leading up to implementation for early financial planning.

Team members should keep current on the status for adoption and maintain a broad understanding of ICD-10-CM and ICD-10-PCS. (See Figure F.2, Web Sites to Watch.)

Preliminary Educational Needs

Another major task in the first stage is education. HIM professionals should educate personnel in their organizations about the impending changes.

Individuals throughout the organization need to be aware of the upcoming changes. (See Figure F.3, Who Needs to Know?)

Figure F.2.   Web sites to watch

Use these Web sites to stay current on the status of the coding systems, as well as the anticipated release dates:

- **NCVHS**   http://aspe.os.dhhs.gov/ncvhs
- **CMS**   www.cms.hhs.gov/providers/pufdownload/icd10.asp
- **National Center for Health Statistics**   www.cdc.gov/nchswww/about/otheract/icd9/abticd10.htm
- **HHS Administrative Simplification**   http://aspe.os.dhhs.gov/admnsimp
  At this site, you can subscribe to the HIPAA-REGS listserv. It will notify you when documents related to the administrative simplification law are published.

Figure F.3.   Who needs to know?

Colleagues throughout the organization need to be aware of the ICD-10 transition team. Remember to provide information on how HIM can help their departments in the transition. Individuals needing to know about the upcoming changes include:

- Senior management
- Clinicians
- IS personnel
- Quality management personnel
- Utilization management personnel
- Release of information personnel
- Ancillary department personnel
- Data quality management personnel
- Data security personnel
- Data analysts
- Researchers
- Billing personnel
- Accounting personnel
- Compliance personnel
- Auditors

It is advisable to briefly review the regulations on electronic transactions and code sets with senior management, paying specific attention to the section on code sets, particularly the process for adoption of new code sets. Senior management should also be briefed on the proposed and final rules regarding adoption of ICD-10-CM and ICD-10-PCS. A short overview of the differences between the code sets might be helpful to justify the time, effort, and resources that will be required to implement the changes.

Because these systems code to a greater degree of specificity, clinical documentation must be examined to ensure that it is comprehensive enough to actually assign a code. HIM professionals should assess the adequacy of medical record documentation to support the assignment of codes from ICD-10-CM and ICD-10-PCS in their healthcare organizations. The need to assess and improve documentation prior to implementation is absolutely critical. This requires HIM professionals to become familiar enough with ICD-10-CM and ICD-10-PCS to be able to review medical record documentation and identify areas where improvement is needed (for example, certain specialties or types of records that are more problematic than others).

The results of this gap analysis would then be used to focus the documentation improvement efforts in the clinician education programs. While the results of a study performed by AHIMA in the summer of 2003 indicate that ICD-10-CM codes could be applied to today's medical records without changing documentation practices, improved documentation would result in higher coding specificity, and therefore higher data quality, in some cases.[1] Therefore, identification of areas in need of documentation improvement and the subsequent clinician education must begin early in order to effect real change in documentation practices. AHIMA plans to publish a clinical documentation assessment tool in 2004 to assist with this evaluation.

The education of IS staff will be vital. IS personnel will need to understand the logic and hierarchical structure of ICD-10-CM and ICD-10-PCS. IS department members will be particularly interested in the specifications of the coding system and may want to address the following questions:

1. How many digits? ICD-10-CM has seven characters, with a decimal point after the third character. ICD-10-PCS has seven characters and no decimal point.

2. Is it alphabetic, numeric, or a combination? Both of the new systems mix alphabetic and numeric characters.

3. Can it be obtained in a machine-readable form? To date, the only distribution has been via the Internet (see the aforementioned Web sites).

4. What coding systems will it replace, and when will it replace them? ICD-10-CM and ICD-10-PCS are slated as replacements for the current uses of ICD-9-CM no sooner than October 2006.

5. Is a crosswalk available? Official sources say these will be developed.

It is essential that IS staff be made aware of these changes, as they will have to implement them into a software application or an interface between two systems. A recommended step is for HIM and IS to work together to identify all systems and software in which ICD-9-CM codes are currently used.

Both IS staff and analysts will need to understand the data comparability issues as data between the two systems are compared over time. Data users will specifically need to understand the definition and composition of categories in the classification. Caution should be used when conducting longitudinal data analysis, as diagnoses and procedures may be classified differently in the two systems or code definitions may have changed, making it easy to misinterpret data.

Others need to know the differences between the code sets, the effect on their work, and the time frames involved in the coming changes. ICD-10-CM maintains many similarities to ICD-9-CM; it has the same hierarchical structure and many of the same conventions. Primarily, changes in ICD-10-CM are in its organization and structure, code composition, and level of detail. The process for selecting a diagnosis code using ICD-10-CM is not expected to change drastically.

ICD-10, as developed by the World Health Organization, does not include a classification for procedures. The US government, specifically the Centers for Medicare and Medicaid Services (CMS), contracted with 3M Health Information Systems to create a procedure coding system, ICD-10-PCS.

Overall, the current drafts of ICD-10-CM and ICD-10-PCS contain a significant increase in codes over ICD-9-CM. The level of specificity in ICD-10-CM and ICD-10-PCS will provide increased clinical detail, addition of information relevant to ambulatory and managed care encounters, enhanced system flexibility, and better reflection of current medical knowledge. Payers, policy makers, and providers will have more detailed information for establishing appropriate reimbursement rates, evaluating and improving the quality of patient care, improving efficiencies in healthcare delivery, reducing costs, and effectively monitoring resource and service utilization.

Two Years Out

The second stage also involves two major tasks: identifying and budgeting required IS changes and assessing, budgeting, and implementing clinician and coder education in the areas identified.

IS Changes

Building on the work in stage one, a more detailed analysis needs to occur in the second year of preparation. A budget for the required changes must also be established. The examination should include the following questions:

- What software changes are needed?

- What changes are required to accommodate multiple systems and applications that use coded data?

- What needs to be done to increase system storage capacity to support both coding systems for an adequate period?

If the facility uses commercial software, HIM professionals should ensure that their software provider is keeping up with the announced changes. This is one area (like the transactions and code sets final rule) in which assuming that someone else is fixing the problem has the potential to do real damage to the facility. Imagine the consequences if your vendor was not prepared and your facility could not submit claims or get reimbursed. Areas to discuss with your vendor include:

- Who will pay for systems upgrades?

- Are the upgrades included in an annual maintenance contract?

- If costs will be incurred by the organization, what are those projected costs and when will they be incurred?

Clinician and Coder Education

Implementation of any new coding system requires educational programs for clinicians responsible for documentation, coders, and a growing number of data users throughout the healthcare industry. The range of users and settings for which programs have to be designed and provided is much wider for ICD-10-CM than ICD-10-PCS.

Using the documentation gap analysis recommended in stage one, focused clinician education continues in those areas in need of improvement. In addition, reanalysis should be done to ascertain success of earlier efforts and assist in refocusing educational programs.

Because ICD-10-CM and ICD-10-PCS allow greater specificity, clinicians must change behaviors in documentation so the appropriate code can be selected (a goal consistent with the industry's goals to eliminate medical error). Clinicians will need to be actively involved in the educational process. This will allow them to understand the importance of complete and accurate documentation to support the level of specificity in ICD-10-CM and ICD-10-PCS.

Initial reports indicate the transition will require an expanded coder knowledge base, specifically in the following areas: detailed knowledge of anatomy and medical terminology; comprehension of operative reports; comprehension, interpretation, and application of standardized ICD-10-PCS definitions; and increased interaction and collaboration with medical staff.[2] It will be necessary to assess the clinical knowledge of the coding staff so that areas of weakness are identified and focused education can occur prior to implementation.

Coder education is a critical step during the third stage, but budgeting will be done in the first stages. Questions to consider when budgeting are:

1. Will you outsource the education or conduct it internally?

2. What are the costs and benefits of these two options?

3. When will the education need to be done?

4. Who will need what level of education?

5. What options (for example, Web-based training) are available for education?

6. How will workload be managed while coders are receiving education?

Although it would be technically possible for coding professionals to use a paper-based version of the ICD-10 systems, given the size and structure of the systems, most coding professionals and healthcare organizations will find them easiest to use in electronic format. Alternatives to manual use of these classification systems should be seriously considered, and the necessary vendors should be contacted.

One Year Out

The third stage involves three major tasks: implementation of required IS changes, follow-up assessment of documentation practices, and intensive education of the organization's coders.

Implement system changes following the detailed analysis of required IS changes that was compiled in stage two. A full reassessment after education should be done one year out to verify that goals are being achieved. A follow-up assessment of documentation practices after the clinician education is complete must be done to determine where improvements have occurred and where enhancements are necessary. Changing clinician documentation patterns will involve continuing education and reinforcement of the ICD-10-CM and ICD-10-PCS requirements for code specificity.

HIM professionals will want to familiarize themselves with the coding systems and any new and revised coding and reporting guidelines. Since ICD-10-CM has the same hierarchical structure and many of the same conventions as ICD-9-CM, experienced coding professionals will not require the same level of extensive education as they would for an entirely new coding system. They will primarily need to be educated in changes in structure, disease classification, definitions, and guidelines. However, ICD-10-PCS does vary from the "look and feel" of ICD-9-CM and will require coders to be educated in its intricacies and guidelines.

Remember that conducting education too far in advance of implementation can adversely affect its effectiveness. Coder education should be provided three months prior to ICD-10-CM implementation, according to 59 percent of respondents to the study conducted by AHIMA on ICD-10-CM.[3]

It is virtually impossible to make changes of this magnitude without encountering some obstacles. The key to managing the process is a good map that establishes "mile markers" to identify steps and priorities early. This method enables everyone to plan and prepare, thus minimizing problems. Watch the *Journal* for further details of AHIMA's strategy for training and provision of tools to facilitate implementation, such as a clinical knowledge assessment (individual practitioner), clinical documentation assessment evaluation (facility or enterprise), and organizational readiness report card (facility). Recommended steps to be undertaken by AHIMA members and other segments of the healthcare industry during each of the years leading up to implementation will also be detailed.

Notes

1. American Hospital Association (AHA) and American Health Information Management Association (AHIMA). "ICD-10-CM Field Testing Project. Report on Findings: Perceptions, Ideas and Recommendations from Coding Professionals across the Nation." Chicago: 2003. Available in the FORE Library: HIM Body of Knowledge at www.ahima.org.

2. Powell, Sharon, Barbara Steinbeck, and Thelma M. Grant. "Will You Be Ready? Preparing Now for ICD-10-PCS Implementation." Paper from the proceedings of the annual conference of the American Health Information Management Association, Chicago, 2002.

3. AHA and AHIMA. "ICD-10-CM Field Testing Project."

Prepared by

AHIMA's Coding Products and Services Team:

Kathy Giannangelo, RHIA, CCS
Susan Hull, MPH, RHIA, CCS
Karen Kostick, RHIT, CCS, CCS-P
Rita Scichilone, MHSA, RHIA, CCS, CCS-P
Mary Stanfill, RHIA, CCS, CCS-P
Sarah D. Wills-Dubose, MA, MEd, RHIA
Ann Zeisset, RHIT, CCS, CCS-P

Acknowledgment

Sue Bowman, RHIA, CCS

Want to learn more about ICD-10? Our new occasional column, "ICD-10: Mapping Our Course," debuts in this issue (March 2004) of JAHIMA.

Source: AHIMA's Coding Products and Services Team. "Destination 10: Healthcare Organization Preparation for ICD-10-CM and ICD-10-PCS" (AHIMA Practice Brief). *Journal of AHIMA* 75, no. 3 (March 2004): 56A–D.

Preparing for the ICD-10 Journey

by Sue Bowman, RHIA, CCS

After years of doubt as to whether ICD-10 was ever going to be implemented in the United States, the journey toward replacement of ICD-9-CM has finally gotten under way. The historic decision of the National Committee on Vital and Health Statistics (NCVHS) to send a letter to the Secretary of Health and Human Services (HHS) recommending the initiation of the regulatory process for the concurrent adoption of ICD-10-CM and ICD-10-PCS begins the process.

Time to Dust off Your ICD-10 Knowledge

The practice brief "Destination 10: Healthcare Organization Preparation for ICD-10-CM and ICD-10-PCS," in this issue, describes the regulatory process required for ICD-10 to be adopted and the ways in which ICD-10 and ICD-10-PCS represent an improvement over ICD-9-CM.

Given the years of uncertainty surrounding ICD-10 implementation, many HIM professionals' interest in and knowledge of ICD-10 have dwindled with time. Now it is time to recall those forgotten memories and refresh our knowledge of the ICD-10-CM and ICD-10-PCS coding systems.

As HIM professionals across the country prepare to lead ICD-10 implementation teams in their organizations, they need to take steps to become "experts" on how ICD-10-CM and ICD-10-PCS differ from ICD-9-CM. The basic understanding HIM managers need to lead implementation efforts is not the same type of knowledge as the in-depth skills in code application that those involved directly in the day-to-day coding function will need.

This article reviews the structure and unique characteristics of ICD-10-CM and ICD-10-PCS. It is not intended to be comprehensive. Use the resources listed in "To Learn More," below, to continue to increase your familiarity with ICD-10-CM and ICD-10-PCS.

How Is ICD-10-CM Different?

ICD-10-CM has many similarities to ICD-9-CM. For example, it has the same hierarchical structure and many of the same conventions, instructional notes, and guidelines. ICD-10-CM will have much the same "look and feel" as ICD-9-CM; however, it includes a number of notable differences:

- ICD-10-CM is entirely alphanumeric (all letters except U are used).

- ICD-10-CM codes may be up to seven characters in length.

- Some chapters have been restructured in ICD-10-CM.

- Some diseases have been reclassified in ICD-10-CM.

- New features have been added to ICD-10-CM.

Conditions with a recently discovered etiology or new treatment protocol have been reassigned to a more appropriate chapter. For example, gout is in the endocrine chapter in ICD-9-CM but in the musculoskeletal chapter in ICD-10-CM. And some conditions have been grouped in a more logical fashion than in ICD-9-CM.

"Excludes" notes were expanded to provide guidance on the hierarchy of chapters and clarify priority of code assignments. Also, two types of Excludes notes are clearly distinguished to eliminate confusion as to the meaning of the exclusion. An early draft of ICD-10-CM referred to three types of Excludes notes, but subsequent system revisions resulted in the use of only two types. An "excludes1" note designates codes that can never be used together. An "excludes2" note is used to clarify that the excluded condition is not a part of or included in the code.

In addition to the alphanumeric structure, ICD-10-CM embodies other differences in code structure. An "x" is used as a placeholder to save space for future expansion. So, for example, there may be a six-character code for which there is no fifth character subclassification at the present time. In this case, an "x" is used in the fifth character position. An example is code S63.8x1a, Sprain of other part of right wrist and hand, initial encounter.

Another change in ICD-10-CM is the use of extensions, which provide additional information in certain circumstances. Extensions are used in the obstetrics, injury, and external cause chapters and always occupy the final (seventh) character position in a code. The example above, code S63.8x1a, includes the extension "a" for "initial encounter." The other applicable extensions for category S63 are "d" (subsequent encounter) and "q" (sequela).

Other notable changes in ICD-10-CM include:

- Injuries are grouped by body part rather than category of injury.

- Factors influencing health status and contact with health services (known as V codes in ICD-9-CM) and external causes of morbidity and mortality (known as E codes in ICD-9-CM) are considered part of the main classification in ICD-10-CM, not "supplementary" classifications.

- Codes for postoperative complications have been expanded and moved to the appropriate procedure-specific body system chapter, and a new concept of "postprocedural disorders" has been added.

- Combination codes have been created for commonly occurring symptoms/diagnoses and etiologies/manifestations.

What about ICD-10-PCS?

ICD-10-PCS was developed specifically as a replacement for ICD-9-CM Volume 3. Four major objectives guided the development of ICD-10-PCS:

- Completeness: a unique code should exist for all substantially different procedures.

- Expandability: as new procedures are developed, the system structure should allow them to be easily incorporated as unique codes.

- Multiaxial: each code character should have the same meaning within the specific procedure section and across procedure sections, to the extent possible.

- Standardized terminology: each term should be assigned a specific meaning, and the coding system should not include multiple meanings for the same term.

ICD-10-PCS has a seven-character alphanumeric code structure. Unlike ICD-9-CM, ICD-10-PCS codes do not exist as "finished" codes in the tabular listing. Rather, they exist as groups of interchangeable coding components called "characters," which must be assembled into a code for each distinct procedure performed. So, in essence, the correct code is "built" for each procedure being coded.

Procedures are divided into 17 sections that relate to the type of procedure. (See Figure F.4, Sections of ICD-10-PCS.) The first character of the procedure code identifies the section.

The medical and surgical section contains 30 root operations. (See Figure F.5, Medical and Surgical Root Operations.) Definitions of these operations can be found in the ICD-10-PCS training manual. (See Figure F.6, To Learn More.) No diagnostic information is contained in ICD-10-PCS codes.

The ICD-10-PCS system contains an index and a tabular listing. The index allows codes to be located by looking up terms alphabetically. The main terms are root operations. However, common operative names, such as hysterectomy, can also be looked up, where a cross-reference directs the coder to the appropriate root operation term. The index provides only the first three or four characters of the procedure code. One must always refer to the tabular listing to obtain the complete code.

The tabular listing is arranged by sections, and most sections are subdivided by body system. There are separate tables for each root operation in a body system. The names of the section, body system, and root operation and its definition are listed at the top of each table. This list is followed by a grid, with the columns representing the last four characters of the code and the rows specifying the allowable combinations of these four characters. As demonstrated

Figure F.4.   **Sections of ICD-10-PCS**

0	Medical and Surgical	B	Extracorporeal Assistance and Performance
1	Obstetrics	C	Extracorporeal Therapies
2	Placement	D	Laboratory
3	Administration	F	Mental Health
4	Measurement and Monitoring	G	Chiropractic
5	Imaging	H	Miscellaneous
6	Nuclear Medicine	J	Substance Abuse Treatment
7	Radiation Oncology		
8	Osteopathic		
9	Physical Rehabilitation and Diagnostic Audiology		

Characters 2 through 7 have a standard meaning within each section but may have different meanings across sections. The characters for the medical and surgical section are:

1 = section	5 = approach
2 = body system	6 = device
3 = root operation	7 = qualifier
4 = body part	

Figure F.5.   **Medical and surgical root operations**

0	Alteration	B	Excision	N	Release
1	Bypass	C	Extirpation	P	Removal
2	Change	D	Extraction	Q	Repair
3	Control	F	Fragmentation	R	Replacement
4	Creation	G	Fusion	S	Reposition
5	Destruction	H	Insertion	T	Resection
6	Detachment	J	Inspection	V	Restriction
7	Dilation	K	Map	W	Revision
8	Division	L	Occlusion	X	Transfer
9	Drainage	M	Reattachment	Y	Transplantation

Figure F.6.   **To learn more**

- The ICD-10-CM draft and ICD-10-CM official guidelines for coding and reporting are available at www.cdc.gov/nchs/about/otheract/icd9/icd10cm.htm.

- "ICD-10-CM Overview: Deciphering the Code" is an Internet-based continuing education course (approved for eight AHIMA continuing education credits) and is available from AHIMA at the following link: campus.ahima.org/campus/course_info/ICD10OVER/ICD10O_info.html.

- The ICD-10-PCS final draft and training manual is available at www.cms.hhs.gov/paymentsystems/icd9/icd10.asp.

- *ICD-10-CM Preview,* by Anita Hazelwood and Carol Venable, can be ordered from the AHIMA Web site: www.ahima.org.

- Six 2004 regional coding community seminars will include a two-hour segment on ICD-10-CM and ICD-10-PCS. More information is available at www.ahima.org/coding/coding_meetings.cfm.

- AHIMA's "Statement in Support of Prompt Adoption of ICD-10-CM and ICD-10-PCS Medical Code Set Standards in the United States" is available at www.ahima.org/dc/positions.

- AHIMA's testimony on ICD-10-CM and ICD-10-PCS before NCVHS is available at www.ahima.org/dc.

- "CodeWrite," the online coding newsletter available to members of the Coding Community of Practice (CoP) and frequently distributed to coding roundtable participants in print form, will feature a regular column on practical application of ICD-10-CM and ICD-10-PCS codes. Members can log in at www.ahima.org.

- The ICD-10 Implementation CoP offers an opportunity to network with colleagues on CD-10 implementation strategies and ensures ready access to a wealth of CD-10 resources. Members can log in at www.ahima.org.

during the testing of ICD-10-PCS by the Clinical Data Abstraction Centers, the format of the tabular listing facilitates bypassing the index entirely and going directly to the tabular listing to assign a code.

Future articles in this column will address implementation strategies organizations should undertake during the next few years to ensure a successful and smooth transition to the new code sets.

Sue Bowman (sue.bowman@ahima.org) is director of coding policy and compliance at AHIMA.

Source: Bowman, Sue. "Preparing for the ICD-10 Journey." (ICD-10: Mapping Our Course column) *Journal of AHIMA* 75, no. 3 (March 2004): 60–62.

Taking the Next Step Forward for ICD-10

by Dan Rode, MBA, FHFMA

In November 2003 the National Committee on Vital and Health Statistics (NCVHS) agreed to recommend that the secretary of Health and Human Services (HHS) adopt the ICD-10-CM and the ICD-10-PCS classification standards as replacement for the ICD-9-CM classification currently used in the US.

The work of many AHIMA volunteers, staff, and other members of the healthcare industry made this professional milestone happen. But the NCVHS agreement is just the beginning. The next step is yours.

Conversion Process Has Roots in HIPAA

Congress passed HIPAA in 1996 to ensure that the healthcare industry would have standards to promote administrative simplification. HIPAA requires that any standard transactions be approved by the secretary of HHS. The secretary must also approve any code sets used in HIPAA transactions—including the eight transaction sets currently in use, such as ICD-9-CM.

HIPAA also established a process for the secretary to approve such code sets. The first step is the advisory process, which NCVHS has just completed. The next step is the regulatory process.

Most HIM professionals who have come into contact with the various elements of Medicare or Medicaid are familiar with the regulatory process. First, the secretary will issue a "notice of proposed rule making" (NPRM) to upgrade the coding systems from ICD-9-CM.

This NPRM will give a history of the issue and explain why these particular rules or regulations are being considered. It will also cite the regulations being proposed and the department's rationale behind them. In addition, it will cite specific sections of HIPAA for reference, name the bodies overseeing the maintenance of the classification systems, and describe potential economic impact. Finally, it will provide a comment period for the public to review the proposed rule and make any recommendations for changes, deletions, or additions. The period for comment will be 30 to 60 days.

Once the comment period is closed, all two-way dialogue between HHS and the public ceases. If the department has a question, it can "fact find" for an answer, but no additional comments can be made or considered, unsolicited, until a final notice is published. The waiting period for a final rule can vary tremendously, as we have seen with other HIPAA regulations. It could be as short as 30 days or it could be years.

The final rule is the last step. It may appear in several iterations, and there may be a version that allows additional comments, should HHS decide to add to the regulation significant changes not considered in the NPRM. The final rule states the final regulations: what they are, how they were reached, and when compliance is required.

Why ICD-10 Can't Wait

AHIMA members know that conversion to the ICD-10-CM and ICD-10-CPS systems is key in the nation's move toward a national health information infrastructure (NHII) and a standard electronic health record. For this conversion to take place, however, every HIM professional must respond to an NPRM. If the industry fails to champion the replacement of ICD-9-CM, the secretary could decide not to move forward in a timely fashion with adoption and implementation of the ICD-10 systems. Any delay in such adoption could mean significantly higher costs for eventual implementation—and we'll be no closer to an NHII or an EHR.

AHIMA has offered testimony in the past, and it continues to work with the coding authorities and others to accelerate an appropriate final rule as soon as possible—ideally, in 2004.

Such a NPRM is likely to include a description of the two classification code set standards (or at least an indicator where the standards can be found); description of the data elements and the impact on known HIPAA transaction standards; how uniform and standardized guidance will be handled, per HIPAA; the maintenance process for both (most likely similar to the coordination and maintenance process we know today); the anticipated implementation process, and the implementation dates.

There will be some differences in implementation between these two classification code set standards and the transaction sets. Namely:

- Conversion or final implementation would be the same date for all covered entities. We expect this to be an October 1 date to coincide with the existing maintenance update.

- The recommended implementation period will probably be two years from the final rule date—coordinated with the October 1 change. Most testimony for conversion indicated a two-year period would be necessary.

- The rule would allow for maintenance to the codes to occur in the classification system during implementation. This has to occur because code sets cannot be frozen during the implementation period and be kept up to date.

What HIM Professionals Can Do to Help

How can HIM professionals help? No matter what your job, your role in this process is important. Here are some things HIM professionals can do to support the process:

- **Get up to speed on ICD-10.** You don't have to know how to code with these classification systems, but you do have to know what the systems achieve, what components of healthcare they affect, why a 30-year-old classification system does not represent 21st-century medicine, and so on. You can find resources describing the issue in the Communities of Practice, the FORE Library: HIM Body of Knowledge, and elsewhere on AHIMA's Web site (www.ahima.org). You can also find articles in past and upcoming issues of the *Journal of AHIMA*. AHIMA will continue to prepare materials to educate its members, but you have to be the authority. Others in the industry will be seeking you out to question this change. Be prepared to discuss the NPRM. Read the rule when it is published, understand how you and your organization will be affected, and lend your voice in support.

- **Know what these classification systems do** and how they will affect your organization or institution. Conversion to ICD-10 will, to some extent, affect everyone. Administrators, information systems managers, financial and billing managers, and doctors will want to know how it will affect computer systems, data collection, documentation, billing, data reporting, and so forth. HIM professionals will need to help their organizations understand how this change will affect the organization and what the benefits are.

- **Comment on the NPRM.** Your expertise and your voice are very necessary for this process. While an association like AHIMA can promote adoption, it can only write one letter. In the face of opposition from groups such as the Blue Cross and Blue Shield Association and the American Association of Health Plans/Health Insurance Association of America, the voice of AHIMA members is particularly needed. These groups have opposed upgrading ICD-9-CM based on cost, but they fail to acknowledge the value of detailed standardized classification of diseases and inpatient procedures. The secretary must see that upgrading ICD-9-CM has the full support of the industry. Your voice must be heard.

Moving Forward: You Won't Go It Alone

You will not be alone in the professional effort to adopt and implement ICD-10-CM and ICD-10-PCS. AHIMA has been very involved in the creation and testing of these two classification systems, and the association intends to be 46,000 members strong in making this change a credit to our profession. Several AHIMA tools are at your disposal regarding the history and arguments for upgrading ICD-9-CM, as well as information and education resources regarding the replacement classification systems.

For instance, a Community of Practice for those interested in ICD-10-CM and PCS implementation has been established. The Coding Roundtables will also offer a means for two-way communication. This is a time for the HIM profession to shine, take the lead, and help bring in these changes in a professional, timely, and efficient manner. Together we can take the next steps.

Dan Rode (dan.rode@ahima.org) is AHIMA's vice president of policy and government relations.

Source: Rode, Dan. "Taking the Next Step Forward for ICD-10." *Journal of AHIMA* 75, no. 1 (January 2004): 14–15.

From V Codes to Z Codes: Transitioning to ICD-10

by Karen M. Kostick, RHIT, CCS, CCS-P

V codes, described in the ICD-9-CM chapter "Supplementary Classification of Factors Influencing Health Status and Contact with Health Services," are often misunderstood in reporting healthcare services. These codes are designed for occasions when circumstances other than a disease or injury result in an encounter or are recorded by providers as problems or factors that influence care.

ICD-9-CM codes such as V01.82, Exposure to SARS-associated coronavirus, and V01.81, Contact with or exposure to anthrax, are examples of how V codes capture significant US healthcare statistics. Although health plans have sometimes been reluctant to accept V codes as justification for reimbursement, these codes play a key role in classifying selected services and capturing important information.

Under ICD-10-CM, these services will be reported under a new set of codes—Z codes—with some significant changes.

V Codes in ICD-9-CM

The official coding guidelines that became effective on October 1, 2002, include coding guidelines for V codes throughout Sections I–IV. Section I C, "Chapter or Disease Specific Coding Guidelines," includes a clarification note for coders and states that unless otherwise indicated, the coding guidelines for this section apply to all healthcare settings. Complete copies of the guidelines are available from the National Center for Health Statistics (NCHS) Web site at www.cdc.gov/nchs.

Section I includes a new section titled "Classification of Factors Influencing Health Status and Contact with Health Service (C-18)." This section provides coding guidelines for frequently used V code categories. V codes reviewed in Section II, "Selection of Principal Diagnosis(es)," and Section III, "Reporting Additional Diagnoses," apply to the inpatient, short-term acute care setting. Section IV, "Diagnostic Coding and Reporting Guidelines for Outpatient Services," provides V code instructions for the outpatient and physician office setting. The outpatient setting includes reporting by home health agencies.

Changes in ICD-10-CM

The selected ICD-9-CM V code coding guidelines included in this article preview coding practices in ICD-10-CM for factors influencing health status and contact with health services. The coding guidelines between the two coding classification systems are the same unless otherwise specified.

A significant change between the two coding classifications is that ICD-9-CM's supplementary codes are incorporated into the main classification in ICD-10-CM. The ICD-10-CM Tabular List categorizes codes to represent reasons for encounters as "Z" codes instead of "V" codes. ICD-10-CM codes in general may have up to seven characters, but Z codes under categories Z00–Z99 consist of three to six character codes. Additional ICD-10-CM information is available for downloading from the NCHS Web site.

Screening, Routine Examination

Screening visits provide healthy patients early detection tests such as a mammogram or a colonoscopy. Screening codes can be used as either a first listed or additional code depending on the reason for the encounter. If the reason for the encounter is specifically the screening exam, the screening code is the first listed code and any condition discovered during the screening may be listed as an additional diagnosis.

A procedure code is required to validate the screening exam. Screening visit codes do not apply when a diagnostic test is ordered for a patient to evaluate a complaint or an abnormality detected by a physician. For these visits, the sign or symptom is used to report the reason for the test. (See "Outpatient Facility-Screening Scenario".)

Routine and administrative examinations are performed without relationship to treatment or diagnosis of an illness or symptom, or performed at the request of third parties such as employers or schools. Routine examination codes should be used as first listed codes only. This category should not be used if the examination is for diagnosing a possible condition or for providing treatment. Instead a sign or symptom code is used to report the reason for the visit.

Codes within ICD-10-CM categories Z00 and Z01, Persons encountering health services for examinations, are available when the encounter is for an examination "with abnormal findings" and "without abnormal findings." A note instructs the coder to use an additional code to identify any abnormal findings based on the results of the examination.

Aftercare Versus Follow-up Visits

Aftercare codes identify specific types of continuing care after the initial treatment of an injury or disease. In 2002, two V code subcategories for orthopedic aftercare (V54.1 and V54.2) were added to specify encounters following initial treatment of fractures. Coding guidelines state that a fracture code from the main classification can only be used for an initial encounter. Subsequent encounters that usually occur in an outpatient, home health, or long-term care facility now have the ability to report the type and site of fractures within the new subcategory sections.

Orthopedic aftercare visit coding guidelines differ in ICD-10-CM in that Z codes should not be used if treatment is directed at the current injury. If treatment is directed at the current injury, the injury code should be reported with an extension as the seventh character to signify the subsequent encounter. The purpose of assigning the extension is to be able to track the continuity of care while identifying the type of injury.

While aftercare codes are used for a resolving or long-term condition, follow-up codes are used for conditions that have completed treatment or for cancer patients to monitor the recurrence of cancer after treatment has been completed. ICD-9-CM coding guidelines state that follow-up codes are listed first unless a condition has recurred on the follow-up visit, then the diagnosis code should be listed first in place of the follow-up code. ICD-10-CM coding guidelines differ in that if a condition is found to have recurred on a follow-up visit, the follow-up code is still used and the diagnosis code is listed second. Personal history codes should be assigned as an additional code with follow-up examinations.

History, Status Codes

Personal and family history codes are important pieces of information that support the need for screening exams and follow-up exams. The Centers for Medicare and Medicaid Services (CMS) requires history V codes when appropriate in conjunction with mammograms, Pap tests, pelvic exams, and colon cancer screenings. You can read the CMS coding policies at: www.cms.hhs.gov/medlearn/womens_health.pdf.

Some status codes support increased healthcare costs, as the status can affect the treatment plans and its outcome as noted in the official coding guidelines. Status codes can also be used to track public health issues. For example, the status codes for infection with drug-resistance microorganism are assigned as an additional code for infectious conditions to indicate the presence of drug-resistance of the infectious organism. It is evident ICD-10-CM offers additional codes and a greater level of specificity to report health status and contact with health services in the revised classification. However, in a couple areas, ICD-9-CM is more specific than ICD-10-CM, as noted in "Inpatient, Acute Care-Status Scenario," with regard to the ICD-10-CM category for infection with drug-resistance microorganisms.

Outpatient Prenatal Visits

An area to pay close attention to when reporting prenatal visits in ICD-9-CM is category V23, Supervision of high-risk pregnancy. Coding guidelines for high-risk prenatal visits instruct that a code from category V23 be assigned as the first-listed or principal diagnosis unless a pertinent excludes note applies. If a V23 category excludes note applies codes from Chapter 11, Complications of Pregnancy, Childbirth, and the Puerperium Chapter (630–677) may be listed as a first-listed or principal diagnosis code.

If appropriate, Chapter 11 codes may be assigned as additional codes with category 23. ICD-10-CM does not include codes for supervision of high-risk pregnancy in the chapter to report factors influencing health status and contact with health services (Z00–Z99). Rather, these codes are incorporated in the chapter for conditions related to pregnancy and childbirth. ICD-10-CM high-risk pregnancy codes are available for patients who have had complications in the past and are categorized by first, second, and third trimester.

Advocating Coding Consistency

The HIPAA standard transactions and code sets regulation includes a requirement that the official coding guidelines are used along with ICD-9-CM for reporting. This represents an important step in the adoption of uniform code reporting requirements across all payers. Coding for reimbursement is addressed in the American Hospital Association's (AHA) 2000 3rd Quarter *Coding Clinic,* including problems that arise between providers and payers in relation to coding guidelines and payer coding policies.

AHA provides helpful tips on how to effectively settle coding conflicts with payers. When payers deny a particular claim, it is recommended that you first identify whether it is really a coding conflict and not a coverage matter. A payer may be using the correct coding guidelines but may not be covering certain services such as a routine or follow-up examination.

If you determine that a health plan reporting policy conflicts with the official coding guidelines, AHA advises you to obtain the payer policy in writing and advocate adherence to official coding guidelines. Coding professionals may influence the fiscal intermediary or carrier to apply official coding guidelines to ensure reliable claims data. These coding practices are also referenced in the AHIMA Standards of Ethical Coding.

Outpatient Facility—Screening Scenario

Asymptomatic 67-year-old female patient presents to the outpatient radiology department for a bilateral mammogram. The physician's order documented breast cancer screening. The radiology report notes clusters of microcalcification in the left breast.

First-Listed Diagnosis	ICD-9-CM:	V76.12 Other screening mammogram
	ICD-10-CM:	Z12.31 Encounter for screening mammogram for malignancy of breast
Additional Diagnosis	ICD-9-CM:	793.81 Mammographic microcalcification
	ICD-10-CM:	R92.0 Mammographic microcalcification found on diagnostic imaging of breast
Procedure	CPT:	76092 Screening mammography, bilateral

Physician Office—Routine Exam Scenario

45-year-old established patient presented to her physician's office for a routine physical exam. During the examination the physician identified an enlarged thyroid. The physician ordered a laboratory test and requested to see the patient in two weeks.

First-Listed Diagnosis	ICD-9-CM:	V70.0 Routine general medical examination at a health-care facility
	ICD-10-CM:	Z00.011 Encounter for general medical examination with abnormal findings
Additional Diagnosis	ICD-9-CM:	240.9 Goiter, unspecified
	ICD-10-CM:	E04.9 Nontoxic goiter, unspecified

Home Health—Aftercare Visit Scenario

74-year-old patient fell at home and sustained a subtrochanteric fracture of the left femur and was discharged home. Physician ordered physical therapy for difficulty in walking and exercise three times a week for one month

First-Listed Diagnosis	ICD-9-CM:	V57.1 Other physical therapy
	ICD-10-CM:	S72.22xd Displaced subtrochanteric fracture of left femur, subsequent encounter for closed fracture with routine healing
Additional Diagnosis	ICD-9-CM:	719.7 Difficulty in walking V54.13 Aftercare for healing traumatic fracture of hip
	ICD-10-CM:	R26.2 Difficulty in walking, not elsewhere classified

Inpatient, Acute Care—Status Scenario

A 54-year-old male is admitted into the hospital with a principal diagnosis of surgical site infection secondary to a recent right side below the knee amputation. Patient is a type I diabetic with diabetic peripheral vascular disease and congestive heart failure. The patient sought treatment when the wound began to exude purulent drainage. On the second day of his hospitalization he had developed nausea, uncontrolled diabetes, and ketoacidosis.

Moist saline dressings were applied twice daily to the wound. Wound culture tested positive for Staphylococcus aureus and was resistant to flucloxacillin. Ciprofloxacin effectively treated the infection. Diabetic ketoacidosis managed well and blood glucose was brought under control. Patient was discharged to a rehabilitation facility for continued wound management.

Principal Dx	ICD-9-CM:	997.62 Amputation stump infection
	ICD-10-CM:	T87.43 Infection of amputation stump, right lower extremity
Additional Dx	ICD-9-CM:	041.11 Staphylococcus aureus V09.0 Infection with microorganisms resistant to penicillins 250.13 Diabetes with ketoacidosis 250.73 Diabetes uncontrolled with peripheral circulatory disorders 443.81 Peripheral angiopathy in diseases classified elsewhere 428.0 Congestive heart failure, unspecified
	ICD-10-CM:	B95.6 Staphylococcus aureus as the cause of diseases classified elsewhere Z16 Infection with drug-resistant microorganisms E10.10 Type 1 diabetes mellitus with ketoacidosis without coma E10.51 Type 1 diabetes mellitus with diabetic peripheral angiopathy without gangrene I50.9 Congestive heart failure, NOS

References

AHA. *Coding Clinic,* 1996, 4th Quarter.

AHA. *Coding Clinic,* 2002, 4th Quarter.

AHIMA's Standards of Ethical Coding are available at www.ahima.org/infocenter/guidelines/standards.cfm.

CMS. Medicare Preventive Services Education Program. "Women's Health." Available at www.cms.hhs.gov/medlearn/womens_health.pdf.

Hazelwood, Anita, and Carol Venable. *ICD-10-CM Preview.* Chicago: AHIMA, 2003.

ICD-9-CM Official Guidelines For Coding and Reporting (Effective October 1, 2002). Available at www.cdc.gov/nchs/datawh/ftpserv/ftpicd9/ftpicd9.htm#guidelines.

ICD-10-CM Official Guidelines. Available at www.cdc.gov/nchs/about/otheract/icd9/abticd10.htm.

Karen Kostick (karen.kostick@ahima.org) is a coding practice manager at AHIMA.

Source: Kostick, Karen M. "From V Codes to Z Codes: Transitioning to ICD-10." *Journal of AHIMA* 75, no. 2 (February 2004): 65–68.

Index

Abandonment or neglect of infants and
   helpless persons, 251
Abbreviations enclosed in square brackets in
   ICD-9-CM, 25
Abbreviations used in ICD-9-CM, NEC and
   NOS, 24–25
Abdominal pain, definition of, 61
ABN. *See* Advance Beneficiary Notice
Abnormal findings, nonspecific, 57–58
Abnormal glucose tolerance (gestational
   diabetes), 102–3
Abnormal weight loss or underweight, 59
Abortion
   classification of, 192–93
   complications of, 194
   fifth digits for, 194–95
   fourth digits for, 193
   habitual or recurrent, 195
   missed, 195
   pregnancy with history of, 195
   resulting in live fetus, 195
   threatened, 195
Accredited Record Technicians, 313
Accuracy of coded data, ensuring, 307
Acid-fast stains, 67
Acidosis, respiratory and metabolic, 163–65
Acquired hemolytic anemias, 128, 129
Acquired immune deficiency syndrome. *See
   also* Human immunodeficiency virus
      disease
   coding, 76–77
   HIV-1 as cause of, 76
   uniform reporting criteria from CDC for, 76
Additional code
   for alcoholism and alcohol abuse, 114
   for chronic kidney disease, 140
   for chronic pyelonephritis, renal agenesis,
      or renal dysplasia, 183
   for complication of pregnancy, 198–99
   for complication or comorbid condition,
      72, 180, 264
   for diabetes mellitus, 103
   for diabetes mellitus late effect
      complication, 100–101
   for disease caused by infectious organism,
      72
   for disorders relating to short gestation
      and low birth weight, 213
   for heart failure, 139
   for hemorrhage caused by anticoagulant
      drug, 130
   for infected burn site, 242
   instructional notation to assign,
      22–23
   for joint replaced by prosthesis, 267
   for long-term use of insulin, 199
   for neoplasm, 88
   for organism causing cystitis, 182
   for residual condition, 120–21, 201
   for urinary incontinence, 183, 187
Additional diagnosis. *See also* Principal
      diagnosis
   for congenital anomaly, 208
   description of causative organism of
      infectious disease using, 71
   general rules for, 381–83
   for HIV disease or AIDS, 76–77
   reason for surgery as, for preoperative
      evaluation, 5
Adult abuse
   fifth digits for, 247
   guidelines for E codes for, 250
Advance Beneficiary Notice, 275
Adverse effects not classified elsewhere,
   246–47
Adverse effects of drugs, 251–54
   causes of, 251
   coding, 251–54
   late effects of, 252
   unspecified, 253–54
Adverse food reactions, 247
Affective disorders, 116
   fifth digits for, 116
Aftercare
   encounter for, 43
   in ICD-10-CM, 402
Agranulocytosis (neutropenia), 130
AHA. *See* American Hospital Association

AHIMA. *See* American Health Information Management Association
AIDS. *See* Acquired immune deficiency syndrome
Alcoholism and alcohol abuse, 114
  fifth digits for, 114
Alkalosis, acidosis versus, 163–65
Allergic reactions, 246
  to drugs, 251
Alphabetic Index to Diseases (Volume 2 of ICD-9-CM codebook), 13–16
  Alphabetic Index to External Causes of Injury and Poisoning (E Codes) in, 16
  Index to Diseases and Injuries in, 13–16
  instructional notes' appearance in, 21
  instructions for coding neoplasms in, 87–88
  neoplasm table in, 16, 85, 87–88
  Table of Drugs and Chemicals in, 16, 251–54
  terms not included in Tabular List but in, 15–16
Alphabetic Index to External Causes of Injury and Poisoning. *See* E codes
AMA. *See* American Medical Association
Ambulatory surgery, coding diagnosis for, 5
American College of Obstetricians and Gynecologists, 195
American Health Information Management Association
  assistance with ICD-9-CM updates by, 3
  Code of Ethics of, 297–305
  Position Statement on Data Quality of, 313–14
  Practice Brief on Data Quality of, 307–11
American Health Information Management Association members, ethical responsibilities of, 297
American Hospital Association, assistance with ICD-9-CM updates by, 3
American Hospital Formulary Service list, 12
American Medical Association
  CMS-1500 claim form approved by, 274
  CPT being revised by, 279
American Public Health Association, 3
Anal fissure and fistula, 173
Anemias
  aplastic, 129
  deficiency, 128
  hemolytic, hereditary and acquired, 128–29
  laboratory tests for, 128
  other and unspecified, 129
Angina pectoris, 141, 143
Angina, unstable (crescendo and preinfaction), 143
Appendices A–E to Volume 1 of ICD-9-CM, 12
Appendicitis, 171
ARTs. *See* Accredited Record Technician
Arterial blood gas results, 163
Arterial embolism and thrombosis of extremities, 149
Arteriosclerosis. *See* Atherosclerosis

Arteriosclerotic heart disease. *See* Ischemic heart disease
Arthritis, 226–28. *See also* Osteoarthrosis and allied disorders
  classification of, 226–27
  Lyme disease with, 227
  rheumatoid, 227–28
  septic (infectious or bacterial), 227
Artificial opening, V codes for status of, 40, 42
Assignment of codes to highest level of specificity, 4, 29
Assignment of Medicare benefits, physician acceptance of, 275
Asterisk * in neoplasm table, 90–91
Asthma, 159–60
  fifth digits for, 160
  fourth-digit subcategories of, 160
Atherosclerosis, 143–44
  of extremities with ulceration, 221
  fifth digits for, 143–44
  of peripheral extremities, 148
Atrial fibrillation, 145
Atrial flutter, 145
Atrioventricular heart blocks, 146
Audit of physician practice, 288

Bacillus bacteria causing human diseases, 69
Bacteremia, 75–76
Bacteria, 66–69
  additional diagnosis to identify causative, 71
  cultures of, 68
  definition of, 68
  shapes of, classifying, 67
  smear and stain examinations of, 66–67
  types of, infections caused by various, 68–69, 181–82
Balanced Budget Act of 1997
  fraud and abuse provisions of, 286
  Medicare Advantage program established under, 274
Bertillon Classification of Causes of Death, 3
Best practices, adopting, 309
Billing practices, audits of physician, 288
Birth weight, low, 213
Bites, 244
Bleeding varices, 150–51
Blood, components of, 128
Blood, diseases of. *See* Diseases of the Blood and Blood-Forming Organs
Blood vessels, injuries to, 244–45
Blue Cross and Blue Shield, 278
Brace } to reduce repetitive wording in coding, 27
Breast disorders, 185–86
Bronchitis, 156
Bronchopneumonia, 158
Burns, 242–43
  coding guidelines for, 242–43
  E codes for, 242
  infected, 242
  multiple, 243
  nonhealing, 242
  residual condition of, 243

CABG. *See* Coronary artery bypass
Calculus of urinary tract, 182
Candida albicans
    causing fungal disease, 70
    prevalence of, 162
    septicemia due to, 73
Candidiasis, 74, 162–63
Carcinoma in situ of cervix, 187
Cardiac defects, congenital, 209–10
Cardiac dysrhythmias, 145–46
Cardiomyopathy, 144–45
Carriers for Medicare Part B, 274–75
Carryover lines in Index to Diseases and
        Injuries, 14
Casts for dislocations, 238
Cataract, 122
    congenital, 122
    snowflake (diabetic), 101
Categories of conditions in Tabular List, 7
Cellulitis, 220–21
Centers for Disease Control, 76
Centers for Medicare and Medicaid Services
    ICD tenth revision reviewed by, 3
    Medicare administered by, 274
Cerebral concussion, 240
Cerebral contusion and laceration, 240
Cerebrovascular accident, 148
Cerebrovascular disease
    acute, but ill-defined, 147
    late effects of, 147, 148
Certain Conditions Originating in the
        Perinatal Period (codebook
        Chapter 15), 211–17
    categories and section titles for, 211
    V codes for, 214–15
Certified Coding Specialists, 313
Cervical dysplasia, 187
Cervical intraepithelial neoplasia, 187
Cervicitis, 186
CHAMPUS. *See* Civilian Health and Medical
        Program of Uniformed Services
Chemotherapy
    adjunct, 91–92
    V codes for, 86–87
Chickenpox, 73
Child maltreatment
    fifth digits for, 247
    guidelines for E codes for, 250
Childhood communicable diseases, 73
Chlamydia, pneumonia due to, 158
Chlamydia trachomatis causing human
        diseases, 69
    additional diagnosis to identify causative,
        71
Chlamydial venereal diseases, 75
Cholecystitis and cholelithiasis, 175
Chronic diseases, coding guidelines for, 5
Chronic kidney disease, 140, 180
Chronic obstructive pulmonary disease, 157
    acute bronchitis with, 156, 157
CIN I, II, III. *See* Cervical intraepithelial
        neoplasia
Circulatory system, diseases of. *See* Diseases
        of the Circulatory System

Civilian Health and Medical Program of
        Uniformed Services, 277
CKD. *See* Chronic kidney disease
Classification systems, early, 3
Cleft lip and cleft palate, 210
Clinical database evaluation, 308
Clostridium difficile, 69
Clostridium perfringens, 69
Clustering service codes, 288
CMS. *See* Centers for Medicare and Medicaid
        Services
CMS-1500 Claim Form
    blank, 293–95
    as universal claim form, 274
Coagulation defects, 129–30
"Code First Underlying Disease" instructional
        notation, 22–23
Code of Ethics (AHIMA), 297–305
    interpreting, 300–305
    preamble to AHIMA Code of Ethics
        describing, 297
    professional values affecting, 297–98
    purpose of, 298
    2004 version of, 299–300
    use of, 298–99
Code verification using Tabular List, 29
Coding
    defined, 2
    ethics in, 297–305
    to greatest specificity through four or five
        digits, 4, 29, 89–94
    of late effects, 50–52
Coding consistency, 403
Coding guidelines for complications of
        surgical or medical care, 265–66
Coding guidelines for E codes, 250
Coding guidelines for symptoms, 56–57
Coding guidelines for V codes used in
        chemotherapy and radiation therapy,
        86–87
Coding guidelines, official
    development of, 4
    exceptions for late effects of, 52
    for hypertensive diseases, 139–41
    for residual condition, 51
    summary of, 4–5
Coding process
    basic steps in ICD-9-CM, 29
    use of health record in, 28–29
Coding professionals, behavioral
        responsibilities of, 310–11
Coding systems
    development of, 2–5
    future of, 279–81
Coexisting conditions, coding, 5
Colon : after word needing modifier
        following it, 26–27
Colony of bacteria on culture, 68
Colostomy, complication of, 173
Commercial coverage for health insurance,
        278
Community of Practice for ICD-10-CM and
        –PCS, 400
Compliance activities, 289

Compliance officer, responsibilities of, 288
Compliance plans
    model, steps in implementation of, 288–89
    to prevent fraud and abuse, 287
Complication or comorbidity
    of abortion, 194
    additional code for, 72
    of colostomy and enterostomy, 173
    of diabetes, 98–100
    of internal prosthetic devices, implants,
        and grafts, 266–67
    of procedure, foreign body inadvertently
        left in operative wound as, 245
    of radiotherapy or chemotherapy, 87
    of reattached extremity or body part, 268
Complications not classified elsewhere, 268,
    269
Complications of Pregnancy, Childbirth, and
        the Puerperium (codebook Chapter 11),
        191–206
    categories and section titles for, 192
    V codes for, 202
Complications of surgical and medical care,
        263–72
    categories and titles for, 264
    coding guidelines for, 265–66
    described as postoperative conditions, 265
    indexed under name of condition and
        under main term Complications, 13
Congenital Anomalies (codebook Chapter
        14), 207–11
Congenital heart defects, 209–10
Connecting word subterms in Alphabetic
        Index, list of, 23–24
Consultations without complaint or sickness, 43
Contraceptive management, V codes for,
        37–38
Contusions with intact skin surface, 244
Convalescence and palliative care, V codes
        for, 43–44
Convulsions or seizures, definition of, 58
COPD. See Chronic obstructive pulmonary
        disease
Coronary artery bypass, 144
Coronary artery disease and coronary
        ischemia. See Ischemic heart disease
Correct coding procedures, 274
Counseling, V code for, 43
CPT. See Current Procedural Terminology
CPT-5, development and phase-in of, 279
Crohn's disease. See Enteritis, regional
        (granuloenteritis)
Cross-references
    in Alphabetic Index, See, See also, and See
        category, 16–18
    following instructions for, during coding,
        29
Crushing injuries, 244
Cultures, specimen, 68
Current Procedural Terminology
    changes in pattern of usage of, 289
    as coding system for E/M services, 274
    as Level I HCPCS codes, 276
    new revision being phased in for, 279

CVA. See Cerebrovascular accident
Cyanotic heart defects, 209–10
Cystic fibrosis, 104
Cystic kidney disease, 211
    fifth digits for, 211
Cystitis, 182

Data collection guidelines, 314
Data integrity, maintaining, 314
Data quality
    AHIMA position statement on, 313–14
    AHIMA practice brief addressing, 307–11
    recommendations by AHIMA for, 309–11
Data quality management and improvement
        initiatives, 308–9
Data quality review results, reporting, 308
DCIS. See Defense Criminal Investigative
        Service
Decubitus ulcer, 221
Defense Criminal Investigative Service, 287
Deficiency anemias, 128
Dementia, 113
Department of Health and Human Services,
        286
Depressive disorder, not elsewhere classified,
        116
Derangement, chronic, old, or recurrent, 239
Dermatitis, 221
Destination 10: Healthcare Organization
        Preparation for ICD-10-CM and
        ICD-10-PCS, 387–93
Developmental disorders, 116
Diabetes mellitus, 98–103
    acute metabolic complications of, 100
    complicating pregnancy, 102–3
    complications and manifestations of,
        98–100
    fifth digits for, 100
    with hyperosmolarity, 100
    incidence of, 98
    with ketoacidosis, 100
    late effect complications of, 100–102
    with neurological manifestations, 101
    in newborn of diabetic mother, 103
    with ophthalmic manifestations, 101
    with other specified manifestations, 102
    with peripheral circulatory disorders,
        101–2
    with renal manifestations, 101
    secondary, 103
    type I, 99–100
    type II , 99–100
Diabetic foot ulcers, 102
Diabetic nephropathy, 101
Diagnoses, coding guidelines for sequencing, 4
Diagnosis, preoperative, corrected with
        postoperative diagnosis, 5
Diagnostic and Statistical Manual of Mental
        Disorders, Fourth Edition (DSM-IV),
        110
Diagnostic services, sequencing, 5
Diagnostic statement
    coding using, 29
    requiring physician clarification, 76

terms classifying secondary malignant neoplasms in, 92–94
Dialysis, V codes for encounters for, 42
Diarrhea, definition of, 60
Dietary surveillance, 43
Digestive system, diseases of. *See* Diseases of the Digestive System
"Direct extension to" in diagnostic statements, 92
Disciplinary standards enforced for compliance plan, 289
Diseases
    eponyms for, 15
    indexed under main term Disease as well as under disease's name, 13
Diseases of arteries, arterioles, and capillaries, 148–49
Diseases of the Blood and Blood-Forming Organs (codebook Chapter 4), 127–33
    V codes for, 131
Diseases of the Circulatory System (codebook Chapter 7), 135–54
    categories and section titles for, 136
    V codes for, 151
Diseases of the Digestive System (codebook Chapter 9), 169–78
    categories and section titles for, 170
Diseases of the ear and mastoid process, 123
Diseases of the Genitourinary System (codebook Chapter 10), 179–90
    categories and section titles for, 180
Diseases of the Musculoskeletal System and Connective Tissue (codebook Chapter 13), 225–33
    categories and section titles for, 226
    fifth digit to describe affected body site for, 7–8
    V codes for, 230
Diseases of the Nervous System (codebook Chapter 6), 119–26
    categories and section titles for, 120
Diseases of the Respiratory System (codebook Chapter 8), 155–68
    categories and section titles for, 156
Diseases of the Skin and Subcutaneous Tissue (codebook Chapter 12), 219–23
    categories and section titles for, 220
Diseases of the tonsils and adenoids, 159
Diseases of the white blood cells, 130
Diseases of veins and lymphatics and other diseases of circulatory system, 149–51
Dislocations, 238–39
Disorders of eye and adnexa, 122
Disorders of menstruation and other abnormal bleeding from female genital tract, 187–88
Disorders of prostate, 184–85
Disorders related to short gestation and low birth weight, 213
Disturbance of skin sensation, 59
Diverticular disease, 171
Dizziness and giddiness, definition of, 58–59
DM. *See* Diabetes mellitus

Doctrine of confidentiality in use and disclosure of information, 299, 300–301
Documentation improvement program, 310
Dorsopathies, 229
Drug abuse or dependence in pregnancy, childbirth, or puerperium, 199
Drugs, adverse effects of or reactions to, 251–54
DSM-IV. See Diagnostic and Statistical Manual of Mental Disorders, Fourth Edition (DSM-IV)
Duodentis, 172–73
Durable medical equipment, certification of need for, 288
Dysphagia, definition of, 60

E codes (Supplementary Classification of External Causes of Injury and Poisoning), 16, 247–51
    additional, for perpetrator in child and adult battering, 250
    for adverse effects not classified elsewhere, 246
    for adverse effects of drugs, 251–54
    for burns, 242
    categories and section titles for, 248
    coding guidelines for, 250
    external cause code with SIRS guidelines for, 250–51
    format of, 11–12
    fourth digits for, 248
    late effect, 243, 249–50, 255–56
    for place of occurrence, 249
    use of, 250
Ear and mastoid process, diseases of, 123
Ectopic pregnancy, 192
    complications of, 194
EKGs. *See* Electrocardiograms
Electrocardiograms, 141–42
Elevated blood pressure, 141
Embolism, definition of, 149
End-stage renal disease, 180
Endocrine, Nutritional, and Metabolic Disorders, and Immunity Disorders (codebook Chapter 3), 97–107
    categories and section titles for, 98
    V codes for, 104–5
Endometriosis, 186
Enteritis, regional (granulomatous), 172
Enterobacteriaceae bacteria, 69
Epilepsy, 121–22
Epistaxis, definition of, 59
Eponyms in Index to Diseases and Injuries, 15
Esophageal and gastric varices, 150–51
Esophagitis, 170
Esophagostomy, 171
ESRD. *See* End-stage renal disease
Ethics, coding, 297–305
    interpreting, 300–305
    preamble to AHIMA Code of Ethics describing, 297

(continued)

Ethics, coding (*continued*)
    professional values affecting, 297–98
    purpose of, 298
    2004 version of, 299–300
    use of, 298–99
Evaluations, sequencing preoperative, 5
Exclusion notes, 19–20
    for chronic obstructive pulmonary disease, 157
    for complications of medical care not elsewhere classified, 269
    for complications of surgical or medical care, 264–65
    in ICD-10-CM, 281
    for mental disorders, 111–12
    for nonspecific findings, 57
    for wounds, 241
"Extension to" in diagnostic statements, 93
Eye and adnexa, disorders of, 122

FBI, fraud investigations by, 287
Federal False Claims Act and Federal False Claims Amendment Act, 286
Fetal abnormality, 200
Fifth digits
    for abortion, 194–95
    for acute myocardial infarction, 142
    for alcohol/drug dependence and abuse, 115
    assignments and instructions at beginning of three-digit category for, 7–9
    for asthma, 160
    for atherosclerosis, 143–44
    for burns, to identify percentage of body surface involved, 243
    for cerebral infarction, 147
    for child and adult maltreatment, 247
    for chlamydial venereal diseases, 75
    for cholecystitis and cholelithiasis, 175
    for cystic fibrosis, 104
    for cystic kidney disease, 211
    for diabetes, 100
    for epilepsy, 122
    for extremity in arterial embolism and thrombosis of extremities, 149
    for glaucoma, 122
    for hypertensive diseases, 139–40
    for hypertrophy (benign) of prostate, 184
    in ICD-10-CM, 281
    instructional notes for, assigning, 21
    for internal injuries, 240–41
    for intracranial injuries, 239
    for mental disorders, 111
    for open wounds, 242
    for osteomyelitis, periostitis, and other infections involving bone, 229
    for peritonitis and retroperitoneal infections, 175
    for pregnancy, 196–97
    for prosthetic device, implant, and graft, 267
    for respiratory problems after birth, 213
    for slow fetal growth and fetal malnutrition, 212–13
    for specificity of coding, 4
    for tuberculosis, 72
    for vesicoureteral reflux, 183
    for viral hepatitis, 74
Fiscal intermediaries for Medicare, 274–75
Follow-up examinations, V codes for, 44
Foreign bodies entering through orifice, effects of, 245
Fractures
    closed, 237
    coding, 237
    defined, 237
    fifth digits for, 238
    fistulas secondary to, 245
    malunion of, 229–30
    multiple, 237–38
    open, 237
    pathologic, 229
    stress, 230
    x-ray report to assign diagnosis code for, 238
Fraud and abuse, 285–89
    agencies investigating, 287
    definitions and examples of, 287
    HIM professional's responsibilities regarding, 311
    legislation addressing, 286
    physician compliance in preventing, steps in, 287–89
Fungi causing infectious diseases, 70

Gastritis, 172–73
Gastroenteritis, 172
Gastrointestinal hemorrhages, 174
Gastrointestinal ulcers, 171
Genital prolapse, 186–87
Genitourinary system, diseases of. *See* Diseases of the Genitourinary System
Geographic practice cost indices, 277
Gestational diabetes, 102–3
Gestational hypertension, 198
Glaucoma, 122
Gonorrhea, 75
Government health programs, 277
    fraud against, 287
GPCIs. *See* Geographic practice cost indices
Gram stain technique, 66–67
    for bacterial pneumonia, 158
Graves' disease, 103
Gynecologic disorders, 186–88

HCPCS. *See* Healthcare Common Procedural Coding System
Health Care Financing Administration (HCFA). *See* Centers for Medicare and Medicaid Services
Health information management knowledge and practice, 300, 303
Health information management profession
    mission of, 297, 298
    representation to public of, 300, 304
Health information management professionals
    assistance in implementing ICD-10 by, 399–400

ethical principles of, 299–305
obligations to reflect values and principles
of, 298
professional values of, 297–98
responsibilities of, performance of, 300,
304
truthfulness about background of, 300,
304
Health Insurance Portability and
Accountability Act, 279, 286
administrative simplification requirements
of, 398
compliance with, 387
official coding guidelines published in
regulations of, 309
Health maintenance organizations, 278
Health record
requirements for, 2
risk areas for fraud in, 288
use in coding process of, 28–29
Healthcare Common Procedure Coding
System, 276
Healthcare data collection, settings for, 2
Healthcare information, functions of, 313
Heart defects, congenital, 209–10
Heart disease
hypertension with, 139
hypertensive, 139
ischemic, 141–44
rheumatic, 136–37
valvular, 136–37
Heart failure
diagnostic tests for, 147
signs of, 146–47
Heartburn, definition of, 60
Heat and light, conditions from effects of,
246
Hematuria, 183
Hemiplegia and hemiparesis, 121
Hemolytic anemias, 128–29
Hemophilia A, B, and C, 130
Hemorrhage
of digestive tract, 174
subdural, subarachnoid, and extradural,
240
Hemorrhagic conditions, 130
Hemorrhoids, 149–50
Hereditary hemolytic anemias, 128–29
Hernias
diaphragmatic (hiatal), 172
obstructed, 172
Herpes simplex, 74
Herpes zoster, 74
HIPAA. *See* Health Insurance Portability and
Accountability Act
History codes in ICD-10-CM, 402–3
Home health routine exam scenario, 404
Human immunodeficiency virus disease,
76–78
code assignment for, 76–77
in pregnancy, childbirth, or puerperium,
76–77
testing for, 77–78
Hydrocele, 185

Hyperplasia of prostate, 184
Hypertension, 137–41
benign, 138, 139
cerebrovascular disease with mention of,
147
essential or NOS, 139
gestational, 198
with heart disease, 139
heart failure due to, 147
malignant, 138–39
official coding guidelines for, 139–41
primary, 138
secondary, 138, 140
secondary to renal disease, 138
transient, 141
Hypertension table of Alphabetic Index, 16,
137–38
Hypertensive cerebrovascular disease, 140
Hypertensive heart and kidney disease, 139–40
Hypertensive retinopathy, 140
Hyperventilation, definition of, 60
Hypoglycemia, 103
Hypotension, 150
Hypothyroidism, 103–4

ICD-9-CM codebook. *See also* individual
volumes
on CD-ROM from U.S. Government
Printing Office, 6
characteristics of, 5–24
conventions in, 16–24, 321–24
ICD-9-CM Official Guidelines for Coding
and Reporting, 315–86
changes in bold text for, 316
chapter-specific, text of, 327–79
conventions, general coding guidelines
and chapter specific guidelines in,
321–79
diagnostic coding and reporting guidelines
for outpatient services in, 383–86
general, 324–27
reporting additional diagnoses in, 381–83
sections of, 316–20
selection of principal diagnosis in, 380–81
ICD-10-CM. *See International Statistical
Classification of Diseases and Related
Health Problems, 10th edition*
ICD-10-PCS. *See* Implementation of
ICD-10-CM and ICD-10-PCS
Ill-Defined and Unknown Causes of
Morbidity and Mortality, 58
Implementation of ICD-10CM and
ICD-10-PCS, 387–405
conversion process needed for, 398
educational requirements for, 391–92
preparation for, 394–97
screening scenario for, 403
Inclusion notes, 19
for complications of medical care not
elsewhere classified, 269
for complications resulting from use of
artificial substitutes or natural sources,
266

(continued)

Inclusion notes *(continued)*
   for conditions originating in perinatal
      period, 211
   for mental disorders, 111–12
Independent practice associations, 278
Indian Health Service, 277
Infantile cerebral palsy, 121
Infections
   descriptions of common, 72–78
   involving bone, 229
   late effects of, 78
   other bacterial, 73
   perinatal, 214
   peritonitis and retroperitoneal, 174–75
   postoperative wound, 221
   primary and secondary tuberculosis, 72
   respiratory, upper and lower, 157, 160
   V codes for, 78
Infections, microorganisms that cause,
      68–71
   drug-resistant, 71–72
Infectious and Parasitic Diseases (codebook
      Chapter 1), 65–81, 120
   categories and section titles for, 66
   coding, health record information for,
      70–71
   combination codes and multiple coding
      for, 71–72
Infectious diseases classified elsewhere
   complicating pregnancy, childbirth, or
      puerperium, 199
   pneumonia in, 158
Infectious diseases, diagnosis of
   by cultured colonies of bacteria, 66–68
   by serologic studies, 68
   by smear and stain examinations, 66–67
Infectious gastroenteritis, 75
Inflammatory disease of female pelvic organs,
      186
Injuries, 236–51
   to blood vessels, 244–45
   classification of, 236
   crushing, 244
   defined, 236
   external causes of, 247–51
   internal, 240–41
   main terms for, 237
   multiple, combination categories for, 238
   to nerves and spinal cord, 245
   primary, 245
   resulting from other and unspecified
      effects of external causes, 245–47
   superficial, 244
   V codes for, 247
Injury, Poisonings, and Adverse Effects
      (codebook Chapter 17), 235–62
   categories and section titles for, 236
Inpatient acute care, ICD-10-CM scenario for,
      404
Instructional notations, 19–21
Instructional notes, 20–21
   section mark to reference earlier, 27
Interdisciplinary collaboration, facilitating,
      300, 304–5

Internal injury of thorax, abdomen, and
      pelvis, 240
   fifth digits for, 240–41
International Classification of Causes of
      Death, first revision of, 3
International Classification of Diseases, 9th
      Revision, Clinical Modification, 2–3
   annual updates to, 3, 6
   comparison of ICD-10-CM to, 280
   introduction to, 1–31
   official addenda to, 3
International Classification 10th Revision
      Procedure Classification System
      (ICD-10-PCS), 279
International Statistical Classification of
      Diseases and Related Health Problems,
      10th edition, 387–405
   comparison of ICD-9-CM to, 280
   educational needs for, 388–90
   implementation plan for, 388
   planned replacement of ICD-9-CM by, 279
   transitioning to, 401–5
Intracranial injuries, excluding those with
      skull fractures, 239–40
   fifth digits for, 240
IPAs. *See* Independent practice associations
Iron deficiency anemia, 128
Ischemic heart disease, 141–44
   chronic, 141, 143–44

Joint Commission on Accreditation of
      Healthcare Organizations, 307

Laboratory tests
   abnormal findings of, reporting, 130
   acute myocardial infarction diagnosed by,
      141
   anemias diagnosed by, 128
   diabetes mellitus diagnosed by, 98
   infectious diseases diagnosed by, 66–68,
      71
   renal failure diagnosed by, 181
Lack of expected normal physiological
      development in childhood, 59
Late effects, 49–54
   of burns, 243
   of cerebrovascular disease, 148
   coding of, 50–52
   of complication of pregnancy, childbirth,
      or puerperium, 201
   defined, 50
   of diabetes mellitus, complications from,
      100–102
   E codes for, 243, 249–51
   of infectious and parasitic diseases, 78
   of inflammatory diseases of central
      nervous system, 120–21
   of poisoning, 255–56
   of unspecified adverse effect, 253–54
LCDs. *See* Local Coverage Determinations
Liveborn infants according to type of birth,
      V codes for, 38–39
   fourth and fifth digits for, 39
   as principal diagnosis, 208

Liver, cirrhosis of, 173–74
LMRPs. *See* Local Medical Review Policies
Local Codes, Level III HCPCS as, 276
Local Coverage Determinations, 278–79
Local Medical Review Policies, 278
London Bills of Mortality, 3
Long-term (current) drug use, V codes for, 43
Low birth weight status for premature babies, 36, 213
Lozenge □ identifying code unique to clinical modification of ICD-9, 28
Lymph nodes, enlargement of, definition of, 59

M (morphology) codes, 85–86
Main terms
    in diagnostic statement, identifying, 29
    in Index to Diseases and Injuries, 13
    located in Alphabetic Index, 29
    requiring V codes, 35
Malignancies. *See* Neoplasms
Mammary dysplasias, benign, 185
Manual of International Statistical Classification of Diseases, Injuries and Causes of Death, revisions of, 3
Maternal causes of perinatal morbidity and mortality, 212
Measles, 73
Mechanical complication of internal orthopedic device, implant, and graft, 266–67
Meconium passage, 213
Meconium staining, 213
Medicaid
    created by Title 19 of Social Security Act, 277
    prosecution of false claims for, 286
Medical examinations, V codes for general, 44–45
Medicare
    fraud for, 287
    funding for, 274
    Part A, 274
    Part B, 274, 275
    Part C, 274
Medicare Carrier Manual, 278
Medicare Conditions of Participation, recording of final diagnoses and procedures required by, 307
Medicare Fee Schedule, 275
Medicare Summary Notice, 274
Medigap insurance coverage, 274
Meningitis, 73, 120
Menopausal and postmenopausal disorders, 188
Mental disorders
    multiple coding of, 110–12
Mental Disorders (codebook Chapter 5), 109–18
    categories and section titles for, 110
    DSM-IV categories listed in, 110
    fifth digits for, 111
    inclusion and exclusion notes for, 111–12
Metabolic disorders, 104

"Metastatic from" and "metastatic to" in diagnostic statements, 92
"Metastatic of one site" in diagnostic statements, 93–94
MFS. *See* Medicare Fee Schedule
Microorganisms that cause infections
    descriptions of, 68–71
    drug-resistant, 71–72
Mitral valve, diseases of, 136–37
Model compliance plan to prevent fraud and abuse, 288–89
Morphology codes. *See* M codes
MSN. *See* Medicare Summary Notice
Multiple codes, assignment of, 22–23
    for cellulitis, 220
    for complications of pregnancy, childbirth, or puerperium, 196
    for disorders relating to short gestation and low birth weight, 213
    for mental disorders, 110–12
    for secondary hypertension, 140
Multiple gestation, 200
Musculoskeletal system, diseases of. *See* Diseases of the Musculoskeletal System and Connective Tissue
Mycoplasma species producing human diseases, 69
Myocardial infarction
    acute, 141
    complications of, 141
    diagnostic tools for, 141–42
    fifth-digit subclassifications for, 142
    fourth-digit subcategories for, 142

National Center for Health Statistics
    abortion codes confirmed by, 195
    ICD tenth revision reviewed by, 3
National codes, Level II HCPCS as, 276
National Committee on Vital and Health Statistics, adoption of ICD-10-CM and ICD-10-PCS advocated by, 387, 398
National Correct Coding Initiative edits, 278
National health information infrastructure, 398
Nausea and vomiting, definition of, 60
NCHS. *See* National Center for Health Statistics
NCVHS. *See* National Committee on Vital and Health Statistics
NEC abbreviation for terms not elsewhere classifiable, 24–25
Neglect, accidental, 251
Neonatal diabetes mellitus, 103
Neoplasm table in Alphabetic Index, 16, 85, 87–88
    asterisk * in, 90–91
    subterms checked in, 94
Neoplasms
    behavior of, 84–86
    benign, 85
    coding, 87–94
    in situ, 85
    of lymphatic and hematopoietic system, 90
(*continued*)

Neoplasms *(continued)*
    malignant, 9, 84, 89–94
    metastatic from and to, 92
    primary, 84, 86–87, 93–94
    primary sites of, classifying, 91–92
    primary site of, determining, 90
    secondary, 84
    secondary sites of, classifying, 92–94
    surgical removal followed by recurrence of, 92
    uncertain behavior, 85
    unspecified nature, 85
Neoplasms (codebook Chapter 2), 83–96
    categories and section titles for, 84
    morphology (M) codes for, 85–86
    V codes for, 86–87
Nephritis, nephrosis, and nephritic syndrome, 180–81
Nephrotic syndrome, 181
Nervous system, diseases of. *See* Diseases of the Nervous System
Neurotic and personality disorders, 112–13
Neutropenia (agranulocytosis), 130
Newborn period, 208, 211
Newborns
    of HIV-positive mothers, 214
    infections specific to, 214
    normal delivery of, 197–98
    other respiratory conditions of, 213
    V codes for, 38–39, 214–15
NHII. *See* National health information infrastructure
Noncovered services, fraudulent billing of, 288
Nonessential modifiers in Index to Diseases and Injuries, 15
Non-PAR physician, Medicare payment to, 275
Nonspecific abnormal findings, 57–58
Normal delivery of infant, 197–98
NOS abbreviation for terms not otherwise specified, 25
Notice of proposed rule making
    HIM professionals' comments on, 399–400
    in regulatory process, 398–99
NPRM. *See* Notice of proposed rule making

OBRA. *See* Omnibus Budget Reconciliation Act
Observation and evaluation, V codes for
    of newborns, 38
    of suspected conditions, 45
Obstetrical conditions, 13
Obstructed labor, 200
Occlusion and stenosis of precerebral arteries, 147
Occlusion of cerebral arteries, 147
Office of Inspector General, 286, 287
    audit recommended by, 288
Official Authorized Addendum to ICD-9-CM, annual editions of, 3
OIG. *See* Office of Inspector General
OM. *See* Otitis media (OM)

Omnibus Budget Reconciliation Act, 276
Open wounds, 241–42
    fistulas secondary to, 245
Operation Restore Trust project, 286
Organ or tissue replacement
    by other means, 40
    by transplant, 39
Organ removal, prophylactic, 41
Organic impotence, 102
Organic Psychotic Conditions subsection, 113
Orthopedic aftercare, 42
Orthopedics, definition of, 226
Osteoarthrosis and allied disorders, 228
Osteomyelitis, periostitis, and other infections involving bone, fifth digits for, 229
Osteopathies, chondropathies, and acquired musculoskeletal deformities, 229–30
Other
    and unspecified anemias, 129
    and unspecified arthropathies, 228
    and unspecified disorders of joint, 228–29
    and unspecified procedures, encounter for, 43
    blood and blood-forming organ diseases, 131
    conditions influencing health status, 41
    dependence on machines, V codes for, 40–41
    diseases of urinary system, 181–84
    disorders of circulatory system, 151
    forms of asthma, 160
    indications for care in pregnancy, labor, and delivery, 200–202
    infection specific to perinatal period, 214
    paralytic syndromes, 121
    respiratory conditions of fetus and newborn, 213
    specified forms of chronic ischemic heart disease, 144, 145
Otitis externa (swimmer's ear), 123
Otitis media, 123
Outcome of delivery, V codes on mother's health record for, 38, 198
Outpatient procedures, CPT used for coding, 6
Outpatient services, diagnostic coding and reporting guidelines for, 393–86
Ovarian cysts, 187

Pacemaker, cardiac, postsurgical, 40
Palpitations, definition of, 59
Paralytic conditions, 121
Parasites, 70
Parentheses ( ) for supplementary words or explanatory information, 25
Percutaneous transluminal coronary angioplasty, 143–44
Perinatal period, congenital anomalies and certain conditions originating in, 207–17
Peripheral vascular disease, 102, 148–49
Peritonitis and retroperitoneal infections, 174–75
Peroxysmal supraventricular tachycardia, 145

Personal health information, 300, 301–2
Personality disorders, 112–13
Phlebitis and thrombophlebitis, 149
Physician billing
    audits of, 288
    volumes 1 and 2 of ICD-9-CM used for, 6
Physician practices
    violations of compliance plan by, 289
    fraud risk areas identified by OIG for, 288
    routine exam scenario for ICD-10-CM for,
        404
Physician queries, 309, 310
Physician reimbursement from Medicare, 275
Physician statement, 71
Pleural effusion, 161
    malignant, 161
Pneumonia
    aspiration, 159
    bacterial, 158
    categories of, 157–58
    due to other specified organism, 158
    in infectious diseases classified elsewhere,
        158
    organism unspecified, 159
    pneumococcal, 158
    viral, 158
Pneumonitis due to solids and liquids
        (aspiration pneumonia), 159
Pneumothorax, 161
Poisonings, 254–56
Polycystic kidney disease, 211
Polycythemia, 131
Postal Inspection Service, fraud investigations
        involving U.S. Mail Service by, 287
Postpartum care, V codes for, 37
Postsurgical states, V codes for, 40
PPOs. See Preferred provider organizations
Practice Brief on Data Quality (AHIMA),
        307–11
Prebirth counseling, V code for, 43
Preferred provider organizations, 278
Pregnancy
    aggravating preexisting condition,
        198–99
    complications of, 198–99
    diabetes mellitus complicating, 102–3
    drug dependence or abuse during, 199
    ectopic, 192, 194
    excessive vomiting in, 198
    fifth digits for, 196–97
    high-risk, 195
    with history of abortion, 195
    incidental, 196
    infectious and parasitic conditions
        complicating, 199
    late, 198
    late effect of complication of, 201
    molar, 194
    normal first, 5
    prebirth counseling during, 43
    preterm, term, and prolonged postterm,
        195–96
    V codes for supervision of normal and
        higher risk, 5, 37

Premature babies, low birth weight status for,
        36, 213
Prenatal visits, outpatient, 5, 403
Principal diagnosis. See also Additional
        diagnosis
    for congenital anomaly, 208–9
    selection of, 380–81
Procedure not carried out, 43
Procreative management, V codes for, 38
Professional values in HIM, 297–98
Prolonged prothrombin time, 130
Prophylactic organ removal, 41
Prostatic hyperplasia, urinary retention
        associated with, 183
Prostatic hypertrophy, benign, 184–85
Prostatitis, 185
Prosthetic devices and implants, fitting and
        adjustment of, 41
Providers, types of Medicare, 275
Provisional diagnoses, 56
Psychoses/neuroses, 112–13
Pulmonary edema, acute or chronic, 162
Punctuation in ICD-9-CM, 25–27
Purpura and other hemorrhagic conditions,
        130
PVD. See Peripheral vascular disease
Pyelonephritis, acute and chronic, 181
Pyloric stenosis, 210–11

Quality healthcare data and information,
        313–14

RA. See Rheumatoid arthritis
Radiation therapy
    adjunct, 91–92
    V codes for, 86–87
Radiological studies, abnormal findings on,
        57–58
RBRVS. See Resource-based Relative Value
        Scale
Reason for encounter, coding first, 4, 5
Reason for surgery as additional diagnosis for
        preoperative evaluation, 5
References and bibliography, 291
Registered Health Information
        Administrators, 313
Reimbursement
    coding systems and, 273–83
    glossary of terms for, 282–83
    by third-party payers, 274
Relative value units for HCPCS codes,
        276–77
Renal failure, 180, 181
Renal (kidney) disease
    chronic, 140, 180
    end-stage, 180
    hypertension secondary to, 138
    hypertensive, 139–40
Residual effects, presence of, 50
Residual subcategories, 10–11
Resource-based Relative Value Scale, 276
Respirator, V codes for dependence on, 165
Respirator failure, 41
Respiratory failure and insufficiency, 161–62

Respiratory infections, upper and lower, 160
Respiratory system and other chest
        symptoms, 59–61
Respiratory system, diseases of. *See* Diseases
        of the Respiratory System
Rheumatic fever, acute, 136–37
Rheumatic heart disease, chronic, 136, 137
Rheumatoid arthritis, 227–28
Rheumatology, definition of, 226
Right to privacy, individual's, 299, 300–301
Rubella (German measles), 73–74
Rule of nines for burns, 243

SCHIP. *See* State Children's Health Insurance
        Program
Schizophrenic disorders, 115–16
Screening examinations
    in ICD-10-CM, 401–2
    for specific conditions and disorders,
        V codes for, 46
Section mark § to indicate footnote or
        references to instructional note, 27
Sections of categories in Tabular List, 7
See, See also, and *See category* cross-
        references in Alphabetic Index,
        16–18
Seizure disorder, 121
Septicemia, 73
Serologic studies, infectious diseases
        diagnosed by, 68
Sexually transmitted diseases, 75
Sick sinus syndrome, 145
Signs and symptoms
    coding guidelines for reporting, 4
    descriptions of common, 58–61
Signs, Symptoms, and Ill-Defined Conditions
        (codebook Chapter 16), 55–63
    categories and section titles for, 56
Sinus tachycardia, 146
Sinusitis, 159
Skin, diseases of. *See* Diseases of the Skin
        and Subcutaneous Tissue (codebook
        Chapter 12)
Skin ulcers, chronic, 220, 221
Slanted (italicized) brackets *[ ]*, 26
Sleep disorders, 121
Slow fetal growth and fetal malnutrition, fifth
        digits for, 212–13
Smear and stain examinations, 66–67
Social Security Act
    Medicaid created by, 277
    Medicare established by, 274
Special investigations and examinations,
        V codes for, 45–46
Spina bifida, 209
Spinal cord injury without evidence of spinal
        bone injury, 245
Sporozoea parasites, 70
Sprains and strains, 239
"Spread to" in diagnostic statements, 93
Sputum specimens
    Gram stain to identify infectious diseases
        using, 67
    for tuberculosis, 72

Square brackets [ ] for synonyms, alternative
        wordings, abbreviations, and
        explanatory phrases, 25–26
Stains of infectious agents, 66–67
Staphylococcus aureus, 68, 69
State Children's Health Insurance Program,
        277
STDs. *See* Sexually transmitted diseases
Stillborns, V codes for, 38
Streptococcal sore throat, 72–73
Streptococcus pyogenes (Group A) and
        pneumoniae (Group C), 68
Subcategories in Tabular List, 7
    residual, 10–11
Subclassifications in Tabular List, 7–10
Subdural, subarachnoid, and extradural
        hemorrhage or hematoma, 240
Subterms
    in Index to Diseases and Injuries, 13–14
    under main terms in Alphabetic Index, 29
Superficial injuries, 244
Supplementary Classification of External
        Causes of Injury and Poisoning. *See*
        E codes
Supplementary Classification of Factors
        Influencing Health Status and Contact
        with Health Services. *See* V codes
Supplementary words or explanatory
        information in ICD-9-CM, 25
Supraventricular tachycardia, 146
Symbols in ICD-9-CM, 27–28
Symptoms, 56–57
    descriptions of common, 58–61
Syncope, definition of, 58
Syndromes indexed under main term
        Syndrome as well as under syndrome's
        name, 13
Synonyms, square brackets in ICD-9-CM to
        enclose, 25–26
Syphilis, classification of, 75
Systemic inflammatory response syndrome,
        250–51
Systemic lupus erythematosus, 226

Table of Drugs and Chemicals (Alphabetic
        Index to Diseases), 16, 251–54
Tabular List of Diseases and Injuries (Volume
        1 of ICD-9-CM codebook), 6–12
    Appendices to, 12
    Classification of Diseases and Injuries in,
        6–7
    instructional notes' appearance in, 21
    instructions for coding neoplasms in, 88–89
    Supplementary Classifications (V Codes
        and E Codes) in, 11
    to verify code selection, 29
TB. *See* Tuberculosis
Temperature, conditions of reduced, 246
Therapeutic services, sequencing, 5
Therapy, V codes for admissions or
        encounters for types of, 42
Third-party payers, 277–79
    commercial, 278
    types of, 274

Thyroid disorders, 103–4
Training and educational programs for
        compliance, 289
Transplant, 39
Trauma to perineum and vulva during
        delivery, 200–201
TRICARE Standard, Extra, and Prime,
        CHAMPUS replaced by, 277
Tuberculosis, 72
    extrapulmonary, 163
    late effects of, 78
    pulmonary, 163

Unbundling of services, 288
Underlying conditions coded first for adverse
        effects not classified elsewhere, 246
Unethical behavior
    guidelines for, 298
    refusal to participate in, 300, 302–3
Unspecified adverse effect of drug, medicinal,
        and biological substance, 246, 253–54
Upcoding of services, 288
Urethral stricture, 183
Urgency of urination, 184
Urinary dysuria, 184
Urinary incontinence
    in benign prostatic hypertrophy, 184
    due to or as result of urethral stricture,
        additional code for, 183
    in genital prolapse, additional code for,
        187
    types of, 184
Urinary obstruction, 183
Urinary tract disorders, 181–84
Urine, retention of, 60
"Use Additional Code, If Desired" instruction
        notation, 22

V codes (Supplementary Classification of
        Factors Influencing Health Status and
        Contact with Health Services), 5,
        33–48
    for artificial opening status, 40, 42
    categories and section titles for, 34
    changed to Z codes in ICD-10-CM, 401
    for circulatory system, 151
    for contraceptive management, 37–38
    for convalescence and palliative care,
        43–44
    for dialysis, 42
    for diseases of blood and blood-forming
        organs, 131
    for diseases of musculoskeletal system and
        connective tissue, 230
    for diseases of respiratory system, 165
    for endocrine, nutritional and metabolic
        disorders, and immunity disorders,
        104–5
    for fitting and adjustment of prosthetic
        devices and implants, 41
    for follow-up care, 44
    for general medical examinations, 44–45
    for infectious and parasitic diseases, 78
    for injury and poisonings, 247
    for liveborn infants, 38–39
    for long-term (current) drug use, 43
    for main terms, 35
    for neoplasms, 86–87
    for newborns, 214–15
    for observation and evaluation of
        newborns, 38
    for observation and evaluation of
        suspected conditions, 45
    for obstetric encounters, 196
    for organ or tissue replaced by other
        means, 40
    for organ or tissue replaced by transplant,
        39
    for orthopedic aftercare, 42
    for other and unspecified procedures and
        aftercare, 43
    for other conditions influencing health
        status, 41
    for other dependence on machines, 40–41
    for outcome of delivery, 38, 198
    for Persons Encountering Health Services
        for Specific Procedures and Aftercare,
        41
    for Persons Encountering Health Services
        in Circumstances Related to
        Reproduction and Development, 36
    for Persons Encountering Health Services
        in Other Circumstances, 43
    for Persons with Condition Influencing
        Their Health Status, 39
    for Persons with Need for Isolation, Other
        Potential Health Hazards, and
        Prophylactic Measures, 36
    for Persons with Potential Hazards Related
        to Personal and Family History, 36
    for Persons with Potential Health Hazards
        Related to Communicable Diseases,
        35–36
    for persons without reported diagnoses,
        44–46
    for physical therapy, speech therapy, or
        occupational therapy, 42
    for postpartum care, 37
    for postsurgical states, 40
    for pregnancy, childbirth, and puerperium,
        5, 202
    for preoperative evaluation, 5
    for presence of artificial opening, 40
    for procreative management, 38
    for screening examinations for specific
        conditions, 46
    for special investigations and
        examinations, 45–46
    for supervision of normal pregnancy, 37
    table of, 370–72
Vaccination not carried out, 43
Valvular heart disease, 136–37
Varicose veins, 149
Venereal diseases, 75
Venous complications in pregnancy and
        puerperium, 201
Ventricular fibrillation, 145
Vesicoureteral reflux, 183

Viral hepatitis, 74
Viruses
    additional diagnosis to identify causative,
        71
    coding, 70–71
    common infections caused by, 70
    pneumonia caused by, 158

WBCs. *See* White blood cells
Weight loss, abnormal, 59
Well-baby care, 214
White blood cells
    diseases of, 130
    granular and nongranular leukocyte, 131
Wolff-Parkinson-White syndrome, 146
Workforce, recruiting and mentoring students
        to strengthen, 300

World Health Organization
    development of ICD-10 by, 390
    responsibility for ICD codebook revisions
        of, 3, 279
Worms classified as parasites, 70
Wounds
    complicated, 241
    fifth digits for, 242
    open, 241–42, 245
    operative, foreign body left in, 245
WPW syndrome. *See* Wolff-Parkinson-White
    syndrome

X-ray report to assign fracture diagnosis, 238

Z codes in ICD-10-CM, 401

Look for These Quality AHIMA Publications at Bookstores, Libraries and Online

Applying Inpatient Coding Skills under Prospective Payment

Basic CPT/HCPCS Coding

Basic ICD-9-CM Coding

The Best of In Confidence

Calculating and Reporting Healthcare Statistics

Clinical Coding Workout: Practice Exercises for Skill Development

Coding and Reimbursement for Outpatient Care

CPT/HCPCS Coding and Reimbursement for Physician Services

Documentation for Acute Care

Documentation for Ambulatory Care

Documentation and Reimbursement for Behavioral Healthcare Services

Documentation and Reimbursement for Long-term Care (book and CD)

Documentation and Reimbursement for Home Care and Hospice Programs

Effective Management of Coding Services

Electronic Health Record

Health Information Management

Health Information Management Technology

Health Information Management Compliance (book and CD)

HIPAA in Practice

ICD-9-CM Diagnostic Coding and Reimbursement for Physician Services

ICD-9-CM Diagnostic Coding for Long-Term Care and Home Care

ICD-10-CM and ICD-10-PCS Preview (book and CD)

Quality and Performance Improvement in Healthcare

More Information

Textbook details and easy ordering are available online at **www.ahima.org/store.** For textbook content questions, contact **publications@ahima.org,** and for sales information contact **info@ahima.org** or **(800) 335-5535.**

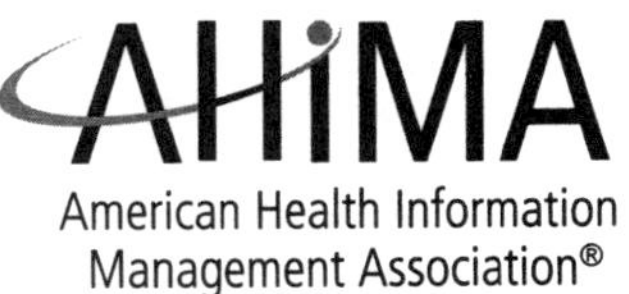